Common Small Animal Diagnoses

AN ALGORITHMIC APPROACH

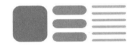

Charlotte Davies, MA, VetMB, Cert VA, MS, MRCVS
Diplomate, ACVIM (Internal Medicine)
Staff Internist, Veterinary Referral and Critical Care LLC
Manakin-Sabot, Virginia

Linda Shell, DVM
Diplomate, ACVIM (Neurology)
Professor, Internal Medicine
Ross University School of Medicine
St. Kitts, West Indies
Formerly Professor, Small Animal Clinical Sciences Department
Virginia-Maryland Regional College of Veterinary Medicine
Blacksburg, Virginia

Terry Lawrence, Illustrator

W.B. SAUNDERS COMPANY
A Harcourt Health Sciences Company
Philadelphia   London   New York   St. Louis   Sydney   Toronto

W.B. SAUNDERS COMPANY

A Harcourt Health Sciences Company

The Curtis Center
Independence Square West
Philadelphia, Pennsylvania 19106

Library of Congress Cataloging-in-Publication Data

Davies, Charlotte.
    Common small animal diagnoses : an algorithmic approach / Charlotte Davies, Linda
Shell ; Terry Lawrence, illustrator.
      p. cm.
    ISBN: 0-7216-8478-5
    1. Dogs—Diseases—Diagnosis. 2. Cats—Diseases—Diagnosis. 3. Algorithms. I. Shell,
Linda. II. Title

SF991.D36 2002
636.7′0896075—dc21   2001049545

Printed in the United States of America

Last digit is the print number: 9   8   7   6   5   4   3   2   1

To our families and friends who endured our many moods while we composed, revised, edited, and agonized over these algorithms

To our peers and students, who continually challenged us to learn, to rethink, and to explain

Charlotte Davies
Linda Shell

Preface

These algorithms are intended as guidelines and as starting points in a problem-oriented approach for the veterinarian. They can never be definitive and should not be followed dogmatically. Only experience, detailed assessment of each case, and regard for the needs of both the client and the patient can allow the clinician to develop an appropriate diagnostic and hence therapeutic plan for an individual. Some diagnostic testing is recommended early on to exclude the most likely underlying causes of clinical signs. Some tests are performed to exclude rare but easily treated conditions or rare but immediately life-threatening problems. This text is intended to provide an outline of the potential approach to a specific problem. However, few patients present for only one problem and even fewer of them "read the textbook" as far as their presentation. We have tried to start with common problems that present to us as practitioners and proceed as logically and safely as possibly toward the final diagnosis.

In evolving these algorithms, our main sources have been *The Textbook of Veterinary Internal Medicine* (4th and 5th Editions, 1995 and 2000) by S. J. Ettinger and E. C. Feldman, *Small Animal Clinical Diagnosis by Laboratory Methods* (3rd Edition, 1999) by M. D. Willard, H. Tvedten, and G. H. Turnwald, as well as our clinical experience. We hope that this text proves helpful in formulating a diagnostic plan for students and clinicians with different degrees of experience and in all walks of life.

Charlotte Davies

Linda Shell

Contents

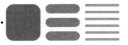

Abbreviations

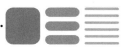

ACE..................Angiotensin converting enzyme
ACH ....Anticholinesterase
ACT..................Activated clotting time
ACTH ....Adrenocorticotropic hormone
ADH ....Antidiuretic hormone
AGIDT ....Agar gel immunodiffusion test
ALP ....Alkaline phosphatase
ALT ....Alanine aminotransferase
ANA..................Antinuclear antibody
APUDoma...........Amine precursor uptake and
                      decarboxylation tumors
ARDS.................Acute respiratory distress syndrome
ARF ....Acute renal failure
ATIII ....Antithrombin III
ATP ....Adenosine triphosphate
ATPase..............Adenosine triphosphatase
AV ....Atrioventricular
BAOS.................Brachycephalic airway obstruction
                      syndrome
BIPs..................Barium-impregnated polyethylene
                      spheres
BMBT ....Buccal mucosal bleeding time
BPH ....Benign prostatic hyperplasia
BPM ....Beats per minute
BSP ....Bromosulfophthalein retention test
BUN ....Blood urea nitrogen
Ca^{2+} ....Calcium
CC.....................Central cyanosis
CDI ....Central diabetes insipidus
CDV ....Canine distemper virus
CK......................Creatine kinase
CLO test.............*Campylobacter*-like organism test

CNS..................Central nervous system
CO_2..................Carbon dioxide
CRF...................Chronic renal failure
CSF ....Cerebrospinal fluid
CT.....................Computed tomography
CVP...................Central venous pressure
DCM..................Dilated cardiomyopathy
DDAVP.............Desmopressin acetate
DIC ....Disseminated intravascular
                      coagulation
DJD ....Degenerative joint disease
DLE..................Discoid lupus erythematosus
DR ....Decremental response
ECG ....Electrocardiogram
ECP ....Estradiol cyclopentylproprionate
EDTA...............Ethylenediaminetetra-acetic acid
EEG..................Electroencephalogram
ELISA ....Enzyme-linked immunosorbent assay
EMG ....Electromyography
EPI ....Exocrine pancreatic insufficiency
FCE ....Fibrocartilaginous embolism
FDP...................Fibrin degradation products
FeLV ....Feline leukemia virus
FePLV ....Feline panleukopenia virus
FeSV ....Feline syncytium-forming virus
FIE ....Feline ischemic encephalopathy
FIP ....Feline infectious peritonitis (feline
                      coronavirus)
FIV ....Feline immunodeficiency virus
FLUTDs ....Feline lower urinary tract disease
FURI ....Feline upper respiratory infection
GDV ....Gastric dilation and volvulus

GFR...................Glomerular filtration rate
GI ....Gastrointestinal
GME ....Granulomatous meningoencephalitis
H&E...................Hematoxylin and eosin
Hb.....................Hemoglobin
HCM..................Hypertrophic cardiomyopathy
HDL...................High density lipoprotein
HE ....Hemorrhagic gastroenteritis
HGE...................Hemorrhagic gastroenteropathy
hpf ....High-power field
IBD ....Inflammatory bowel disease
IBS ....Irritable bowel syndrome
IFA ....Immunofluoresent antibody assay
IgG ....Immunoglobulin G
IgM ....Immunoglobulin M
IMHA.................Immune-mediated hemolytic anemia
IMT ....Immune-mediated
                       thrombocytopenia
IV......................Intravenous
IVU ....Intravenous urogram
K^+ ....Potassium
LDL...................Low density lipoprotein
LI ....Large intestinal or large intestine
LMN..................Lower motor neuron
LRT...................Lower respiratory tract
LS ....Lumbosacral
Mb ....Methemoglobin
MCHC ....Mean cell hemoglobin
                       concentration
MCV...................Mean cell volume
MI ....Mitral insufficiency
MNCV.................Motor nerve conduction velocity

MRI	Magnetic resonance imaging
Na$^+$	Sodium
NCS	Nerve conduction studies
NDI	Nephrogenic diabetes insipidus
NSAIDs	Nonsteroidal anti-inflammatory drugs
PaCo$_2$	Partial pressure of carbon dioxide
PaO$_2$	Partial pressure of oxygen
PC	Peripheral cyanosis
PCR	Polymerase chain reaction
PCV	Packed cell volume
PD	Polydipsia
PDA	Patent ductus arteriosus
PIVKA	Proteins induced by vitamin K antagonism
PLR	Pupillary light response
PP	Psychogenic polydipsia
PPP	Periosteal proliferative polyarthritis
PT	Prothrombin time
PTE	Pulmonary thromboembolism
PTH	Parathyroid hormone
PTHrP	Parathyroid hormone–related polypeptide
PTT	Partial thromboplastin time
PU	Polyuria
RA	Regenerative anemia
RAS	Reticular activating system
RAST	Radioallergosorbent test
RBCs	Red blood cells
RCM	Restrictive cardiomyopathy
Rh factor	Rheumatoid factor
RMSF	Rocky Mountain spotted fever
RPI	Reticulocyte production index
RSAT	Rapid slide agglutination test
SA	Sinoatrial node
SBA	Serum bile acids
SI	Small intestinal or small intestine
SIBO	Small intestinal bacterial overgrowth
SLE	Systemic lupus erythematosus
SPE	Serum protein electrophoresis
SSS	Sick sinus syndrome
T$_3$	Triiodothyronine
T$_4$	Thyroxine
TAT	Tube agglutination test
TEN	Toxic epidermal necrolysis
TI	Tricuspid insufficiency
TLI	Trypsin-like immunoreactivity
TMJ	Temporomandibular joint
TP	Total protein
TSH	Thyroid-stimulating hormone
UMN	Upper motor neuron
usg	Urine specific gravity
URT	Upper respiratory tract
UTI	Urinary tract infection
VLDL	Very low density lipoprotein
VPCs	Ventricular premature contractions
VPM	Ventilation-perfusion mismatch
VSD	Ventricular septal defect
vWD	von Willebrand disease
vWF	von Willebrand factor
vWFAg	von Willebrand factor antigen
WBCs	White blood cells

SECTION ···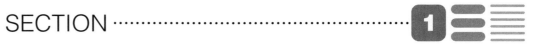

Generalized Disorders

1 Pain is defined as the perception of an unpleasant sensation that begins from a specific body part. Pain is initiated by stimulation of nociceptors (free nerve terminals of afferent fibers). Pain receptors are most numerous in tissues that interact with the environment (skin, muscles, and joints). Pain originating from these structures is called *somatic pain* and is usually distinct and well localized. *Visceral pain* originates from internal organs and is more difficult to localize, probably because fewer nociceptors are associated with abdominal viscera. Pain is a clinical sign, not a diagnosis. Dogs and cats cannot verbally describe pain or discomfort; however, one can infer pain from their behavior. Lameness, behavioral changes, lethargy, whining, reluctance to move or play, and hyporexia all are potential signs of pain. Acute pain is associated with injury, surgery, diagnostic manipulation, or an acute-onset, painful disease such as disc herniation or pancreatitis. Chronic pain is pain that has been present for months and is usually associated with disease processes that can be managed but not cured.

2 Both the history and the physical examination can help to localize a site of discomfort. If the patient is reluctant to go up and down stairs, a musculoskeletal or spinal problem is likely. If the patient cries when picked up, the spine and abdomen are possible sources of pain. Lameness suggests an orthopedic or neurological source. If the patient is sore and reluctant to move when first arising but improves as ambulation proceeds, degenerative joint disease is likely.

3 Muscle pain manifests as reluctance to move or vocalization when muscles are gently palpated. Affected muscles may be atrophied, hypertrophied, or swollen. Creatine kinase (CK) is an enzyme released from muscle. If it is elevated in serum, myositis or myopathy should be suspected. However, normal CK concentrations do not eliminate muscle as a source of the pain.

4 Abdominal pain can cause splinting or crying out on abdominal palpation. Pain localized to the right anterior abdominal quadrant suggests pancreatitis. Pain localized dorsally near the caudal ribs and sublumbar area suggests renal or spinal pain. Differential diagnosis of abdominal pain includes trauma, foreign body impaction, inflammation (hepatic abscess, peritonitis, pancreatitis), ischemia (bowel torsion), and passage of urethral or ureteral calculi. Abdominal tumors are a less likely cause of pain, except for renal tumors.

5 A cryptorchid dog with acute abdominal pain and a firm abdominal mass may have an ischemic testicle due to torsion.

6 Bone or joint pain often produces lameness. Usually the more severe the problem, the less weight is borne on the affected limb. If the lameness shifts from one limb to another, possibilities include polyarthritis, panosteitis, and degenerative joint disease affecting multiple joints. Radiographs of the affected limb usually yield the diagnosis.

7 If radiographs are normal or if joint effusion is present, cytological evaluation and aerobic/anaerobic culture of synovial fluid help to determine if joint disease is causing the pain. These tests also can help distinguish immune-mediated, degenerative, and infectious arthritis.

8 Spinal pain is detected by palpation over each dorsal spinous process, starting near the lumbosacral area and moving cranially to the caudal cervical area. In the cervical spine, palpate the lateral processes of each vertebra and then gently move the neck from side to side and up and down. Avoid manipulation of the spine if trauma or atlantoaxial luxation is suspected. Thoracolumbar pain is often confused with abdominal pain and vice versa.

9 If pain is found on opening the mouth, palpate carefully for temporomandibular joint (TMJ) disease, TMJ fracture or luxation, retrobulbar abscess, or look for an oral foreign body. Muscles of mastication are swollen in the acute stage of masseter myopathy and atrophied chronically. Palpate around the ears and evaluate for otitis externa that could have spread to the middle ear. Evaluate the teeth for abscesses.

10 Craniomandibular osteopathy is a nonneoplastic, noninflammatory, proliferative bone disease in growing dogs. It affects the mandibles, as well as occipital and temporal bones. Terrier breeds as well as larger breeds of dog are predisposed to this disease.

11 If the temporalis and masseter muscles are atrophied or enlarged or if the jaw cannot be opened, then masticatory muscle myositis is likely. Skull radiographs rule out bony abnormalities. Serum and muscle biopsy sections can be evaluated for antibodies against masticatory muscle Type 2M proteins.

12 If the pain cannot be localized, begin evaluation with a hemogram, serum chemistries, urinalysis, and CK measurement.

13 Pancreatitis can be associated with hyporexia, vomiting, fever, abdominal pain, and leukocytosis. Elevation of lipase and amylase is supportive evidence. Pancreatitis can be especially difficult to diagnose in cats.

14 Urinary tract inflammation is not usually associated with pain unless pyelonephritis is present. Finding pyuria and/or white blood cell (WBC) casts on urine sediment examination supports a diagnosis of pyelonephritis. Abdominal imaging and urine culture are indicated in such cases.

15 If the minimum database does not contribute to a diagnosis, the next step is to image the abdomen or spine, depending on which area appears to be the more likely site of the pain. A dachshund over 2 or 3 years of age with nonlocalizable pain is more likely to have intervertebral disc disease/herniation than an intra-abdominal problem.

16 If abdominal imaging does not yield an answer, evaluate spinal radiographs.

17 Discospondylitis usually manifests as spinal pain before there is radiographic evidence of the problem or neurological signs develop. If the patient is painful and febrile (especially a young male dog), and if spinal pain is repeatable but radiographs are normal, treat for discospondylitis and repeat radiographs at 4- and 8-week intervals.

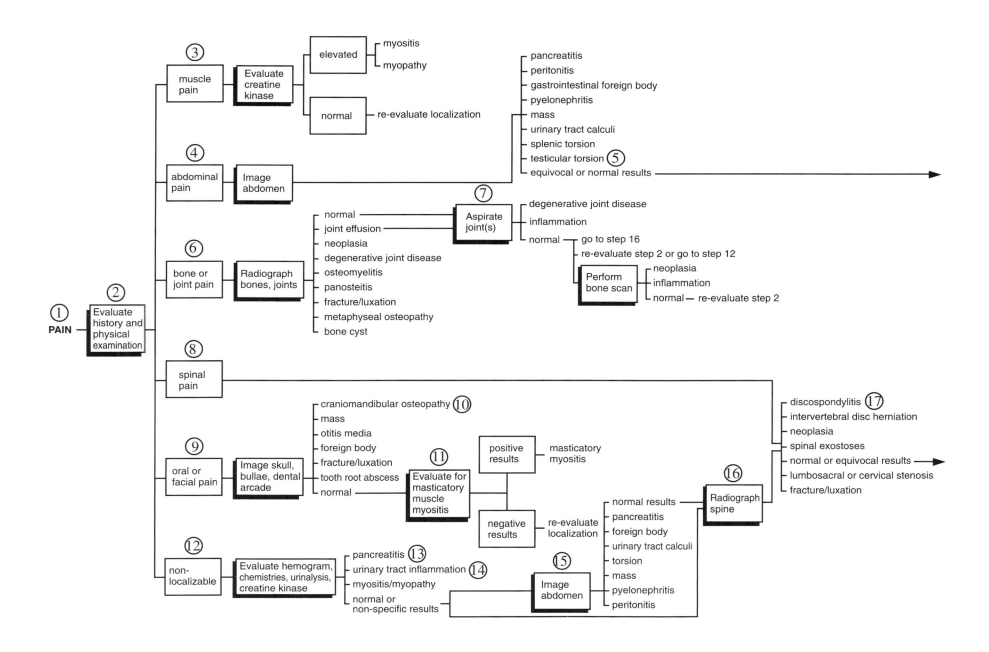

① **PAIN**

② Evaluate history and physical examination

③ muscle pain → Evaluate creatine kinase
- elevated
  - myositis
  - myopathy
- normal → re-evaluate localization

④ abdominal pain → Image abdomen
- pancreatitis
- peritonitis
- gastrointestinal foreign body
- pyelonephritis
- mass
- urinary tract calculi
- splenic torsion
- testicular torsion ⑤
- equivocal or normal results →

⑥ bone or joint pain → Radiograph bones, joints
- normal
- joint effusion
- neoplasia
- degenerative joint disease
- osteomyelitis
- panosteitis
- fracture/luxation
- metaphyseal osteopathy
- bone cyst

⑦ Aspirate joint(s)
- degenerative joint disease
- inflammation
- normal
  - go to step 16
  - re-evaluate step 2 or go to step 12

Perform bone scan
- neoplasia
- inflammation
- normal — re-evaluate step 2

⑧ spinal pain

⑨ oral or facial pain → Image skull, bullae, dental arcade
- craniomandibular osteopathy ⑩
- mass
- otitis media
- foreign body
- fracture/luxation
- tooth root abscess
- normal

⑪ Evaluate for masticatory muscle myositis
- positive results → masticatory myositis
- negative results → re-evaluate localization

⑯ Radiograph spine
- discospondylitis ⑰
- intervertebral disc herniation
- neoplasia
- spinal exostoses
- normal or equivocal results →
- lumbosacral or cervical stenosis
- fracture/luxation

⑫ non-localizable → Evaluate hemogram, chemistries, urinalysis, creatine kinase
- pancreatitis ⑬
- urinary tract inflammation ⑭
- myositis/myopathy
- normal or non-specific results

⑮ Image abdomen
- normal results
- pancreatitis
- foreign body
- urinary tract calculi
- torsion
- mass
- pyelonephritis
- peritonitis

18 If abdominal pain is present but abdominal radiographs/ultrasound have not yielded conclusive results, reevaluate the hemogram, chemistry profile, and urinalysis. Elevation of serum lipase and amylase suggests pancreatitis, pyuria or WBC casts in urine can indicate pyelonephritis, and elevated liver enzymes suggest hepatitis or cholangiohepatitis.

19 If a conclusive result is not obtained, consider contrast radiographic studies. A barium series may be needed to diagnose radiolucent gastrointestinal foreign bodies and some masses. Contrast excretory urography may be needed to diagnose some disorders of the urinary tract. Ultrasound can help diagnose urinary tract problems, but it is not always as useful for the gastrointestinal tract because intraluminal gas can block the ultrasound beam.

20 In patients with spinal or nonlocalizable pain and in which spinal radiographs are nondiagnostic, the next steps are either
  A) Joint aspiration and synovial fluid analysis or
  B) Cerebrospinal fluid aspiration and analysis.
The procedure selected depends on which area appears most likely to be involved in the disease process and on the risks of the procedure to the patient.

21 Polyarthritis usually causes fever, reluctance to move, the appearance of "walking on eggshells," and shifting leg lameness. Some patients have neck pain due to inflammation in the vertebral articulations. Thus clinical signs often suggest meningitis rather than polyarthritis.

22 Degenerative joint disease usually manifests with a chronic and sometimes progressive history of patient discomfort. It is most common in middle-aged and older patients, especially if they are obese. If multiple joints are affected, lameness may change from one limb to another over months. Cats do develop degenerative joint disease but less frequently than dogs.

23 Meningitis is very painful and often makes patients reluctant to move. The diagnosis is based on evaluation of spinal fluid. Typically there will be increased fluid protein and a raised WBC count. Causes of meningitis include infectious (rickettsial, bacterial, fungal, protozoal, and viral) and immune-mediated conditions. In young to maturing large breeds of dogs (especially males), a steroid-responsive meningitis has been described. In young beagles, there is a specific syndrome of pain, often called *beagle pain syndrome* or *necrotizing vasculitis*. This syndrome has a relapsing course, but clinical signs may be ameliorated with prednisone. In cats, meningitis is most commonly associated with feline infectious peritonitis (FIP) and feline immunodeficiency virus (FIV) infections.

24 If cervical, spinal, or nonlocalizable pain is still present and a diagnosis has not been obtained, spinal imaging can be performed to look for disc herniations, mass lesions, subtle spinal fractures/luxations, stenosis of the vertebral canal, and hydromyelia. Imaging is via myelography or epidurography (depending on the region affected) or computed tomography (CT) and magnetic resonance imaging (MRI) scans. If joint fluid has not been evaluated, joint disease should be excluded prior to performing more invasive and costly spinal imaging studies. Finally patients can have cervical pain due to thalamic and brainstem masses. A CT or MRI scan is required to make the diagnosis.

25 Hydromyelia is an enlarged spinal central canal filled with spinal fluid. Syringomyelia is characterized by fluid-filled cavities within the spinal cord. These conditions are congenital or acquired and have been associated with pain. In the cavalier King Charles spaniel, signs reported consist of scratching at the neck/shoulder area, crying out as if in pain, and reluctance to have the ears, neck, or forelimbs touched. Antemortem diagnosis of such conditions is usually best made via MRI studies.

26 Thalamic pain syndrome is caused by a brain tumor located in the thalamus. Neck pain is a common manifestation. The thalamus is thought to be one of the main areas of the brain responsible for receiving and interpreting pain. However, exactly why a mass in this area causes neck pain is unknown.

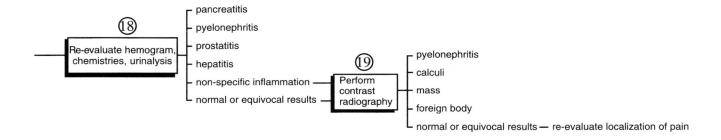

pancreatitis

pyelonephritis

prostatitis

hepatitis

non-specific inflammation

normal or equivocal results

⑱ Re-evaluate hemogram, chemistries, urinalysis

⑲ Perform contrast radiography

pyelonephritis

calculi

mass

foreign body

normal or equivocal results — re-evaluate localization of pain

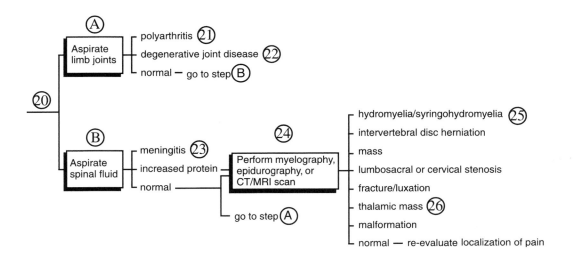

Ⓐ Aspirate limb joints

polyarthritis ㉑

degenerative joint disease ㉒

normal — go to step Ⓑ

⑳

Ⓑ Aspirate spinal fluid

meningitis ㉓

increased protein

normal

㉔ Perform myelography, epidurography, or CT/MRI scan

go to step Ⓐ

hydromyelia/syringohydromyelia ㉕

intervertebral disc herniation

mass

lumbosacral or cervical stenosis

fracture/luxation

thalamic mass ㉖

malformation

normal — re-evaluate localization of pain

1 Elevated body temperature in dogs and cats is defined as a rectal temperature above 102.5°F. Mild elevations are not harmful to the patient and can represent an appropriate response to a physiological situation. For example, it is not uncommon for dogs to have a body temperature between 103°F and 105°F during exercise or periods of stress.

2 If body temperature is greater than 105°F in a resting patient, steps should be taken to lower it. This should not be done if the temperature elevation appears to be due to infection, in which case the patient's body temperature set point in the hypothalamus has been reset and attempts to cool the patient will lead the body to strive to recover the heat lost. Methods for cooling hyperthermic patients include surface cooling with cold water or alcohol, followed by the use of a fan to enhance conductive heat loss. If the temperature is greater than 106°F, both external and internal cooling techniques should be considered. Ice water baths and enemas, sedation with phenothiazines to reduce shivering, oxygen administration, antipyretic drugs, and administration of cooled, isotonic, polyionic crystalloid intravenous fluids are all possible treatments. The more severe the hyperthermia, the more aggressive the cooling techniques required.

3 Review the history and physical examination findings to determine whether elevated body temperature is associated with underlying infectious disease, heat exhaustion or heat stroke, drug administration, exercise, or stress. Note any respiratory difficulty since dyspnea and upper airway obstruction increase body temperature due to failure to thermoregulate. Pyometra, prostatitis, and *Brucella canis* orchitis should be considered in intact patients.

4 Chorioretinitis and anterior uveitis often are associated with systemic infections with canine distemper virus (CDV) and FIP virus, as well as fungal, protozoal, and rickettsial diseases, FIV, and feline leukemia virus (FeLV). Serum or blood tests/titers, polymerase chain reaction (PCR), or immunofluoresence (IFA) techniques can help diagnose many of these diseases.

5 Lymphadenopathy in a febrile patient suggests inflammation (infectious/immune-mediated) or neoplasia. See the algorithm for lymphadenopathy.

6 Joint effusion in a febrile patient suggests immune-mediated/infectious joint disease or, less commonly, neoplasia.

7 Heat exhaustion is associated with mild elevations of body temperature, whereas heat stroke is associated with marked increases. Cellular damage starts to occur when body temperature reaches 108°F, at which point oxygen delivery to tissues can no longer keep pace with increased oxygen consumption.

8 Malignant hyperthermia is a rapid, progressive increase in body temperature associated with exercise, excessively nervous or abnormally muscled patients, or administration of certain anesthetic agents. Abnormal intracellular calcium metabolism results in excessive metabolic heat production. Therapy includes aggressive cooling and administration of dantrolene sodium (at a rate of 2.5–10 mg/kg intravenously).

9 Endocarditis and/or septicemia should be considered if a heart murmur is auscultated in a febrile patient. Vegetative valvular lesions on an echocardiogram suggest endocarditis.

10 If an echocardiogram does not suggest the diagnosis, blood cultures can diagnose bacterial causes of septicemia, especially if three samples are taken in a 24-hour period and when the patient is hyperthermic. Urine cultures also can be useful, often growing the same organism as blood cultures.

11 Prolonged muscle exertion, such as that occurring during seizure activity/status epilepticus and hard exercise, often results in elevated body temperature.

12 Dyspnea and upper airway obstruction result in the inability of the canine or feline patient to thermoregulate. Dyspnea or hyperpnea also produces increased muscular exertion. In such cases, anxiety also contributes to the temperature elevation.

13 Drugs such as phenothiazines and antihistamines inhibit cutaneous vasodilation and thereby may increase body temperature. Drug therapy also can idiosyncratically produce malignant hyperthermia

14 Large-breed dogs undergoing general anesthesia can develop body temperature elevations if the patient is breathing fully humidified gas, is well covered with surgical drapes, and is in a light anesthetic plane allowing development of some muscle tension.

15 If neck pain and fever are present, infection of bone (osteomyelitis), vertebral joint spaces (discospondylitis), meninges (meningitis), joints, or muscle is possible. Spinal or bone radiographs can indicate discospondylitis or osteomyelitis lesions. Meningitis is diagnosed via cerebrospinal fluid analysis.

16 If the initial history and physical examination do not yield clues to the cause of the elevated body temperature, repeat these steps and continue to monitor body temperature. If the temperature becomes normal at rest, consider anxiety or stress as possible underlying causes. If temperature elevation is cyclic (i.e., occurring every few days to weeks), then a sterile inflammatory or immune-mediated process is likely.

17 In a cat exposed to other cats, a cat-bite abscess should be considered as a possible cause of fever. An abscess may not be evident on initial evaluation, but within a few days a draining area is likely to appear. If respiratory signs are present, consider underlying pyothorax.

18 If there is no response to appropriate treatment for an abscess, then evaluate the patient's FeLV and FIV status even if test results were negative in the past.

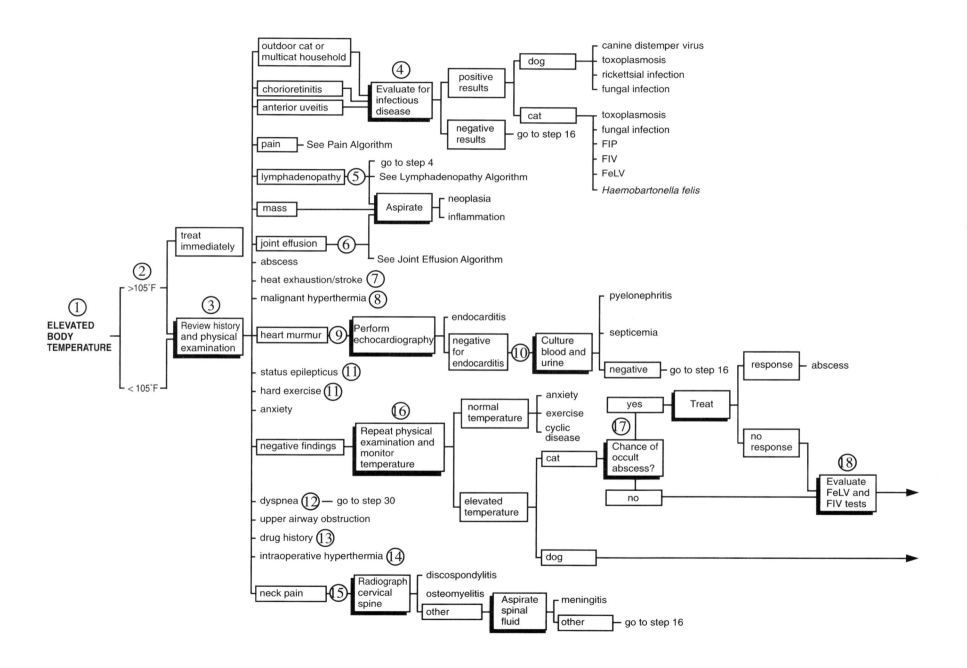

19 If the cat is FeLV/FIV negative or if the patient is a dog, the next step is to evaluate the results of a hemogram, a serum chemistry profile, and urinalysis for evidence of an infectious, immune-mediated, or neoplastic process.

20 Pyuria and bacteriuria in a urine sample collected by cystocentesis suggest urinary tract infection. Fever more often is associated with pyelonephritis or prostatitis than with cystitis.

21 Azotemia does not produce temperature elevations per se. However, diseases that cause azotemia also might cause fever. Examples include pyelonephritis, pancreatitis, and inflammatory or neoplastic conditions that lead to dehydration and/or renal failure.

22 Hyperglobulinemia often is associated with FIP in cats but can also be due to abscesses, other infectious diseases, and neoplasia. In dogs, consider neoplasia and rickettsial infections.

23 Increased liver enzymes themselves do not produce an increase in body temperature. However, inflammatory diseases (cholecystitis, FIP) or hepatic neoplasia that cause elevated liver enzymes can also cause elevations in body temperature.

24 Increased lipase and/or amylase in conjunction with elevated body temperature suggests pancreatitis or gastrointestinal disease. Abdominal imaging should be pursued initially. In primary gastrointestinal disease, endoscopy or exploratory surgery may be needed to obtain stomach and small intestinal biopsy specimens to achieve a definitive diagnosis.

25 If results of the minimum database are negative or nonspecific, evaluate CK if this is not usually part of the serum chemistry profile. Elevated CK is associated with muscle injury or inflammatory/infectious disease (myositis). However, normal CK does not eliminate myositis as an underlying cause of fever/hyperthermia.

26 Hemolytic anemia, either due to autoimmune hemolytic anemia or to infectious diseases, often is associated with fever. *Haemobartonella felis* is a common infectious cause of fever and hemolytic anemia in the cat.

27 Thrombocytopenia due to immune-mediated or infectious diseases (rickettsial infections, FIP) is often associated with fever.

28 Neutropenia in conjunction with fever should raise the suspicion of panleukopenia virus infection in the cat and parvovirus or CDV infection in the dog. The fever may be due to the viral infection itself, secondary infection, or generalized sepsis because the patient is neutropenic or generally immunosuppressed.

29 Leukocytosis with a left shift suggests an infectious process. Blood or urine cultures may be positive for bacterial infections in septicemic patients.

30 If the serum CK concentration is normal, start looking for radiographic evidence of infection. Thoracic radiographs can show evidence of neoplasia, pneumonia, intrathoracic lymphadenopathy (due to fungal or neoplastic causes), pleural effusion (due to FIP or pyothorax), or other abnormalities that might suggest an underlying cause of the fever. If normal ventilation is restricted by the intrathoracic changes, the patient can become hyperthermic.

31 If thoracic radiographs do not yield a diagnosis, the next step is to
A) Image the abdomen or
B) Evaluate joint and/or spinal fluid.
The clinician must select the test that appears to be most appropriate for a particular patient/clinical presentation.

32 If testing to this stage has not yielded a cause of the fever or hyperthermia, a central nervous system (hypothalamic) lesion may be present. Other neurological signs (behavior changes, seizure activity, endocrine abnormalities) may exist. Imaging the brain via CT or MRI scans could reveal a hypothalamic lesion. Repeated testing, beginning with step 3, is another means of approaching a patient with persistent fever/hyperthermia.

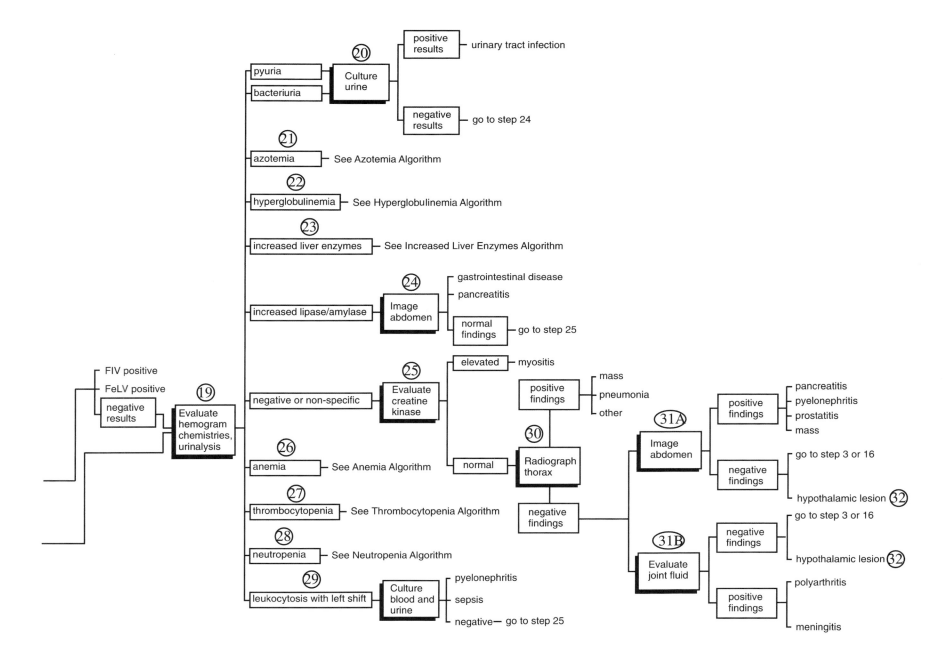

1 Polyuria (PU) occurs when urine output is greater than 50 ml/kg body weight per day. Polydipsia (PD) is defined as when water intake exceeds 100 ml/kg body weight per day.

2 Even though PU and PD occur together, clients often report only one or the other. PU may manifest as inappropriate urination, increased frequency of urination, nocturia, or increased litter box weight in indoor cats. PD may be reported as having to fill the water bowl with increased frequency, or the patient's begging for water or drinking out of toilets and sinks. The history should include the type of diet (e.g., excessive salt content, high protein level), preexisting diseases, current medications, and other clinical signs. The owner should be asked to measure the amount of water consumed by the patient in a 12- to 24-hour period at home.

3 Preexisting disorders or abnormalities that cause PU/PD include diabetes mellitus, renal insufficiency or failure, hyperadrenocorticism, hyperthyroidism (cats), hypercalcemia, and liver disease.

4 Drugs that can cause PU/PD include glucocorticoids, phenobarbital, phenytoin, potassium bromide, primidone, ethanol, and diuretics. Glucocorticoids affect antidiuretic hormone (ADH) release from the pituitary and its action on renal tubules.

5 Lymphoma may cause hypercalcemia and hence PU/PD. It also can affect renal function or cause PU/PD as a result of hepatic dysfunction.

6 Pyometra causes PU/PD as a result of *Escherichia coli* endotoxin deposition in renal tubules, which interferes with sodium and chloride reabsorption and results in loss of medullary hypertonicity.

7 Hyperthyroidism in cats causes PU/PD by stimulating increased water intake or by decreasing medullary hypertonicity via increased renal blood flow. Clinical signs include weight loss, gastrointestinal signs, polyphagia, irritability, and hyperactivity.

8 If pain is present on renal palpation and the patient is febrile, suspect pyelonephritis. Inflammation and infection of the renal pelvis may destroy the countercurrent concentrating mechanism of the medulla, causing dilute urine and PU/PD. Pyelonephritis is diagnosed by finding an inflammatory urine sediment, a positive urine culture, and pyelonephritis on renal imaging.

9 Small kidneys in a patient with PU/PD should raise the suspicion of chronic renal insufficiency/failure.

10 Overt polyuria is not a commonly reported sign of hypoadrenocorticism (Addison's disease), but if bradycardia, weakness, collapse, or gastrointestinal signs also are present, hypoadrenocorticism should be suspected. PU is due to chronic renal sodium wasting, resulting in medullary washout. Hypercalcemia also may be present and contributes to PU/PD.

11 If the patient is a middle-aged or older dog with signs of truncal alopecia, pendulous abdomen, comedones, or hepatomegaly, hyperadrenocorticism (Cushing's disease) is a differential diagnosis for PU/PD.

12 If the history and physical examination are normal or nonspecific, evaluate the urine specific gravity. If this is less than 1.035 in dogs or less than 1.045 in cats, or if there is documented PD, evaluate a hemogram, urinalysis, and chemistry screen. These tests will exclude many common causes of PU/PD.

13 If the urine specific gravity is greater than 1.035 in dogs or greater than 1.045 in cats, the historical report of PU/PD may be incorrect. Have the owner document the 12- to 24-hour water intake at home for 3 to 5 days before other testing is done.

14 Diabetes mellitus results in hyperglycemia, and renal loss of glucose exceeds the renal tubular capacity for reabsorption. Glucose in the urine acts as an osmotic diuretic, leading to PU and consequent PD.

15 Hypercalcemia interferes with the ability of renal tubules to respond to ADH, inactivating the transport of sodium and chloride into the renal medullary interstitium and inhibiting reabsorption of water. Calcium precipitation in renal tubules also can occur, resulting in renal failure. Common causes of hypercalcemia include neoplasia (lymphoma, anal sac adenocarcinoma, plasma cell myeloma) and chronic renal failure. Rarer causes include hyperparathyroidism, hypoadrenocorticism, and hypervitaminosis D.

16 Renal insufficiency/failure is one of the most common causes of PU/PD in dogs and cats. Nephron loss results in inability of renal tubules to reabsorb fluid and solutes, causing osmotic diuresis and decreased renal medullary hypertonicity. If uremia is present, ADH antagonism also may occur. Diagnosis of renal failure (greater than 75% renal function loss) is based on finding increased blood urea nitrogen, serum creatinine, and phosphorus concentrations in conjunction with fixed/low urine specific gravity (1.008 to 1.020). Renal insufficiency (66–75% renal function loss) is harder to diagnose and requires documentation of reduced glomerular filtration rates (e.g., by iohexol, creatinine, or inulin clearance measurement).

17 Renal glycosuria is an uncommon condition that occurs occasionally in dogs with acute or chronic renal failure, Fanconi syndrome, or hepatorenal disease or in those with primary renal glycosuria. Fanconi syndrome is characterized by multiple renal tubular reabsorptive defects. It is seen most frequently in the basenji but also occurs in other breeds. Primary renal glycosuria has been reported in Scottish terriers, mixed-breed dogs, and Norwegian elkhounds. Differentiation of primary renal glycosuria from Fanconi syndrome is based on finding reabsorptive defects for other solutes.

18 Hypokalemia (potassium values below 3.5 mEq/l) may cause the terminal portions of the nephron to be less responsive to ADH. This results in partial nephrogenic diabetes insipidus due to impaired renal tubular transport and reduced medullary hypertonicity. Hypokalemia also may interfere with normal pituitary release of ADH. See the algorithm for hypokalemia.

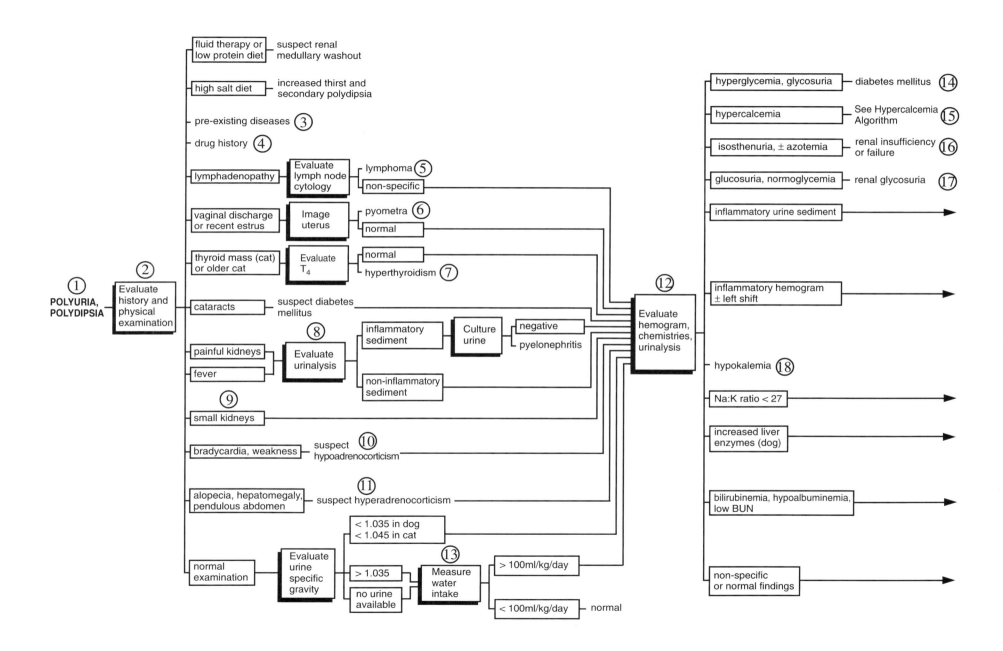

19 If WBCs or WBC casts are observed in a sample of urine obtained by cystocentesis, pyelonephritis should be suspected as a cause of PU/PD. Urine cultures should be performed.

20 An inflammatory leukogram on the hemogram in conjunction with PU/PD should raise the suspicion of pyometra, pyelonephritis, or prostatitis. Abdominal radiographs or ultrasound may help to confirm the diagnosis.

21 Laboratory features of hypoadrenocorticism include hyperkalemia, hyponatremia, hypercalcemia, prerenal azotemia, metabolic acidosis, and lymphocytosis. The Na:K ratio usually is less than 27. These findings should prompt ACTH stimulation testing. Increased liver enzymes, especially increases in alkaline phosphatase (ALP), may be seen with hyperadrenocorticism in dogs. These findings in a middle-aged or older dog with PU/PD also warrant an ACTH stimulation test.

22 Dilute urine and PU/PD are common in dogs and cats with chronic liver disease. Impaired hepatic function may delay clearance of endogenous aldosterone (causing sodium retention, thirst, and hence PD) and cortisol (causing PU). Decreased renal medullary hypertonicity results from decreased urea production from ammonia. Signs of liver disease often include gastrointestinal problems, episodic salivation, depression or other neurologic signs, ascites, hypoalbuminemia, low blood urea nitrogen, or hyperbilirubinemia. Evaluation of pre- and postprandial bile acids, fasting ammonia or ammonia challenge tests, or measurement of sulfobromophthalein (BSP) retention can confirm liver dysfunction. Ultrasound-guided liver aspiration or biopsy may yield a diagnosis.

23 If laboratory results are nonspecific or normal, then PD must be documented by having the owner measure 12- to 24-hour water consumption over a 3- to 5-day period. If PD is documented in any dog, urine should be cultured at some point to ensure that pyelonephritis is not causing PU/PD.

24 If PD is documented in a dog over 8 years of age, hyperadrenocorticism should be considered even if the physical examination and laboratory findings are not typical of this condition. An ACTH test is recommended.

25 If PD is documented in a cat older than 8 years of age, hyperthyroidism is a consideration and the serum thyroxine (T_4) concentration should be measured.

26 Even if the urinary sediment is unremarkable, a urine culture should be evaluated before the next cycle of testing is initiated. Cultures should be quantitative or on a sterile urine sample obtained by cystocentesis.

27 Finally, if a diagnosis of PU/PD has not yet been made and the glomerular filtration rate (GFR) has been measured in an isosthenuric patient (see step 16) to exclude the possibility of subclinical renal dysfunction, a modified water deprivation/ADH response test can be performed. It is *vitally* important to obtain the GFR and to know that renal function is normal first. Failure to determine that renal function is normal prior to performing this test may be considered negligent. The modified water deprivation test determines whether a patient can release endogenous ADH in response to dehydration and whether the kidneys can respond to ADH. It differentiates central and nephrogenic diabetes insipidus and primary (psychogenic) polydipsia (PP). Contraindications include dehydration, diabetes mellitus, renal disease, and most of the previously discussed diseases. Performing the water deprivation test without excluding previously described conditions may cause confusing results and misdiagnosis at best and may result in significant patient morbidity or mortality at worst. Consult a veterinary medical textbook for more details before performing this test.

28 If the patient's urine concentrates to more than 1.035 in dogs and more than 1.045 in cats, the diagnosis is PP. Compulsive water drinking is found more commonly in young, hyperactive, large breeds of dog. Stress, lack of sufficient exercise, fever, and pain are some underlying factors. Rarely, PP is associated with a hypothalamic lesion (trauma, mass, infection). Brain imaging is needed to exclude such underlying causes. Hepatic encephalopathy causing behavioral changes such as PP also should be excluded if hepatic function testing has not previously been performed.

29 If urine does not become concentrated during modified water deprivation testing and the patient has lost 5% of its initial body weight, the differential diagnosis is central or nephrogenic diabetes insipidus. To distinguish the two, ADH (in the form of DDAVP/vasopressin) is administered either as an injection or by conjunctival instillation.

30 If urine becomes concentrated after ADH administration, the diagnosis is central diabetes insipidus (CDI). This uncommon condition results from a complete or partial deficiency of ADH synthesis or secretion in the pituitary. Although head trauma, pituitary or hypothalamic masses, and congenital brain deformities can cause CDI, most cases do not have a known cause. Onset is commonly acute in middle-aged dogs. Only a partial ability to concentrate urine may be seen in response to ADH administration in CDI due to renal medullary washout.

31 If the patient's urine does not become concentrated after ADH administration, the diagnosis is nephrogenic diabetes insipidus (NDI), which implies that the renal tubules are insensitive to ADH. Renal insensitivity to ADH occurs most commonly secondary to many of the metabolic conditions already discussed (renal insufficiency/failure, hyper- and hypoadrenocorticism, pyometra, pyelonephritis). It also can occur with administration of glucocorticoids, anticonvulsants, and ethanol. If none of these conditions have been identified and if the algorithm has been followed to rule out all such conditions, then the diagnosis becomes primary NDI. This is an uncommon congenital renal abnormality. Renal biopsy may further characterize this abnormality.

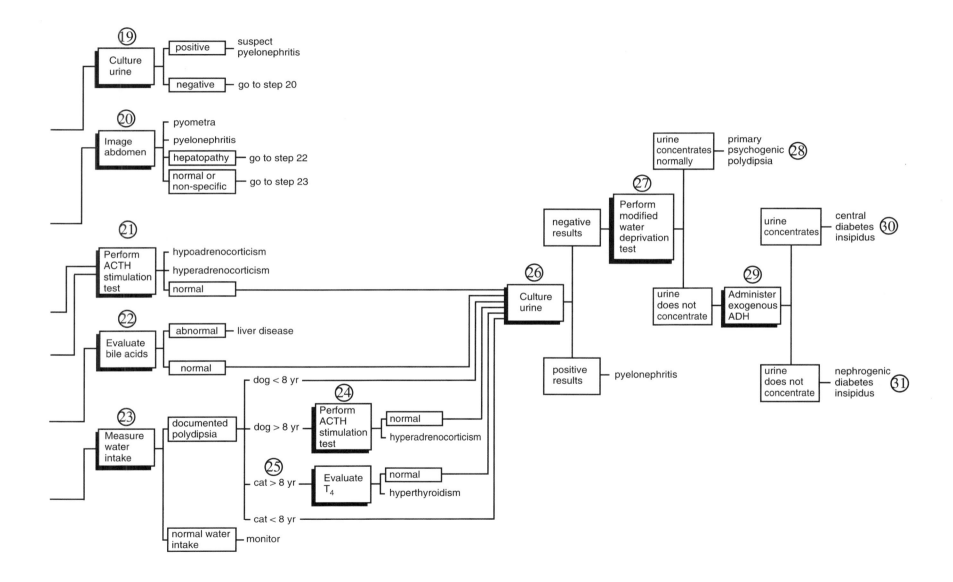

1 In patients demonstrating exercise-induced weakness, strength and gait are initially normal. With exercise, weakness develops as the animal expends energy. The pelvic limbs usually are most affected. Weakness may progress slowly or rapidly to a state of collapse. The animal goes from standing to lateral or sternal recumbency and remains there long enough for the owner to notice. The animal may or may not struggle to rise. Consciousness may or may not be affected, depending on the underlying cause. Syncope or fainting is a form of collapse in which there is sudden, transient loss of consciousness due to reduced oxygen or glucose in the systemic circulation, causing impaired cerebral metabolism.

2 There are numerous causes of collapse and exercise-induced weakness. The history and physical examination are necessary to determine the initial focus of the investigation.

3 Syncope may be the result of an acute decrease in cardiac output associated with arrhythmias, cardiac muscle disease, or valvular disease. If cardiac disease is suspected, based on abnormal pulses or thoracic auscultation, a cardiac evaluation is needed. This generally consists of an electrocardiogram (ECG), a heartworm test, and thoracic radiographs initially. If more information is needed, an echocardiogram will be required.

4 Cats and dogs with pericardial effusion often present with severe weakness and collapse, pale oral mucous membranes, and right-sided heart failure (abdominal effusion in dogs and pleural effusion in cats).

5 Heartworm disease can cause weakness if it results in right-sided heart failure or pulmonary thromboembolic disease. Syncope can develop secondary to pulmonary hypertension.

6 Congenital and acquired valvular heart diseases cause weakness if they result in congestive heart failure. Cardiomyopathy (a cardiac muscle problem) also causes profound weakness.

7 Tachycardia and bradycardia reduce cerebral, coronary, and peripheral blood flow and consequently can produce weakness or syncope. Pheochromocytoma is a rare cause of tachyarrhythmias that can result in collapse.

8 Disorders of skeletal muscle that produce weakness or collapse also affect the canine esophagus because this contains skeletal muscle. Esophageal dysfunction often is associated with regurgitation. Overt dilation of the esophagus may be diagnosed on plain thoracic radiographs and, if necessary, a contrast esophagram can be obtained. Common causes of esophageal dysfunction, combined with weakness and collapse, include myasthenia gravis and polymyositis. Hypothyroidism and hypoadrenocorticism rarely also can produce these signs in the dog; therefore, routine laboratory findings should be assessed before testing for myasthenia gravis and polymyositis.

9 Clients may confuse pain and reluctance to move with weakness, especially if stifle or hip joints are diseased. A complete orthopedic examination should eliminate or confirm joint disease (see the algorithm for joint effusion).

10 Organophosphate or carbamate intoxication can produce generalized weakness and cervical ventroflexion, especially in cats. Signs also can be restricted to the nervous system. A low serum cholinesterase concentration confirms the diagnosis, but a normal concentration does not eliminate organophosphate toxicity. Thus, if there is a history of exposure to organophosphates, the animal should be treated and routine laboratory work performed to eliminate metabolic causes of weakness (step 15).

11 Pale mucous membranes in an animal that is weak or having episodes of collapsing are due either to hypoperfusion (e.g., cardiac problems) or to anemia. Sudden-onset weakness and syncope usually are associated with acute blood loss. Long-standing anemia produces progressive or episodic weakness. With chronic anemia, weakness does not usually occur until the hematocrit drops to less than 20% in the dog and 10–15% in the cat.

12 Splenomegaly or ascites in a middle-aged or older dog with a history of collapse or weakness can suggest a splenic mass (usually a hemangiosarcoma) with acute rupture and bleeding. Abdominal ultrasound is more helpful than radiographs for finding discrete splenic, hepatic, or other organ masses. Exploratory laparotomy

and histopathological evaluation of abnormal tissue is required to confirm the diagnosis.

13 If the patient collapses when food is presented or with excitement (e.g., when the owner enters the room), narcolepsy should be a consideration. Owners can perform and videotape a food-elicited cataplexy test at home since signs may not be reproducible in a hospital setting. If the pet collapses while picking up pieces of a favorite food placed in a row about 30 to 50 cm apart, the narcolepsy complex is very likely. Normal dogs take less than 45 seconds to eat all pieces, while affected dogs may take 25 minutes or more.

14 Scotty cramp is a hyperkinetic syndrome associated with episodes of a "goose-stepping" gait, spasticity, and collapse. Severely affected animals may collapse and curl up into a ball. The syndrome is associated with anxiety, disease, and stress. Drugs (e.g., antiprostaglandins, such as phenylbutazone and flunixin, and penicillin) exacerbate signs. A disorder of serotonin metabolism is the likely underlying cause.

15 Evaluation of a hemogram, serum chemistries, and a heartworm test will rule in or out many metabolic causes of collapse or exercise-induced weakness.

16 If the hematocrit is low, a reticulocyte count is performed to determine if the anemia is regenerative or not.

17 If the serum potassium concentration is high-normal or elevated and the serum sodium concentration is low-normal or below normal, calculate the $Na:K^+$ ratio. If the ratio is less than 27:1 in a dog, evaluate an ACTH test for hypoadrenocorticism. Most patients with adrenal insufficiency have a ratio of less than 23:1.

18 An increased serum cholesterol concentration in conjunction with historical or physical examination findings suggestive of hypothyroidism in a canine patient with collapse or exercise-induced weakness should lead to an evaluation of serum thyroid hormone concentration.

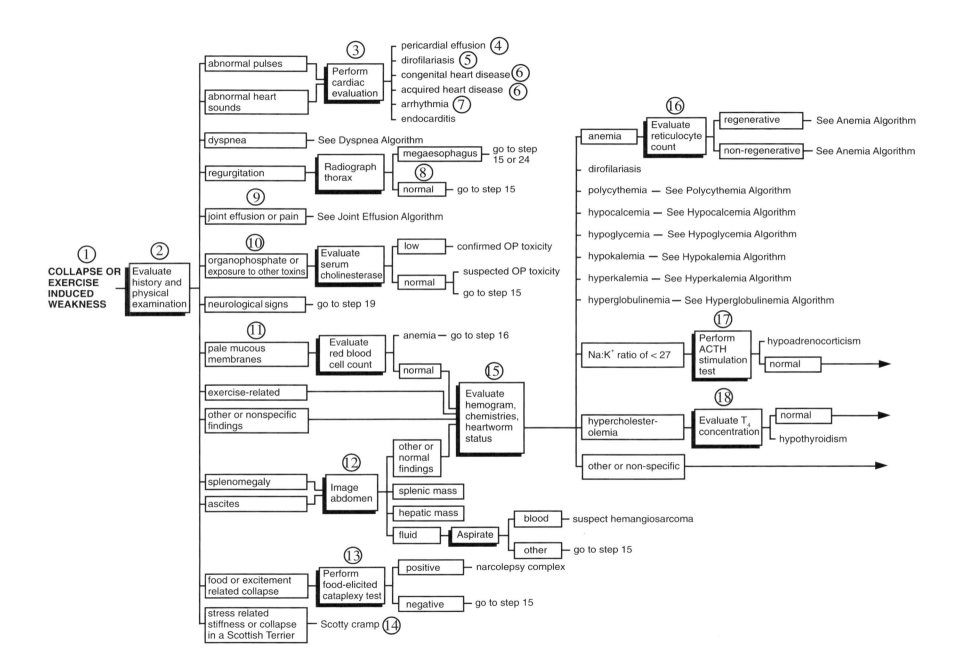

19 By this stage in the algorithm, prior evaluation should have excluded cardiac, respiratory, metabolic, and toxic causes of collapse and exercise-induced weakness. This leaves neurological causes to be investigated. A complete neurological examination is the next step.

20 It is uncommon for lumbosacral (LS) disease to cause collapse or exercise-induced weakness. However, if other causes have been eliminated, LS disease should be considered, especially if hyperpathia is found on palpation or if there are other signs of LS disease (urinary/fecal incontinence, reduced tail tone, conscious proprioceptive deficits). Radiographs or CT scans of the area are helpful in making a diagnosis of instability, discospondylitis, or disc herniation.

21 If spinal limb reflexes are reduced (hyporeflexia) or there is muscle pain, hypertrophy, or atrophy, evaluate serum CK. This is often elevated in polymyositis.

22 If CK is elevated, check antinuclear antibody (ANA) titers for immune-mediated causes.

23 If the history suggests potential exposure to *Toxoplasma gondii* or *Neospora caninum,* assess titers for these diseases. Both affect peripheral nerves and/or muscles but are not common causes of collapse. Acute infections may not cause increased serum titers, and these should be rechecked 3 weeks after the initial presentation.

24 If the CK concentration is normal or if the physical/neurological examination shows dysphagia or facial weakness in addition to exercise-induced weakness/collapse, evaluate a serum titer for acetylcholine receptor antibodies (myasthenia gravis titers).

25 If the myasthenia gravis titer is negative, review all information obtained to date to decide whether weakness could be due to intermittent cardiac disease, neuromuscular junction disease, or an unusual form of seizure disorder. Weakness that worsens with exercise is usually due to a neuromuscular junction disorder. Therefore, unless there are strong reasons to suspect cardiac disease or a seizure disorder, it may be best to pursue neuromuscular junction problems first.

26 Collapse associated with intermittent cardiac problems may be due to acquired or congenital heart disease or underlying arrhythmias. Physical examination may be normal or may indicate tachycardia, bradycardia, cyanosis, coughing, or abnormal lung sounds.

27 An intermittent arrhythmia leading to collapse can be difficult to diagnose unless the patient is undergoing continuous ECG monitoring. The ECG should be assessed during an episode of collapse.

28 In order to diagnose most neuromuscular junction disorders, electromyography, nerve conduction studies, and nerve/muscle biopsy are required. Electrodiagnostic tests are usually available only through specialty practices or teaching hospitals. However, anyone can perform a muscle biopsy and send the sample to a laboratory that processes and stains such samples. Routine H&E staining is helpful in diagnosing myositis, but it will not distinguish myofiber atrophy from neurogenic or myopathic causes. Histochemical staining is required for such differentiation. Contact the laboratory to determine how the sample should be processed and packed before performing the biopsy.

29 Type II myofiber deficiency is a specific disease of young Labrador retrievers. Signs range from minimal to severe and are often more noticeable during periods of stress or in cold weather. Stiffness of gait, reluctance to exercise, muscle atrophy of the proximal limbs and pelvic girdle are common signs. The disease is not treatable. This deficiency is inherited as an autosomal recessive.

30 Myotonia is excessive muscle tone. Causes can be congenital or acquired. Affected animals may have a slow, stiff gait and may not be able to tolerate exercise. Proximal limb muscles may be hypertrophied. Percussion of muscles may result in a "dimple," an indentation that lasts long after the muscle body is percussed.

31 Polymyositis has many causes. There are two main reasons for generalized muscle inflammation: infectious and immune mediated. Exercise-induced weakness and megaesophagus can develop with either underlying cause. Elevated serum CK is a helpful finding, but this is not always present with polymyositis.

32 Many breed-specific myopathies are congenital or inherited. Weakness with exercise often occurs with such disorders. Myopathy secondary to untreated hyperadrenocorticism also can cause weakness and even collapse.

33 Most neuropathies do not cause collapse but they can cause generalized weakness, especially if associated muscle wasting is severe.

34 Seizures occasionally manifest as sudden "dropping" or collapse of the pelvic limbs. Narcolepsy also is a consideration (see step 13) if excitement precipitates collapse.

35 Most patients with epilepsy manifest generalized or partial seizure activity.

36 Encephalitis and intracranial masses are unusual causes of collapse and weakness unless clinical signs are seizure activity that is mistaken for weakness or collapse. Some brain infections and masses may cause bradycardia or other cardiac arrhythmias that could result in exercise-induced weakness.

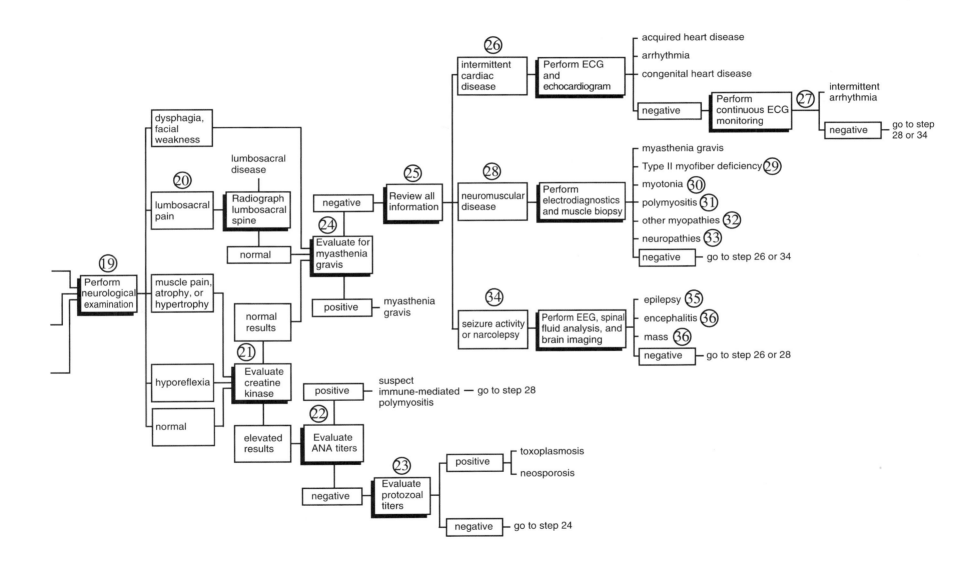

1 Abdominal enlargement may be due to organ enlargement, fluid accumulation, gaseous distention of hollow viscera or of the peritoneal cavity, or reduced abdominal muscle tone. Abdominal enlargement often develops insidiously. However, it also may be acute or dramatic, as with gas accumulation in the stomach in gastric distention and volvulus (GDV) or bleeding from a ruptured splenic hemangiosarcoma. Acute abdominal enlargement is likely to be more immediately life-threatening than chronic progressive enlargement, either because of the severity of the underlying disease (e.g., hypovolemia from abdominal bleeding) or compromise of venous return to the heart by increases in intra-abdominal pressure. Occasionally, abdominal enlargement may seem acute (e.g., ascites secondary to hypoalbuminemia), although the underlying disease is obviously more chronic.

2 If the patient is relaxed and not obese, abdominal palpation may detect intra-abdominal masses, organomegaly, gas, or fluid accumulation.

3 With ascites, a fluid wave often can be balloted through the abdominal wall in the standing patient (unless only small amounts of fluid are present). Radiographically, fluid accumulation obscures intra-abdominal structures, including any masses that might be the underlying cause. Ultrasound may be more useful for identifying changes in solid structures within the abdomen, potential sources of fluid, and mass lesions.

4 Progressive wasting and weakening of abdominal musculature commonly occurs due to high levels of glucocorticoids in the circulation (hyperadrenocorticism) or severe debilitation. Hyperadrenocorticism also causes hepatic enlargement as a result of glycogen accumulation in the liver. Muscle wasting and hepatic enlargement combine to produce the classical pot-bellied appearance in the patient. This is a major presenting complaint with hyperadrenocorticism, along with bilaterally symmetrical hair loss, thin skin, comedones, prominent abdominal blood vessels, and excessive panting.

5 Asymmetrical distention of the abdomen or tympany on percussion suggests air accumulation, either within a viscus or within the peritoneal cavity. Abdominal radiographs are the imaging method of choice for patients with suspected air accumulation (bowel obstruction, torsion, ileus, or other causes of gaseous distention of a viscus or peritoneal gas accumulation) because gas blocks the ultrasound beam. If both left and right lateral radiographs as well as ventrodorsal views are obtained, the majority of gastric dilations and GDVs will be identified.

6 The abdomen can be imaged by a variety of methods (plain and contrast radiographs, ultrasound, or CT/ MRI scans of the abdomen). Abdominal ultrasound is probably the highest-yielding test if ascites or organomegaly is present, if hyperadrenocorticism is suspected, or if no abnormalities are detected on physical examination. It can document whether diffuse organ enlargement is present (with infiltrative conditions such as diffuse neoplasia, abnormal accumulation of metabolic products, or inflammatory cells) versus focal or mass-like lesions (benign or malignant neoplasia, hematomas, abscesses, cystic lesions, or hepatic nodular regeneration). Abnormal areas, once identified, may be aspirated for cytology and culture or biopsied to obtain a histopathological diagnosis once adequate precautions (e.g., coagulation panels, cross-match, assessment of renal function) have been taken. If the abdominal ultrasound scan is normal or inconclusive, plain or contrast radiographs may be considered (for the conditions described above).

7 Patients with normal or inconclusive abdominal imaging results, hepatomegaly or bi-/unilateral adrenomegaly should be tested for hyperadrenocorticism by means of an ACTH stimulation test. If that test is negative, it may be because the patient does not have hyperadrenocorticism or because it is one of the 15–20% of patients with hyperadrenocorticism that do not test positive on an ACTH stimulation test. If clinical signs are still suggestive of hyperadrenocorticism, it may be worthwhile to test the patient further with a low-dose dexamethasone suppression test or a urine cortisol : creatinine ratio. While these tests are more sensitive than the ACTH stim-

ulation test in detecting hyperadrenocorticism, they are also less specific and may be influenced by other current diseases (e.g., diabetes mellitus, seizure disorders, phenobarbitol therapy).

8 If all of these screening or diagnostic tests for hyperadrenocorticism are negative, the patient needs to be evaluated for other causes of muscle wastage (e.g., malnutrition, severe inflammatory bowel disease and malabsorption, neoplasia, polyneuropathy, other neuromuscular diseases, autoimmune conditions).

9 If the ACTH test is positive, then combine the findings of a high-dose dexamethasone suppression test and/ or previous abdominal ultrasound findings to determine whether the condition is adrenal or pituitary in origin.

10 Patients with focal masses or diffuse organomegaly should have fine-needle aspiration or biopsy of the tissue(s) involved in an effort to identify the underlying abnormality (e.g., neoplasia, inflammation, and immune-mediated disease). Cytology is less invasive than biopsy for histopathology, does not require general anesthesia, and usually does not require a coagulogram. However, although it may allow assessment of the cell types present, it will not identify structural changes in an organ such as fibrosis, cirrhosis, dysplasia, or hyperplasia, and it does not permit diagnosis of neoplasia if the tissue involved does not exfoliate.

11 If a diagnosis has not been reached via cytology in a patient with focal or diffuse organomegaly, pursue excisional or incisional biopsy either percutaneously or via exploratory celiotomy (the method selected depends on the patient's clinical condition, the structures involved, and whether or not complete excision can be performed). All biopsies of intra-abdominal structures are likely to require general anesthesia. Biopsy may be required to confirm the diagnosis or to treat conditions that may be diagnosed confidently with ultrasound (e.g., hydronephrosis, pyometra, paraprostatic cysts, perirenal cysts).

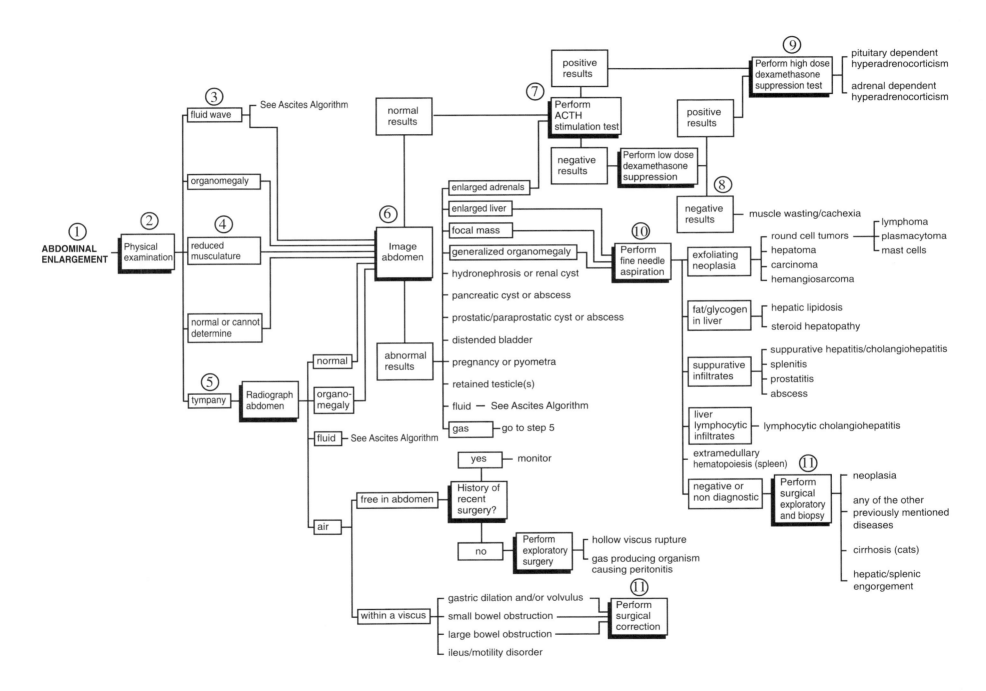

1 Ascites is accumulation of fluid in the abdominal cavity. It must be distinguished from other conditions that cause abdominal distention (e.g., muscle wastage, organomegaly). Moderate amounts of fluid may be found by ballotment of a fluid wave. Small amounts are best detected by ultrasound.

2 Abdominocentesis (step 3) is the most useful initial test for evaluating abdominal effusion. Few contraindications exist, the most important being underlying coagulopathy (e.g., due to coumarin-based rodenticides, disseminated intravascular coagulation [DIC], or severe thrombocytopenia). If these conditions are suspected, abdominocentesis should not be performed because of the risk of further bleeding. Coagulation times, platelet count, and possibly fibrin degradation products (FDPs) should be measured. It also may be appropriate to bypass abdominocentesis and proceed to ultrasound to look for intra-abdominal masses, thoracic radiographs for primary/metastatic neoplasia or concurrent pleural effusion, or other tests.

3 Perform abdominocentesis if there is no history of a coagulation abnormality or if the benefits of obtaining a sample outweigh the risks. The procedure can be performed "blind" at the most dependent region of the abdomen in recumbent patients or from the lowest portion of the ventral abdomen in standing patients. The spleen should be avoided during blind procedures, because aspiration of this organ leads to misdiagnosis of hemoabdomen. Ultrasound may be needed for small amounts of fluid and where fluid is confined to pockets within the abdominal cavity.

4 Fluid should be evaluated for cell counts (including the packed cell volume if appropriate) and total protein. Later, fluid chemistries (e.g., cholesterol, triglycerides, creatinine, bilirubin, glucose), titers for specific diseases (e.g., FIP), and cytology of smears or concentrated preparations may be evaluated (see step 25). Abdominal effusions are divided into transudates (low-protein, low-cellularity fluid), modified transudates, and exudates (high-protein, high-cellularity fluid). However, there is considerable overlap between the categories in terms of protein concentrations and cell counts (see below).

5 Transudates are low-protein fluids (<2.5 g/dl) with low cell counts (<1000 nucleated cells/mm^3). They form in association with conditions that cause low serum protein (especially decreased albumin) and hence reduced plasma oncotic pressure (e.g., liver failure, protein-losing nephropathy, protein-losing enteropathy, severe malnutrition, large cutaneous burns). They also may develop in association with neoplasia, especially lymphoma. For a transudate to form as a result of decreased plasma oncotic pressure alone, serum albumin must be less than 1.5 g/dl. However, serum albumin concentrations of 1.8–2.0 g/dl may result in transudate formation if other factors affecting intravascular pressure are present (e.g., portal hypertension). Transudates are modified over time as a result of inflammation due to the presence of fluid in the abdominal cavity.

6 Modified transudates generally have protein contents between 2.5 and 3.5 g/dl and variable cellularity (most often less than the cell counts of exudates). Some conditions are associated with either exudates or modified transudates, depending on the duration of fluid accumulation in the abdomen eliciting an inflammatory response. Therefore, considerable overlap exists between causes of these types of abdominal effusion. Conditions that can result in both exudates and modified transudates include chylous effusions, bile and urine peritonitis, and some neoplastic effusions.

7 Abdominal modified transudates are common in dogs with right-sided heart failure. Cats are more likely to form pleural effusions with this condition. Right-sided heart disease is suspected if patients have a right-sided cardiac murmur, jugular pulses extending more than one-third of the way up the neck, hepatojugular reflux, or pitting edema of the extremities. Pulmonic stenosis, patent ductus arteriosus, tricuspid valve insufficiency, ventricular septal defects, heartworm infestation, or chronic pulmonary disease may lead to right-sided heart failure. Thoracic radiographs can show right-sided cardiac enlargement, increased sternal contact of the heart, arterial pruning that suggests heartworm infestation, venous distention, or diaphragmatic rupture. They also can show chronic pulmonary disease or suggest biventricular heart failure (pulmonary edema in addition to right-sided signs) or pleural effusion. An echocardiogram may be needed to determine the extent of underlying heart disease.

8 If a modified transudate is not secondary to heart disease, a serum chemistry profile should be evaluated. Hyperproteinemia can be associated with underlying neoplasia, FIP, or immune-mediated disease. Ascites accompanying azotemia may result from urinary tract rupture or fluid overload with oliguric/anuric renal failure. Elevated serum bilirubin is seen with underlying hepatic neoplasia or biliary tract rupture. Evidence of sepsis secondary to peritonitis also may be picked up (elevated ALP, low albumin, low glucose).

9 If the serum chemistry profile is nonspecific, abdominal imaging (particularly ultrasound, since fluid obscures detail on radiographs) may identify focal masses, diffuse lesions such as carcinomatosis, walled-off abscesses, or cysts that might lead to the formation of modified transudates.

10 An occult heartworm test should be performed in patients with modified transudates, especially in endemic areas and if there is a questionable history of heartworm prevention. Severe heartworm infestation may result in extension of worms into the caudal vena cava (vena caval syndrome), posthepatic portal hypertension, and abdominal fluid accumulation.

11 If no other underlying cause of a modified transudate has been identified, posthepatic portal hypertension must be considered. This requires the presence of a constrictive or obstructive lesion located between the liver and the right side of the heart (i.e., in the caudal vena cava). Such lesions are rare unless they are due to vena caval syndrome, but they have been identified via thoracic ultrasound and venography. Causes include neoplasia in the caudal mediastinum, thrombosis, or trauma to the caudal vena cava.

12 Exploratory celiotomy and biopsy of multiple tissues are required to prove idiopathic peritoneal effusion (step 35). Some effusions are suspected of being immune-mediated (e.g., in systemic lupus erythematosus [SLE]), but this is difficult to prove. Finding inflammation on biopsy specimens with no obvious underlying cause, a positive ANA titer, and involvement of other body systems (e.g., protein-losing nephropathy, immune-mediated hemolytic anemia) are helpful in confirming the SLE-related effusion. The amount of fluid formed is generally small.

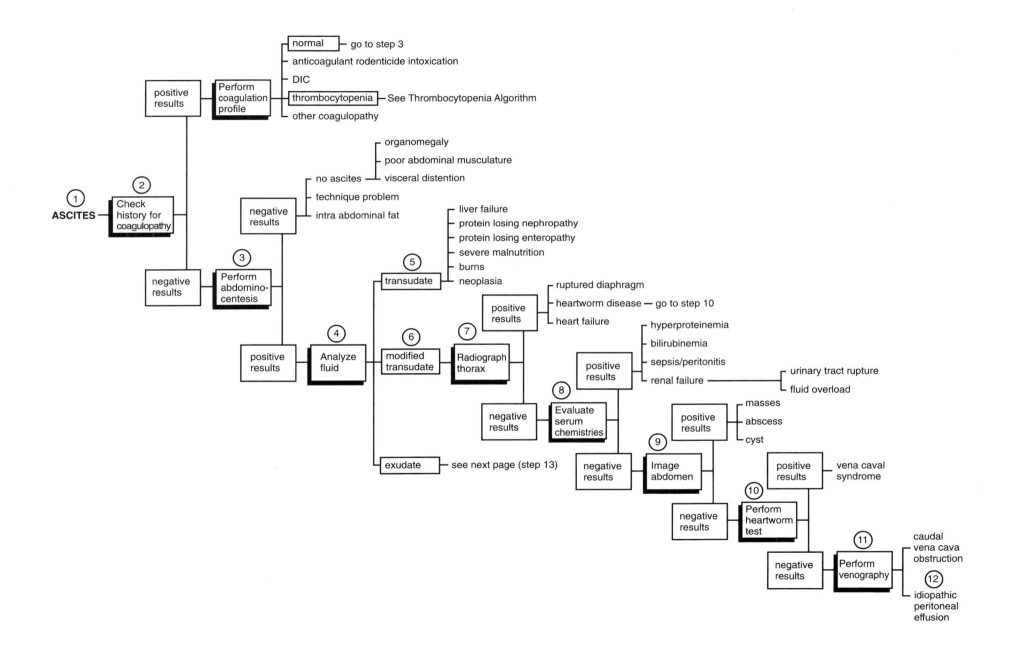

ASCITES

1 ASCITES

2 Check history for coagulopathy

positive results — Perform coagulation profile
- normal — go to step 3
- anticoagulant rodenticide intoxication
- DIC
- thrombocytopenia — See Thrombocytopenia Algorithm
- other coagulopathy

negative results

3 Perform abdomino-centesis

negative results
- no ascites
  - organomegaly
  - poor abdominal musculature
  - visceral distention
- technique problem
- intra abdominal fat

positive results

4 Analyze fluid

5 transudate
- liver failure
- protein losing nephropathy
- protein losing enteropathy
- severe malnutrition
- burns
- neoplasia

6 modified transudate

7 Radiograph thorax

positive results
- ruptured diaphragm
- heartworm disease — go to step 10
- heart failure

negative results

8 Evaluate serum chemistries

positive results
- hyperproteinemia
- bilirubinemia
- sepsis/peritonitis
- renal failure
  - urinary tract rupture
  - fluid overload

negative results

9 Image abdomen

positive results
- masses
- abscess
- cyst

negative results

10 Perform heartworm test

positive results — vena caval syndrome

negative results

11 Perform venography
- caudal vena cava obstruction

12 idiopathic peritoneal effusion

exudate — see next page (step 13)

13 Exudates are defined as fluid accumulations with total protein greater than 3 g/dl and cell counts greater than or equal to 5000 nucleated cells/mm^3. Exudates have a wide variety of appearances and underlying causes.

14 With sanguinous or serosanguinous exudates, the packed cell volume (PCV) of the effusion should be checked by spinning a sample in a hematocrit tube. The result can be compared to the patient's peripheral blood PCV. If the two are similar or the PCV of the abdominal fluid is greater than that of peripheral blood, intra-abdominal bleeding has occurred.

15 A sample of sanguinous intra-abdominal fluid may be held in a glass tube to see whether or not a fibrin clot forms. If it does, bleeding has been very recent (usually fibrin is deposited on peritoneal surfaces very quickly after a bleeding episode, depleting the abdominal fluid of fibrinogen and preventing it from clotting) or the spleen has been aspirated.

16 In patients with sanguinous abdominal fluid, coagulography should be performed unless there is a definite history of trauma and no suspicion of complicating underlying conditions such as hepatic disease. Patients with a definite history of trauma should either be treated symptomatically and supportively, and evaluated frequently for deterioration, or testing should proceed to abdominal ultrasound (step 20).

17 Positive FDPs are probably the least sensitive but most specific indications of DIC. They form when fibrinolytic pathways in the body break down large numbers of fibrin clots. If FDPs are found in conjunction with prolongation of the prothrombin time (PT) and the activated partial thromboplastin time (PTT), as well as a low platelet count, DIC is very likely to be the underlying cause of abdominal bleeding. Causes of DIC include neoplasia, sepsis, toxin, heat or cold exposure, and severe pancreatitis. However, the evaluation may be confused because deposition of fibrin in the peritoneal cavity also will lead to elevation of FDPs as the body breaks down the clots formed on peritoneal surfaces.

18 Markedly prolonged PT and activated PTT values (greater than 60 seconds) are seen most commonly in patients with exposure to coumarin-based products and DIC. Smaller elevations are seen in association with liver disease/liver failure.

19 Thrombocytopenia is an uncommon cause of body cavity bleeding unless it occurs in association with DIC or there is a history of trauma. Thrombocytopenia generally results in cutaneous bleeding and bruising, bleeding from mucosal surfaces, petechial hemorrhages, hemoptysis, and epistaxis. Spontaneous bleeding generally arises with platelet counts less than 20 to 30,000/μl. Thrombocytopenia also may be the result rather than the cause of excessive bleeding. However, in those circumstances, platelet counts rarely go below 50 to 80,000/μl.

20 Patients with intra-abdominal bleeding and a normal coagulogram and patients suspected of having hepatic disease or DIC should be further evaluated as appropriate. Abdominal ultrasound may prove useful to evaluate for intra-abdominal masses (e.g., hepatic, splenic, renal tumors), masses eroding into major blood vessels (e.g., adrenal tumors), evidence of trauma, or splenic torsion. On occasion, further imaging techniques may prove necessary, including abdominal CT and MRI scans. Exploratory laparotomy may be needed to further define and treat underlying conditions.

21 Serosanguinous, serous, cloudy, opaque, or obviously purulent exudates should be submitted for aerobic and anaerobic culture and antimicrobial sensitivity testing. A cytological preparation should be Gram stained to allow preliminary identification of bacteria, especially intracellular organisms that are unlikely to be contaminants.

22 Patients with a positive culture or intracellular bacteria or cytological examination from an abdominal exudate have septic peritonitis, and an underlying cause should be sought. Note that a septic abdominal exudate is almost always an indication for exploratory laparotomy to attempt to diagnose and remove the underlying cause

and lavage the abdomen. Therefore, it may be appropriate to bypass the next few diagnostic steps and go straight to exploratory laparotomy (step 35) unless diffuse, inoperable neoplasia is suspected.

23 Abdominal radiographs are useful for identification of bowel obstructions or bowel rupture. These will be visible despite the presence of abdominal fluid. Bowel obstruction will manifest as excessive gaseous and fluid distention of bowel proximal to the obstruction. Radiodense foreign bodies also will be seen. The distinction between bowel masses, intussusceptions, and radiolucent foreign bodies leading to obstruction cannot usually be made. Bowel rupture will appear as free gas within the abdominal cavity (best seen just behind the diaphragm). Penetrating abdominal wounds also may result in free air in the abdomen as well as formation of a septic exudate. However, there will be historical and physical evidence of such a wound. Patients who have undergone exploratory celiotomy in the last 7 to 10 days may still have free air in the abdomen. Contrast abdominal radiographs may be needed to identify urinary tract rupture (intravenous urography for renal and ureteral damage and contrast urethrocystography for the urethra and urinary bladder).

24 Abdominal ultrasound is useful for identifying lesions in solid tissues such as abscesses (prostatic, hepatic, pancreatic), cysts (renal, prostatic, paraprostatic), solid tissue masses (benign or malignant neoplasms of almost any tissue), pyometra, trauma to the biliary system and lower urinary tract, and some urinary tract obstructions. The last three may not be obvious on ultrasound and may require exploratory surgery or contrast studies to make a diagnosis. Additionally, ruptured abscesses originating in any tissue may not be obvious on abdominal ultrasound since the abnormal area no longer has obvious boundaries to define it.

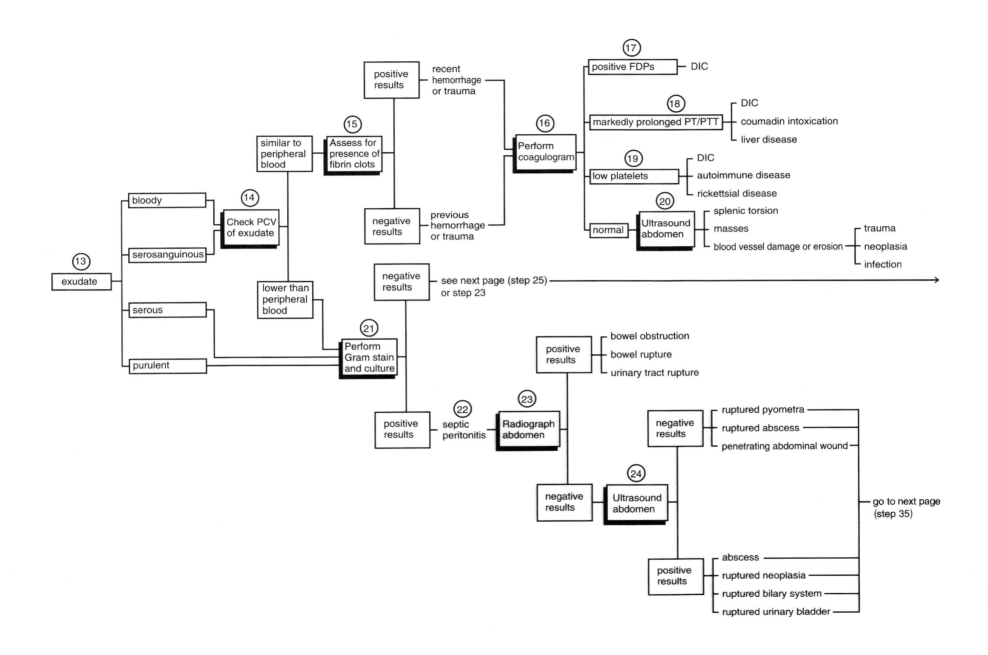

25 When an exudate is neither sanguinous nor septic, the next step is to evaluate it more specifically, including gross appearance (chyle, bile), chemistries, serology, and cytology.

26 Milky white/opaque fluid should be assessed to determine if it is chylous. Chyle contains large chylomicrons, clears in ether, and fluid triglyceride concentrations are greater than fluid cholesterol concentrations. A chylous abdominal effusion results from rupture or obstruction of abdominal lymphatics. The patient's history should be reviewed for trauma or surgery leading to lymphatic disruption or right-sided heart disease causing backward heart failure affecting the thoracic duct. Patients also should undergo abdominal ultrasound to evaluate for masses. Mesenteric root adenocarcinoma is particularly associated with chyloabdomen in cats, while lymphoma may be an underlying cause in both dogs and cats. An echocardiogram is used to evaluate for right-sided heart failure in patients with appropriate clinical signs or when no other cause of a chylous abdominal effusion has been found.

27 Patients with negative results may need exploratory celiotomy to investigate further for causes of chylous effusion. Intra-abdominal problems with lymphatic drainage (e.g., secondary to neoplasia) are most likely. Young animals may have congenital malformation or absence of lymphatics. Intestinal lymphangiectasia generally results in loss of chylous fluid into the bowel lumen, hypoalbuminemia, and a low-protein transudate. However, occasionally the cause of lymphangiectasia is generalized inflammation/granuloma formation around intra-abdominal lymphatics, in which case chylous effusions form.

28 If there is peripheral hyperglobulinemia and the total protein concentration of an abdominal effusion is greater than 4.5 g/dl, underlying neoplasia is possible in dogs and cats and FIP should be suspected in cats. In FIP, fluid is straw-colored, cells consist of macrophages and small lymphocytes, and the patient has a history of fever and hepatic, renal, or gastrointestinal signs. Titers for FIP are not conclusive but may aid the diagnosis in patients with an appropriate history, clinical signs, and cytological indications. Positive titers indicate exposure to and an immunological response to feline coronavirus, but this does not mean that the patient has FIP. Negative titers indicate lack of an exposure or lack of an immunological response. Titers also may be run on abdominal effusions. Histopathological examination of the liver or kidney is needed for confirmation (step 35).

29 Neoplastic cells in an abdominal effusion may identify the tissue type, if not the source. Be careful not to identify reactive mesothelial cells shed from the peritoneal lining as neoplastic cells. Further imaging of the abdomen (ultrasound, CT, or MRI scans) may identify neoplastic masses and assess potential for biopsy or resection.

30 Bile peritonitis results from gallbladder or intra/extrahepatic biliary system rupture (traumatic or secondary to inflammation/obstruction). Signs develop slowly unless there is a biliary infection (bacterial cholecystitis). Patients develop lethargy and progressive abdominal distention over as many as 10 days. An exudate forms due to peritoneal irritation. Abdominocentesis can yield unmistakable green-staining fluid because of bilirubin and biliverdin. However, fluid also may be icteric and cannot be distinguished from abdominal fluid in patients with high serum bilirubin due to other causes. Fluid cytology may show bilirubin crystals. Since bilirubin is a small molecule, its concentration in abdominal fluid quickly equilibrates with peripheral blood concentrations, and bilirubin in blood and fluid rises over time because of failure to excrete bilirubin in feces. Ultrasound can identify some biliary ruptures, calculi, and mass lesions. However, surgery is required to locate and treat ruptures.

31 Urine peritonitis develops secondary to rupture of the urinary bladder, urethra, or terminal ureters. Most of the ureters, the urethra, and the kidneys are enclosed in the retroperitoneal space, and damage results in accumulation of urine in that area. Retroperitoneal ruptures cause less abdominal distention and more external signs of bruising and exudation. Urinary tract ruptures generally are traumatic, although partial/complete obstructions by calculi and neoplasia anywhere may lead to rupture. With bladder rupture, abdominal distention develops 3 to 5 days later. Clinical signs take longer to develop if urine is sterile. The fluid is a modified transudate/exudate, depending on the concentration of the urine and the amount of irritation it induces. Patients develop postrenal azotemia due to failure to excrete blood urea nitrogen (BUN) and creatinine. Fluid BUN concentrations equilibrate with blood quickly because urea is a small molecule and crosses membranes easily. Therefore, fluid creatinine concentrations may be more reliable for diagnosing urinary tract rupture. Abdominal ultrasound can distinguish retroperitoneal and abdominal fluid, mass lesions, and some calculi and identify changes in bladder shape suggestive of rupture. However, a contrast study (either a urethrocystogram or an intravenous urogram) will be needed to identify the location of the leak. Exploratory surgery is needed to repair any damage.

32 If an abdominal exudate is identified but there is no obvious cause, the differential diagnosis includes benign or malignant neoplasia, abscesses, cysts, diaphragm rupture (this usually causes a modified transudate unless there is organ entrapment/necrosis), immune-mediated disease (e.g., SLE), pancreatitis, other vasculitides, and steatitis. Imaging the abdomen, usually by ultrasound, can be helpful.

33 Amylase and lipase concentrations can be higher in fluid than in peripheral blood with pancreatitis. Increased fasting serum trypsin-like immunoreactivity also can increase the suspicion of pancreatic inflammation. Amylase and lipase concentrations also increase with pancreatic abscesses or neoplasia; therefore, concentrations need to be interpreted in light of the ultrasound findings.

34 If negative results are obtained to this point, vasculitis should be considered. Causes of vasculitis include rickettsial disease (especially Rocky Mountain spotted fever), FIP, steatitis, and SLE. Titers can be obtained for acute rickettsial disease and should be reevaluated 3 weeks later for significant increases. Feline coronavirus (FIP) titers on peripheral blood and abdominal fluid may suggest infection, but tissue biopsy is needed to confirm the diagnosis. Steatitis is inflammation of subcutaneous/intra-abdominal fat. It occurs particularly in cats and may cause pain, fever, and abdominal effusion. It also requires biopsy of affected tissue to make a diagnosis. ANA titers help to confirm the presence of SLE, but other criteria need to be fulfilled and other immune-mediated diseases can cause vasculitis.

35 Exploratory surgery and tissue biopsy may be required to make or confirm many of the diagnoses above or to exclude all underlying causes and reach a diagnosis of idiopathic effusion. Surgery should be performed at any stage in the diagnostic algorithm at which it appears appropriate.

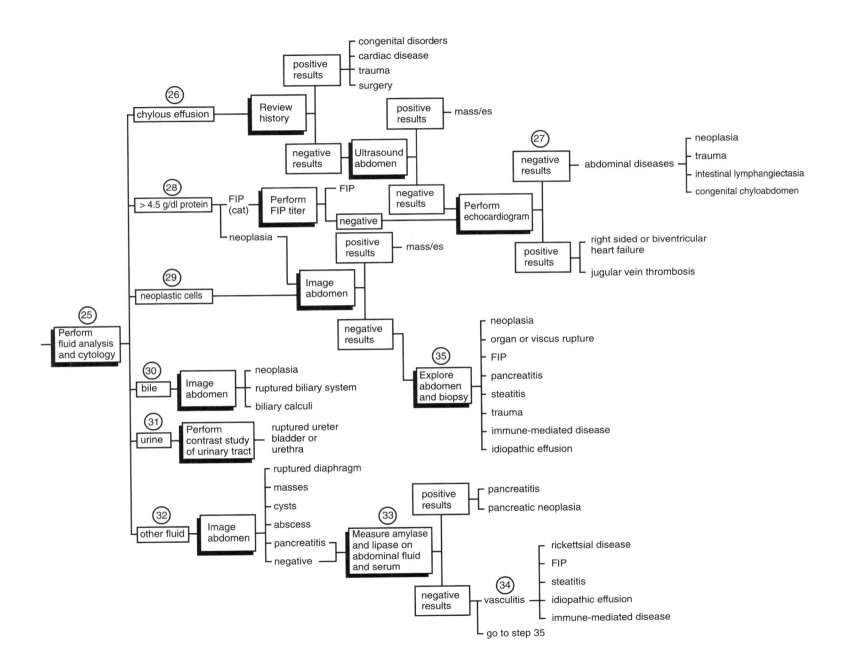

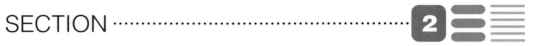

Musculoskeletal Problems

1 Lameness is an abnormal gait characterized by stiffness, shortened stride, and altered weight bearing. It may be due to mechanical problems (e.g., fracture malunion, angular limb deformity) or an attempt to decrease weight bearing on a limb in response to pain (e.g., enostosis, immune-mediated polyarthritis, neoplasia).

2 The history is important. Acute-onset, single-limb, weight-bearing lameness is often due to minor trauma or muscle and tendon strains that usually resolve within a week. Current therapy for unrelated diseases is important since lameness is a common sign of drug-induced polyarthritis. Sulfa-containing drugs, macrolides, and penicillin-like antibiotics all have been associated with inflammatory polyarthritis. Joint luxations and bone fractures are associated with more severe trauma and manifest with non-weight-bearing or severe weight-bearing lameness. Immediate progression to radiographs is appropriate with non-weight-bearing lameness.

3 The causes of lameness vary with the patient's age (immature vs. mature) and the affected limb (forelimb vs. hindlimb). In young, growing dogs, lameness is frequently found in association with enostosis (panosteitis), bone cysts, and metaphyseal osteopathy (hypertrophic osteodystrophy). In mature large or giant-breed dogs with one affected limb, osteosarcoma should be considered. Hip dysplasia is seen most frequently in large-breed dogs, whereas patellar luxation is most common in toy breeds. Young toy and small-breed dogs can also have aseptic necrosis of the femoral head (Legg-Calvé-Perthes disease). Elbow dysplasia is common in rottweilers, Labrador retrievers, and Bernese mountain dogs. Young male Persian cats can develop periosteal proliferative polyarthritis.

4 A thorough physical examination is performed next. If the patient is allowed to roam in areas with thorn bushes, splinters, cacti, or other sharp elements, the clinician should look for foreign bodies between the toes. Orthopedic examination begins with observation of the gait at a slow walk and then a trot. Careful palpation of the affected limb's muscles, joints, and bones in con-

junction with signalment and history taking allows the formation of an initial differential diagnosis list. Sedation allows a more thorough examination of the affected limb, especially if the patient has pain or is unruly. Once the diagnosis of lameness is made, based on the severity of the clinical signs, the time of onset, and the owner's concerns and finances, the algorithm may stop. However, important information often is obtained by radiographing the affected limb or area.

5 If radiographs do not show a reason for the lameness, if more than one limb is affected, if the lameness shifts from one limb to another, or if systemic signs are present, it is appropriate to pursue joint diseases and arthrocentesis (see the algorithms for joint effusion and pain).

6 If lameness is acute and affects only one limb, if the physical examination does not suggest systemic illness, and if radiographs are normal or show only minor soft tissue damage/injury, it is prudent to restrict the patient's activity and reevaluate in 5 to 7 days.

7 If the radiographs are normal but lameness is chronic or progressive, the patient should be evaluated for infectious diseases common in the environment or in areas of previous travel. These include a variety of rickettsial diseases (borreliosis, Rocky Mountain spotted fever, and ehrlichiosis). Arthrocentesis should be considered even if joint pain or effusion is not obvious on physical examination because the results of synovial fluid analysis may help to identify joint disease and classify it as inflammatory versus degenerative.

8 An ANA titer is an indirect immunofluorescence test that documents the presence of serum antibodies with specificity for nuclear antigens. A positive ANA titer can be found in SLE, as well as some other immune-mediated disorders.

9 It has been estimated that about 75% of dogs with SLE will exhibit polyarthritis at some time during the disease. The mean age of dogs with SLE is about 6

years. Shetland sheepdogs, collies, Afghan hounds, beagles, Irish setters, Old English sheepdogs, poodles, and German shepherds may be overrepresented in this category. Arthrocentesis should be performed if lameness is thought to be due to inflammatory arthritis. Cytological analysis shows increased cell counts consisting mainly of nondegenerate neutrophils, some mononuclear cells, and no bacteria. Synovial fluid has decreased viscosity. Criteria other than an inflammatory, noninfectious joint effusion are needed to diagnose SLE. These include ANA titers and evidence of involvement of other body systems (skin, red blood cells [RBCs], platelets, kidneys, etc.). Isolated immune-mediated polyarthritis also can be a cause of lameness with inflammatory joint cytology. In this case, there will be no other criteria for the diagnosis of SLE.

10 If diagnostic testing to this point has not shown indications of bone or joint disease to explain the clinical signs, then a neurological basis for the lameness must be considered. Neurological examination reveals changes in spinal reflexes, areas of hyperpathia, or atrophy of specific muscle groups, all of which suggest a possible neurological basis for the disease. Occasionally, muscle inflammation causes lameness; thus, a serum CK evaluation should be considered.

11 Even if the general neurological examination is normal, a focal neurological cause for the lameness remains possible. Careful palpation of areas where the nerves travel along the limb may reveal an area of pain or discomfort. Ultimately, specialized imaging will probably be needed to diagnose peripheral nerve involvement completely. Nerve sheath neoplasia occurs most commonly in the front limbs, producing chronic lameness that becomes more severe over a period of months.

12 If an abnormal area is detected using radiographs or advanced imaging techniques, the next step is surgical exploration and biopsy of abnormal tissue.

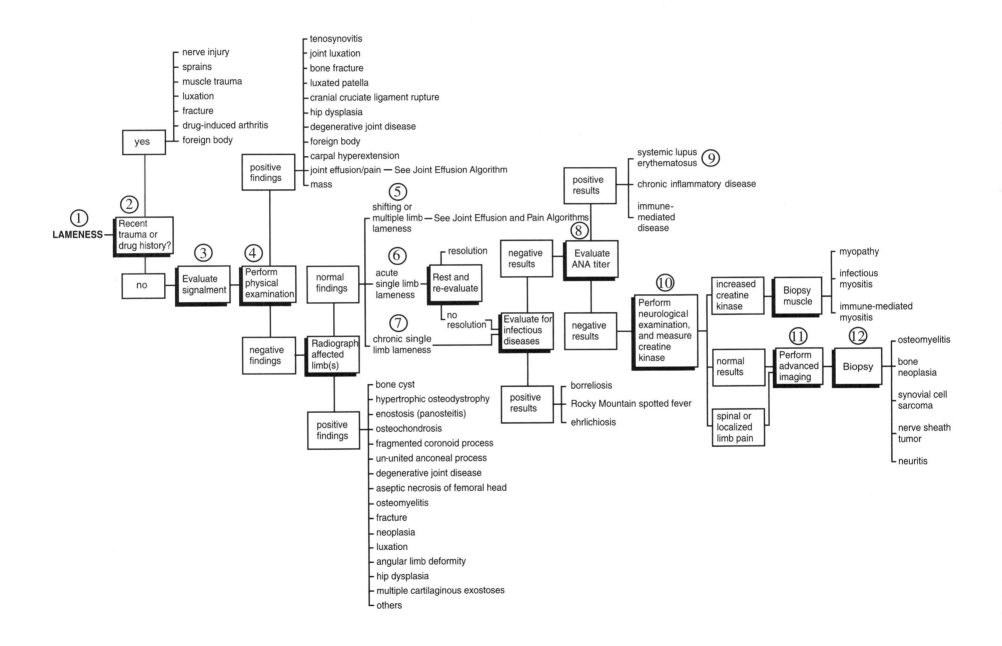

1 Joint effusion is distention of the joint capsule caused by inflammation of the articular (arthritis) and periarticular tissues. Affected joints are usually palpably warm and painful, with decreased range of motion. Dogs are affected more frequently than cats. Arthritis is generally classified as noninflammatory or inflammatory. Noninflammatory joint disease is characterized by degenerative changes in joint cartilage, absence of inflammation in the synovium or synovial fluid, and lack of systemic signs such as leukocytosis or fever. Inflammatory joint disease is either infectious (septic) or immune-mediated in origin. It is characterized by inflammatory changes in the synovium or synovial fluid and by the presence of systemic signs such as leukocytosis or fever. Immune-mediated arthritis is further classified as erosive or nonerosive based on the presence or absence of joint cartilage destruction and bone erosion that is visible on radiographs. Arthritis is monoarticular when one joint is involved and polyarticular when more than one joint is involved.

2 Neonatal, immature, and immunocompromised patients are more likely to have inflammatory arthritis due to infectious agents. Mature and older animals, especially obese ones, may have a noninflammatory joint effusion associated with degenerative joint disease (DJD). Immune-mediated arthritis can be seen in patients of any age. Erosive arthritis occurs most often in cats and young to middle-aged small-breed dogs, while idiopathic polyarthritis is seen in puppies and young, large breeds of dogs. Check the patient's history for tick exposure, penetrating wounds or trauma, generalized skin disease, or drug usage (sulfa drugs, macrolides, and penicillin-like antibiotics). Drug-induced polyarthritis in dogs and cats is rare, but it has been noted most commonly with trimethoprim-sulfadiazine use. Regardless of the underlying etiology, signs of immune-mediated arthritides often include cyclic fever, malaise, hyporexia, and lameness that may shift from one limb to another.

3 The most important diagnostic tools for determining the cause of joint effusion are arthrocentesis and analysis of synovial fluid. Arthrocentesis of multiple joints is recommended because a sample from a single joint may not be diagnostic. This is especially true if systemic, infectious, or immune-mediated disease is suspected or if there is a history of fever or shifting leg lameness. Since effusion often is associated with pain, sedation or anesthesia is recommended for the procedure, but sometimes arthrocentesis can be accomplished without sedating the patient. After a surgical clip and preparation, the affected joint is aspirated using a 25- or 22-gauge needle attached to a small-volume syringe. Fluid should be retained for bacterial culture if cytological evaluation indicates inflammation.

4 Joint distention can occur with synovial cell sarcoma. If cells are suspicious for neoplasia, proceed to radiograph the joint (step 7).

5 Noninflammatory joint diseases include DJD and hemarthrosis. Synovial fluid in DJD cases is often slightly turbid, with a nucleated cell count between 1000 and $5000/\mu l$. In hemarthrosis cases, fluid is red in color because of red blood cells (RBCs), and the nucleated cell count is between 3000 and $10,000/\mu l$, with 50–75% of cells consisting of polymorphonuclear cells. Hemarthrosis is associated with trauma and coagulopathies (see the bleeding/coagulopathy algorithm).

6 A nucleated cell count greater than $5000/\mu l$ indicates inflammation associated with either infectious or immune-mediated diseases. A bacterial culture of joint fluid is always indicated in such cases, and a blood culture should be considered if sepsis or bacterial endocarditis is suspected. Other causes of infectious arthritis include rickettsial organisms and spirochetes. Immune-mediated polyarthritides include rheumatoid arthritis, SLE-associated arthropathy, feline periosteal proliferative (chronic progressive) arthritis, and idiopathic polyarthritis.

7 Radiography of affected joint(s) is done primarily to distinguish erosive from nonerosive disease and to evaluate for neoplasia. Radiographs can be taken before or after arthrocentesis.

8 Erosive changes are associated with rheumatoid arthritis in the dog and periosteal proliferative polyarthritis (PPP) in the cat (specifically, male cats between 1.5 and 4.5 years of age). Because PPP has been associated with FeLV- positive cats, an FeLV test should be performed. All cats with PPP are serologically and virologically positive for feline syncytium-forming virus (FeSFV).

9 A semierosive arthritis in greyhounds less than 30 months of age most frequently affects the proximal interphalangeal, carpal, tarsal, elbow, and stifle joints. Peripheral lymph nodes may be enlarged and reactive.

10 Nonerosive arthritis is most likely due to infectious or immune-mediated diseases.

11 Puppies and kittens that develop fever, reluctance to move, pain, shifting leg lameness, and joint effusion within 2–4 weeks of vaccination may have vaccine-induced polyarthritis. The condition responds to corticosteroids. Sometimes signs appear to be more like those of meningitis (fever, pain, and reluctance to move).

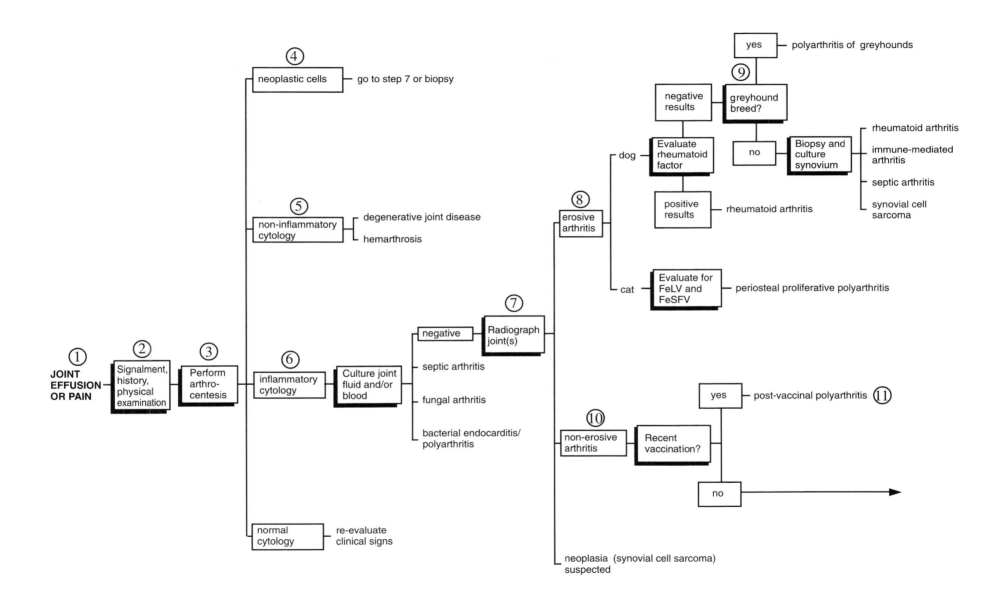

12 If patients have not been recently vaccinated, evaluate for infectious diseases endemic to the area where they live or have traveled. Serological and other testing of dogs (and, more rarely, cats) for heartworm disease, borreliosis, systemic fungal infections, Rocky Mountain spotted fever, ehrlichiosis, and leishmaniasis may be appropriate.

13 If infectious diseases have been eliminated from the list of differential diagnoses, consider evaluating an ANA titer. Since nuclear antigens are exposed in many inflammatory diseases, a positive test is not specific for SLE. However, a positive ANA titer suggests an immune-mediated condition that could respond to appropriate immunosuppressive treatment. SLE is reportedly more common in female dogs and in German shepherds, collies, Shetland sheepdogs, beagles, and poodles. There is no age predilection. Protein-losing nephropathy, hemolytic anemia, thrombocytopenia, and vasculitis may be seen concurrently with polyarthritis in dogs with SLE. A diagnosis of any of these conditions in a dog with nonerosive polyarthritis and a positive ANA titer is strongly suggestive of SLE.

14 If the ANA titer is negative, evaluate serum CK. An elevated CK concentration in conjunction with nonerosive polyarthritis is found most often in spaniel breeds and has been given the name *polyarthritis-polymyositis syndrome*. Multiple muscle biopsies may be required to demonstrate the polymyositis.

15 A variety of underlying illnesses can be associated with polyarthritis. Some are breed related (see steps 17 and 19 to 21). Some breeds have concurrent meningitis or myositis causing overlap and confusion with other syndromes.

16 Idiopathic polyarthritis is the most common disorder of dogs with immune-mediated polyarthritis. It is termed *idiopathic* because there is no evidence of an underlying cause or disease. It occurs mostly in pure-breed dogs between 1 and 6 years of age. The history often includes a cyclic fever associated with lameness, stiffness, malaise, and anorexia. Lymphadenopathy can be seen, and when the condition is most severe, leukocytosis with neutrophilia and hyperfibrinogenemia may be present.

17 Rheumatoid arthritis occurs most commonly in small-breed dogs between 2 and 6 years of age. It is a chronic, progressive, deforming polyarthritis affecting the more distal weight-bearing joints (carpus and tarsus) first and most severely. Early in the course of the disease, there may be no radiographic or systemic signs. Discomfort or pain on rising or walking is common, and joints are often hot and painful to the touch. As the disease progresses, lymphadenopathy, splenomegaly, cyclic fever, and muscle wasting may develop. Joint radiographs show significant joint erosion or destruction. Rheumatoid factor is positive in about 70% of dogs with erosive polyarthritis but false positives do occur, especially in dogs with other inflammatory arthritides (e.g., SLE, idiopathic polyarthritis, and lymphocytic-plasmacytic arthritis).

18 Sjögren's syndrome is an uncommon immune-mediated disorder that is associated with dry eyes, dry mouth, and erosive or nonerosive polyarthritis.

19 Large-breed dogs (e.g., Weimaraners, German shorthaired pointers, Bernese mountain dogs, boxers) and cats may have concurrent polyarthritis and meningitis. Affected dogs often are young. Many respond to corticosteroids, but long-term treatment with slow weaning may be necessary to treat the disease. Recurrences are common.

20 Intermittent fever and swollen joints (particularly the hock joint) in Chinese shar-peis are associated with deposition of amyloid in several organs, especially the kidneys. Spontaneous recovery from arthritis occurs, but signs are recurrent.

21 Peripheral lymphadenopathy, fever, polyarthritis, and lethargy in young Akitas are associated with a heritable polyarthritis and carry an unfavorable prognosis. Meningitis may also be noted.

22 Polyarthritis is a common feature of polyarteritis nodosa but most frequently presents as meningitis (neck pain), especially in beagles. Other names for this condition include *beagle pain syndrome* and *necrotizing vasculitis*. Some beagles respond to aspirin or prednisone, but recurrences are common. The final diagnosis is by histological examination of affected tissues.

23 A nonerosive arthritis has been associated with subacute bacterial endocarditis, pyometra, discospondylitis, chronic *Actinomyces* species infections, chronic salmonellosis, heartworm disease, urinary tract infections, and severe peridontitis. Usually only one or two joints are affected, and the carpal and tarsal joints are predisposed to disease. Since the organisms involved in the primary process cannot be identified in synovial membrane biopsies, the joint disease is probably immune-mediated in origin.

24 Enteropathic arthritis is associated with colitis and enteritis. Hepatopathic arthropathy has been reported in dogs with chronic active hepatitis and cirrhosis.

25 A sterile polyarthritis occasionally occurs in both dogs and cats with neoplasia. Signs of polyarthritis may precede or follow the diagnosis of neoplasia.

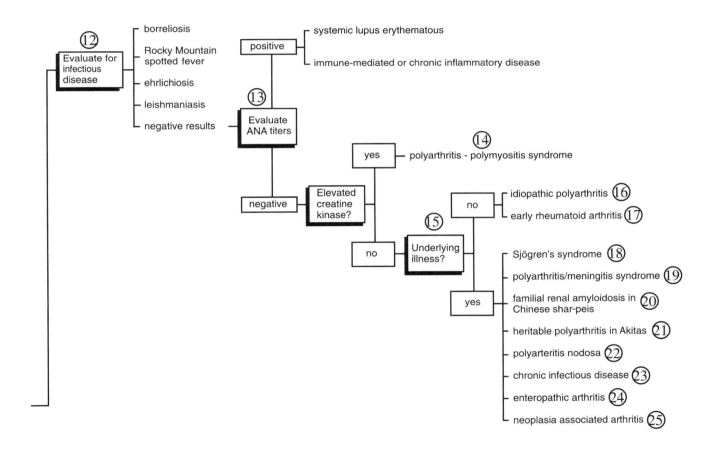

Neurological Problems

1 A seizure, fit, or convulsion is a transient dysrhythmia of brain cells that is sudden in onset and ceases spontaneously. Seizures occur because of structural or functional damage to the cerebrum, especially the frontal and temporal lobes. The clinical appearance of a seizure varies with the location and severity of the dysrhythmia. Generalized seizures are associated with changes in or loss of consciousness; tonic, clonic, or tonic-clonic (paddling) limb activity; and loss of bowel and bladder control. Partial seizures often manifest as abnormal movements on one side of the body. An accurate description of the event is crucial to differentiate a seizure from syncope. Usually syncope does not cause autonomic signs (e.g., urination, defecation) or excessive involuntary motor activity (paddling). If hypoxia associated with a syncopal episode lasts long enough, urination, defecation, or paddling can occur, making it difficult to distinguish syncope from seizures.

2 The history and physical examination (looking for fractures, scleral hemorrhage, generalized abrasions, etc.) are important in establishing whether head trauma is a possible cause of the seizure. Evidence of toxin exposure often can be elicited via a thorough history (e.g., insecticide use, chewing on foreign objects) and a physical examination (e.g., detecting a chemical odor on the patient's haircoat). A neurological examination should be done to look for other neurological signs that might suggest a multifocal or diffuse disease process (step 11).

3 Finding a dome-shaped head or palpable open fontanelle in a young animal increases the suspicion of congenital hydrocephalus. Remember, however, that seizure activity could be caused by other conditions common in small-breed dogs (e.g., portosystemic shunts, juvenile hypoglycemia). Congenital hydrocephalus often can be diagnosed by ultrasonography of the lateral ventricles through the fontanelle.

4 Because intracranial neoplasia is the main consideration in an older dog or cat with a first seizure, the clinician should progress quickly to step 14 in such cases.

5 In 1- to 7-year-old pug dogs presenting with seizures, pug dog encephalitis is the main consideration. This disease often has electroencephalographic (EEG) and spinal fluid changes consistent with encephalitis. Thus, the initial diagnostic evaluation should consist of an EEG and analysis of cerebrospinal fluid (CSF). A CT or MRI scan also might be appropriate prior to CSF analysis.

6 Head trauma can produce immediate seizure activity or cause brain damage leading to the development of a focus of abnormal electrical activity, manifesting as seizures. In human beings, seizures can develop up to 2 years after the initial traumatic incident.

7 In cats, exposure to flea control products is the most common cause of seizures secondary to intoxication. There are many toxins that free-roaming animals can encounter. Many of these seizures can be treated successfully by withdrawal of the toxin and supportive measures. Organophosphate and lead intoxication can be easily confirmed via blood tests. Both can be treated once they are diagnosed.

8 Finding severe cardiac arrhythmias or pulmonary problems should alert the clinician to the possibility that these problems are causing brain damage and subsequent seizures or hypoxia and seizure-like activity.

9 If the patient is a toy-breed dog, especially one under 1 year of age, juvenile hypoglycemia should be suspected as a cause of seizure activity, along with portal systemic shunts and congenital hydrocephalus. Evaluating the serum glucose concentration during a seizure is important. Note that in affected toy breeds, resting serum glucose may be very low even if the patient appears clinically normal.

10 The results of a hemogram and a serum chemistry screen can eliminate or verify many extracranial causes of seizures including hypocalcemia, hypoglycemia, renal failure, polycythemia, and hyperlipidemia. Marked hyperlipidemia has been reported to cause seizures and other neurological signs in miniature schnauzers and cats. Liver disease is suspected if BUN is low or if hypoalbuminemia, hypocholesterolemia, and hypoglycemia are present; however, liver function tests (BSP retention testing, pre- and postprandial bile acids, fasting serum ammonia concentration) and possibly a liver biopsy are required to diagnose liver disease. Note that hypoglycemia cannot be excluded as a cause of seizure activity if blood glucose is normal unless the sample was drawn during the seizure. In dogs over 5 years of age, an insulin-secreting tumor (usually of the pancreas or liver) can cause hypoglycemia, weakness, and seizures. Evaluating several fasting blood glucose concentrations may increase the chance of diagnosing hypoglycemia.

11 A neurological examination should be performed in every seizure patient after the patient has recovered completely from the seizure (i.e., is in the interictal state). The findings of the neurological examination are more likely to be abnormal with structural central nervous system disease (e.g., neoplasia, trauma, infection) than with functional disease (e.g., primary epilepsy, metabolic or toxic disorders).

12 If a reason for the seizure has not been found at this stage, repeat the physical and neurological examinations. If these are normal and no further seizures have occurred, assume that the event is transient and have the owner monitor the patient for other signs or more seizures. If examinations are abnormal, assume that structural brain disease exists and proceed with the diagnostic algorithm.

13 If the patient is middle-aged or older and has not had prior seizures, intracranial or extracranial neoplasia is a possibility. Evaluating the thorax and abdomen is often easier and less invasive initially for the patient than evaluating the brain. Left and right lateral and ventrodorsal thoracic radiographs exclude metastatic or primary pulmonary neoplasia that could have spread to the brain. Abdominal ultrasound is beneficial for detecting neoplastic masses of the liver, kidney, and spleen that also could have metastasized to the brain. Occasionally, pancreatic masses (insulin-secreting beta cell tumors that result in hypoglycemic seizures) are found using ultrasound.

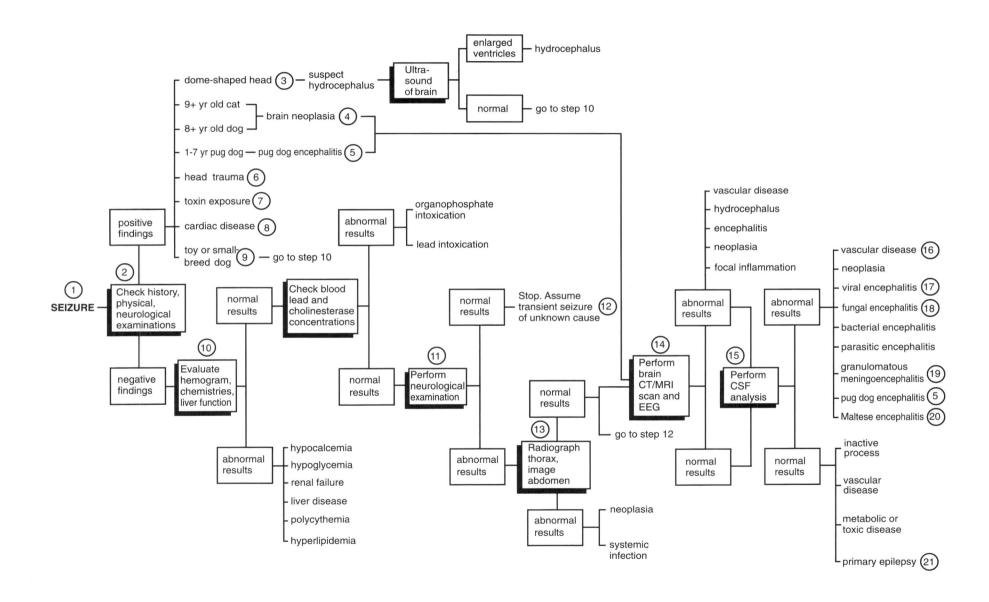

14 If blood tests and radiographs or ultrasound scans do not suggest a reason for seizure activity, the clinician should proceed to more invasive procedures or stop (step 12) and wait to see what happens. The choice depends on the age and breed of the patient and what disease process is most likely. For example, if the patient is a 1- to 4-year-old Labrador retriever, Irish setter, German shepherd, poodle, cocker spaniel, or another breed of dog with a propensity for primary (idiopathic or genetic) epilepsy, it would be suitable to wait at step 12. However, if the patient is a 12-year-old cat or a dog that has never had a seizure before, the chances of intracranial neoplasia are greater. Obviously, client concerns and finances also help determine how rapidly one proceeds to a CT/MRI scan. General anesthesia is required for CT or MRI scans of the brain; for this reason, a hemogram and a chemistry screen should be reviewed first. Such scans do not always yield the specific diagnosis but can reveal the presence or absence of structural brain disease. For example, an intracranial mass may be identified, but whether it is neoplastic or a granuloma requires histopathological evaluation of the lesion. Another test that might be of benefit in seizure patients is an EEG. This can be used to detect asymmetrical brain activity or to increase the index of suspicion for encephalitis.

15 The risks and benefits of a CSF tap must be weighed for each patient. If a CT or MRI scan shows a mass effect (falx shift, evidence of cerebral edema), the risks of a CSF tap might outweigh the benefits. If the scan is normal, then spinal fluid analysis is needed to detect inflammatory disease. CSF analysis can yield a specific diagnosis (e.g., cryptococcal meningitis). However, many diseases have similar CSF findings, making a specific diagnosis difficult.

16 Vascular central nervous system disease occurs more commonly in cats (feline ischemic encephalopathy [FIE]) than in dogs. It may be idiopathic or associated with aberrant migration of *Cuterebra* spp. larvae. A sudden onset of behavioral changes, seizures, or asymmetric neurological deficits in a cat, especially an outdoor cat in the summer months, increases the index of suspicion for this disorder.

17 Viral encephalitis is most commonly caused by CDV infection in the dog and FIP in the cat. However, there are numerous other viruses that can infect the brain and cause seizure activity. Unfortunately, the diagnosis of most viral encephalitides is based on characteristic histopathological findings at necropsy. Spinal fluid titers for certain viral diseases can be evaluated, but interpretation of results is difficult if the blood-brain barrier is broken or if the spinal fluid was contaminated with peripheral blood during collection.

18 The most commonly diagnosed fungal brain infection is cryptococcosis (usually in cats). Often the organisms can be seen in the spinal fluid. Other fungal agents are seen occasionally.

19 Granulomatous meningoencephalitis (GME) is nonsuppurative inflammation of the canine brain. The cause is unknown. A dog of any breed and age can be affected. Lesions can be large and appear like a mass on CT or MRI scans. They also can be microscopic and focal or multifocal and diffuse. Thus, GME can look like neoplasia or encephalitis on scans. Spinal fluid analysis, signalment, and the history are used to increase the suspicion of GME antemortem.

20 Maltese encephalitis is very similar to pug dog encephalitis in terms of presentation and histopathological findings. The cause is unknown.

21 Primary (idiopathic) epilepsy cannot be diagnosed in a dog or cat with a history of just one seizure. However, if other seizures occur within months of the first seizure, if the age and breed fit well, if the animal is normal between seizures and has a normal neurological examination, and if all other diagnostic tests have essentially normal results, the diagnosis, by exclusion, is primary epilepsy.

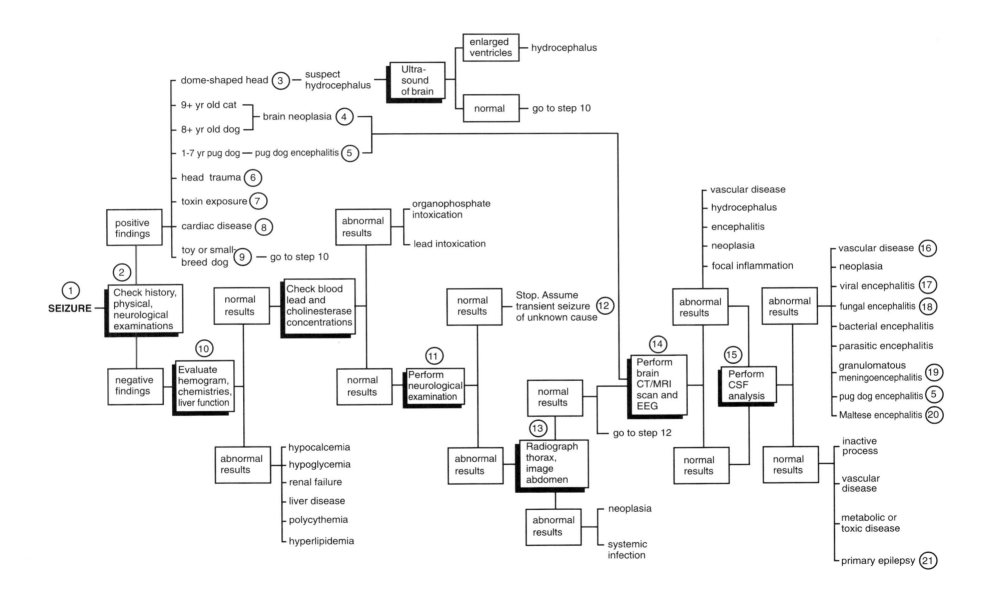

1 Consciousness is controlled primarily by the brainstem ascending reticular activating system (RAS). Conditions affecting consciousness involve the cerebrum (metabolic disease, toxins) or RAS. Changes in consciousness often are abrupt but can develop gradually. The most severe changes are stupor and coma. Stupor is a poorly conscious state that can be overcome by vigorous or noxious stimuli. Comatose patients cannot be aroused even with noxious stimuli. The prognosis is more guarded for coma than for stupor.

2 The history and physical examination findings (lacerations, shock, fractures, scrapes) help to establish head trauma as a potential cause of stupor or coma. Previously identified medical conditions (renal, hepatic, or cardiac disease, diabetes mellitus, hypothyroidism) can be identified from the history. A history of drug administration (sedatives, antitussives, antihistamines, various controlled substances, anticonvulsants) should be ascertained because these agents affect the patient's level of consciousness.

3 A hemogram, serum chemistry, and urinalysis should be obtained on any stuporous or comatose patient. If test results are not going to be available immediately, do simple, rapid tests (packed cell volume, total protein, blood glucose, Azostix, urine dipstick) for anemia, uremia, hyperviscosity, polycythemia, and hypo/hyperglycemia.

4 Severe hypercholesterolemia in a dog with changes in mentation should increase the suspicion of severe hypothyroidism (*myxedema coma*). Other clinical signs include hypothermia, bradycardia, hypotension, and apparent peripheral edema. Obtain serum for evaluation of the thyroid concentration and immediately start supplementation orally or intravenously.

5 A patient with diabetes mellitus that has received an excessive dose of insulin could develop hypoglycemia and become comatose. Likewise, a ketoacidotic diabetic patient could present with stupor or coma due to hyperosmolality.

6 The brain relies upon glucose as its primary source of energy; thus, hypoglycemia affects the patient's level of consciousness. Causes of hypoglycemia in young, small-breed dogs can include juvenile hypoglycemia, liver disease, and heavy hookworm infestation. In middle-aged and older dogs, an insulin-secreting neoplasm (pancreatic beta cell tumor) is most likely. Hypoglycemia is not a common cause of stupor or coma in cats.

7 End-stage renal disease or oliguric acute renal failure can cause stupor or occasionally coma. Such patients have a very poor prognosis.

8 Thoracic radiographs can be helpful, especially in older patients with a higher risk of neoplasia. Various systemic tumors (e.g., hemangiosarcoma) can metastasize to the brain, increasing intracranial pressure, causing herniation of brain tissue at the midbrain or medullary brainstem level, and causing coma. Physical signs of systemic neoplasia such as cachexia, palpable organomegaly, or abdominal masses are not always present at the time that the brain becomes involved. Brain tumors do not usually spread outside the central nervous system (CNS). Skull radiographs are relatively low in yield unless neoplastic or infectious processes invade overlying bone or there are fractures secondary to trauma.

9 Severe hepatic disease can produce stupor or coma. If the liver malfunctions and does not degrade toxic substances (e.g., ammonia) from gastrointestinal protein breakdown, these toxins enter the circulation and reach the brain. Liver enzymes often are normal in patients with congenital portosystemic shunts or with cirrhosis and acquired shunts. Liver function testing (pre- and postprandial bile acid concentrations, fasting ammonia and ammonia challenge testing, or BSP retention) helps to diagnose hepatic encephalopathy. Young dogs and cats usually have congenital shunts, while older animals are likely to have acquired shunts or cirrhosis.

10 A CT or MRI brain scan is likely to be necessary if metabolic, traumatic, and neoplastic causes have been excluded based on the history, results of the physical examination, laboratory tests, and thoracic and skull radiographs.

11 With the advent of MRI and CT scanning, cerebrovascular disease is being diagnosed more often than in the past. Clinical signs are usually sudden in onset and can improve over time. A specific syndrome, FIE, has been reported in cats. It may be associated with aberrant migration of *Cuterebra* spp. larvae. In dogs, evaluate for system illnesses and metastatic neoplasia as potential causes of cerebrovascular disease. Arteriovascular malformations also can be found on scans.

12 Some intracranial masses are curable or can be palliated by surgical intervention or radiation. However, if stupor or coma is the presenting problem, the prognosis is very poor. In some cases, the mass itself does not cause stupor or coma, but signs develop secondary to elevated intracranial pressure and/or brainstem herniation.

13 If a brain scan does not yield sufficient information to make a diagnosis, then a CSF tap should be considered. The danger of brainstem herniation following a CSF tap should be discussed with the owner, especially if the scan shows a falx shift or if elevated intracranial pressure is suspected. The CSF analysis can help to diagnose neoplasia, bacterial, viral, or fungal encephalitis, or GME, but it may not yield a specific diagnosis.

14 If the brain scan and CSF results are normal, then toxin exposure should be suspected. The clinician should reevaluate the history for information that might suggest a toxic etiology.

15 Rarely, severe hypothyroidism can cause mental depression and coma. The serum chemistry profile can show elevated triglycerides and cholesterol, and there may be other historical or physical signs. Serum thyroid hormone concentrations should be evaluated.

16 There are many different causes of encephalitis (infectious and inflammatory). Inflammation in the brain can cause elevated intracranial pressure and mental depression. Subsequent brain herniation can cause stupor or coma. GME and fungal encephalitis are relatively common inflammatory causes of stupor.

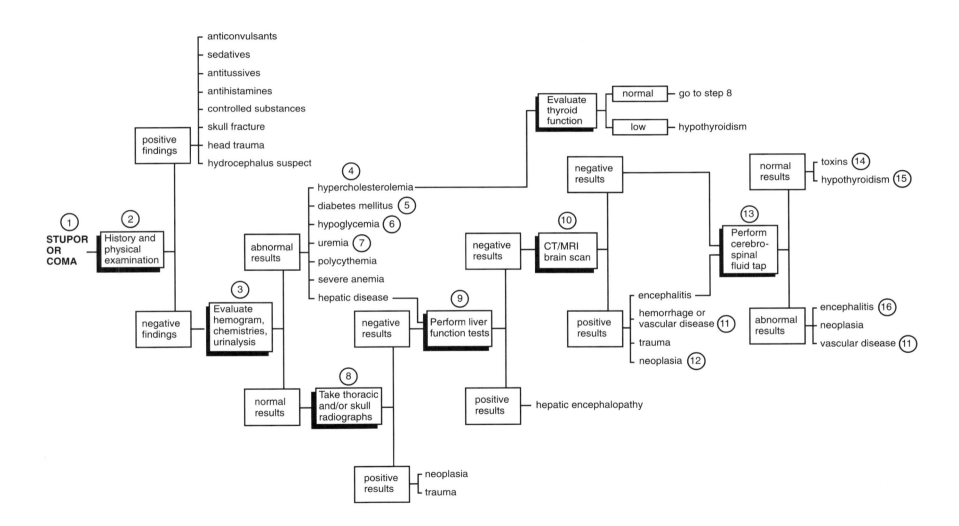

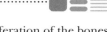

1 A head tilt (ear pointed toward the ground) or head turn in conjunction with nystagmus (spontaneous jerking motion of the eyes) indicates dysfunction of the vestibular system. Patients also can lean, circle, fall, or roll, usually to the affected side. Nystagmus can be spontaneous (i.e., present while the clinician views the patient) or positional (i.e., present only when the head or body is placed in positions such as lateral recumbency). Nystagmus can be in a horizontal, vertical, or rotary direction. Vertical nystagmus most often is associated with central (brainstem) lesions.

2 A good history will exclude trauma, recent ear cleaning or ear disease, and systemic or topically ototoxic drugs as possible causes of head tilt/nystagmus.

3 Streptomycin, gentamicin, erythromycin, and tobramycin can affect vestibular function regardless of the route of administration. Signs may or may not resolve if the agent is discontinued. Many topical agents, including drug vehicles such as propylene glycol, can be ototoxic and cause vestibular signs if they contact middle ear structures (i.e., if the tympanic membrane is disrupted).

4 Metronidazole crosses the blood-brain barrier readily, and toxicity has been reliably associated with doses of over 66 mg/kg/day. The mechanism of CNS intoxication is unknown. Signs of metronidazole-induced toxicosis include ataxia, weakness, seizures, head tilt, and nystagmus.

5 Untreated hypothyroidism can cause central or peripheral vestibular signs. Affected dogs may or may not have classical signs of hypothyroidism, including obesity, haircoat thinning, cold sensitivity, lethargy, and hypercholesterolemia.

6 A dog presenting with vestibular signs during the tick season and with a history of tick exposure should be evaluated for rickettsial infection, especially in endemic areas. Clinical signs often progress rapidly unless treatment is initiated with appropriate agents (doxycycline, tetracycline, and fluoroquinolones) while waiting for rickettsial titers to be assessed.

7 Otic examination is necessary to determine if otitis externa or otitis media is present. Otitis media produces a head turn or tilt, but if nystagmus is present, it is likely that the infection has spread to the inner ear as well. Horizontal nystagmus suggests middle ear disease, and vertical nystagmus with conscious proprioceptive deficits suggests inner ear problems. One sign of otitis media is a discolored, swollen, or ruptured tympanic membrane. In cats, nasopharyngeal polyps can extend into or originate from the middle ear, producing signs of middle and even inner ear disease.

8 A neurological examination is necessary to determine whether vestibular signs are peripheral (outside the brain) or central (within the brain). Head tilt, falling, leaning, ataxia, and nystagmus are common signs at both locations. Signs of limb weakness, conscious proprioceptive deficits, intention tremors of the head, hypermetria, and multiple cranial nerve deficits are associated with a central location of the lesion. Disorders such as hypothyroidism and rickettsial vasculitis can produce both peripheral and central vestibular signs. Rickettsial vasculitis may produce paradoxical vestibular disease.

9 If peripheral signs are present and the external ear examination is normal, reevaluate patient signalment. In older dogs, sudden onset of severe vestibular signs can be due to a condition known as *old dog vestibular disease*. The cause is unknown, but clinical signs usually improve within days and resolve almost completely within weeks. A similar *vestibular syndrome* also occurs in cats of any age and may be a manifestation of FIE.

10 If the neurological examination indicates peripheral vestibular disease, middle and inner ear problems (infection and neoplasia) should be considered. Radiographs or a CT scan of the middle ear (tympanic bullae) may be needed to make the diagnosis. General anesthesia is required to obtain good-quality radiographic views.

11 Radiographs/scans of the bullae may show sclerosis or fluid within the middle ear cavity that suggest otitis media. Scans are more sensitive than radiographs.

12 Destruction and/or bony proliferation of the bones around the middle or inner ear suggest a neoplastic process. However, exploratory surgery and biopsy are required to confirm the diagnosis.

13 Cats with nasopharyngeal polyps tend to be younger (1 to 5 years old) but cats of all ages are susceptible, especially if there is a prior history of upper respiratory disease. Radiographic changes include a rounded soft tissue density in the nasopharynx or the middle ear cavity.

14 If central vestibular signs are present, evaluate a hemogram (including the platelet count) and serum chemistry profile. It would be unusual for these tests to result in a specific diagnosis to explain the vestibular signs, but they are an important preliminary to anesthesia and more extensive testing. Rarely, another disease process is identified on these tests, affecting the decision to pursue vestibular signs.

15 Hypercholesterolemia on routine laboratory evaluation should increase the index of suspicion for hypothyroidism in canine patients. Evaluation of a baseline serum T_4 concentration or a full thyroid profile (including free T_4 by equilibrium dialysis) should be the next diagnostic step.

16 A low-normal or low platelet count in a dog with central or vestibular signs evaluated during the tick season in an endemic area should increase the suspicion of Rocky Mountain spotted fever or possibly ehrlichiosis. The correlation between vestibular signs and borreliosis is less clear. Treatment for suspected rickettsial infection should begin immediately while waiting for titers to be determined. Some dogs will have negative rickettsial titers but respond to tetracycline or doxycycline, suggesting either very acute infection (recheck titers in 3 weeks) or other, as yet unknown, rickettsial organisms as the underlying cause.

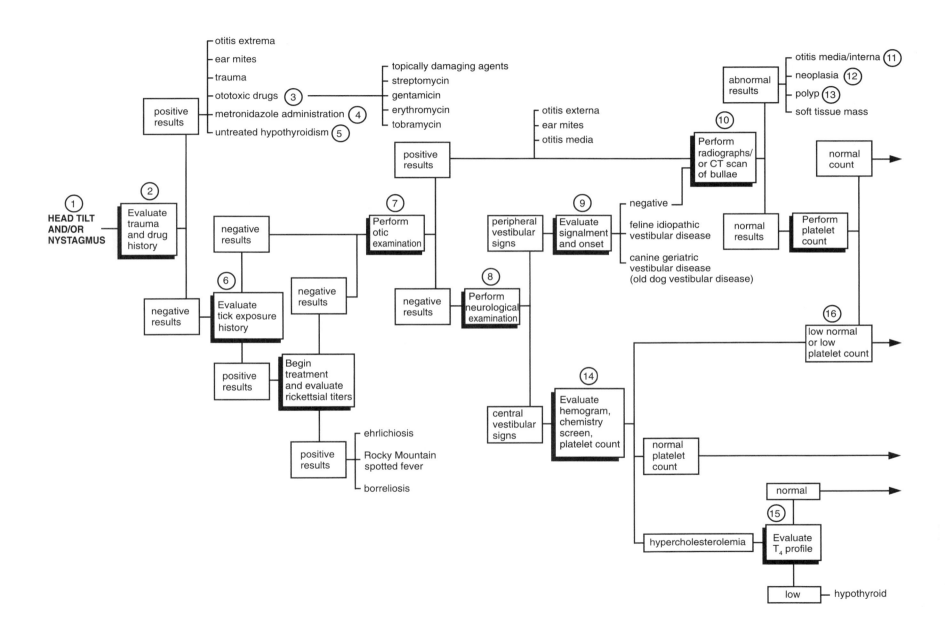

17 Not all cases of otitis media/interna produce radiographic or even CT changes. If an infection is suspected, then a prolonged trial of oral antibiotics with good penetration into the middle ear (cephalosporins or enrofloxacin) should be attempted. If no response is noted, exploratory bulla surgery is a consideration.

18 Vestibulocochlear nerve neoplasia is an uncommon diagnosis. However, with CT and MRI scanning becoming more widely available, peripheral nerve tumors are being found more frequently prior to necropsy examination. In an older dog or cat with persistent peripheral vestibular signs, a nerve sheath tumor should be considered.

19 Patients with central vestibular signs for which a diagnosis has not been made require a brain scan (either a CT or MRI scan). The vestibular area in the brainstem is small and is situated in the caudal fossa, where bone densities can obscure subtle or small abnormalities on CT scans. The best way to image this area is with an MRI scan.

20 Lesions of the cerebellopontine angle that are suspected to be neoplastic can be detected on some CT scans and on most MRI scans. The most common early presentation in patients with brainstem neoplasia includes acute and progressive vestibular signs. Patients with meningiomas in this area tend to survive longer than those with intraparenchymal neoplasia (e.g., astrocytoma) or metastatic neoplasia (e.g., hemangiosarcoma). Mass lesions at the cerebellopontine angle may produce paradoxical signs. With paradoxical vestibular syndrome, the head tilt and/or circling will be away from the side of the mass. Signs also can shift from one side to the other. Usually the mass is located on the side of the body with the most obvious conscious proprioceptive deficits or weakness.

21 GME is an inflammatory CNS condition found in many breeds of dog, usually between 1 and 8 years of age.

Female toy breeds may be predisposed. Nonsuppurative inflammatory lesions occur anywhere within the brain or spinal cord, but there seems to be a predilection for the cerebrum and the cerebellopontine angle. Lesions can be focal, multifocal, or diffuse. The diagnosis cannot be based on the CT or MRI appearance of the lesions, but it can be suspected based on the information above. Spinal fluid analysis increases the suspicion of GME if the spinal white blood cell count and protein in the spinal fluid are elevated. On cytological evaluation, spinal fluid is found to consist of about 60–80% lymphocytes. In some cases, large, anaplastic-looking mononuclear cells are present and are considered diagnostic for the condition. Protein also is elevated in spinal fluid, with significant increases in IgG on electrophoresis. The diagnosis is confirmed by brain biopsy or at necropsy. The prognosis generally is guarded, since the condition tends to be progressive despite treatment with immunosuppressive drugs (prednisone) or cerebral radiation.

22 Encephalitis is suspected if CT or MRI brain scans show diffuse or multifocal densities within the parenchyma of the brain. Spinal fluid analysis may be the method of choice for diagnosis of CNS inflammation, along with tissue biopsy.

23 A CSF tap with spinal fluid analysis is the best way to diagnose inflammation around or sometimes within the brain. The spinal tap can be done at the cerebellomedullary cistern or in the lower lumbar region. Always shave and surgically prepare the site and use aseptic technique for sample collection.

24 CDV and fungal organisms (especially *Cryptococcus neoformans*) often affect the cerebellopontine angle and produce vestibular signs. Spinal fluid should be cultured, and titers for both CDV and *Cryptococcus* spp. can be determined on peripheral blood and spinal fluid samples.

25 Cerebellar and vestibular signs can be found with storage diseases such as gangliosidosis. Spinal fluid protein may be elevated. The diagnosis requires biopsy or necropsy. Patients usually are less than 3–5 years of age, and clinical signs are progressive.

26 Neoplasia can cause an increase in CSF protein concentrations. A significant number of brain neoplasms (especially meningiomas and choroid plexus tumors) cause an inflammatory CSF response with elevated WBC counts. Unless neoplastic cells are observed in the spinal fluid (as they can be in CNS lymphoma), a specific diagnosis of neoplasia cannot be made on the basis of CSF analysis.

27 If the underlying cause of vestibular signs has not been diagnosed and if serum thyroid concentrations have not been measured previously, they should be measured at this point. Hypothyroidism is a treatable condition, and although only a few cases of head tilt and nystagmus are actually due to hypothyroidism, this problem should never be overlooked.

28 CNS vascular injury may have a variety of underlying causes, including neoplasia, CNS infection, aneurysms, atherosclerosis, arteriovenous malformations, cardiogenic emboli, vasospasm, atrial fibrillation, mitral stenosis, hematological disorders, polycythemia, hyperviscosity syndrome, DIC, and vasculitis. Vasculitis can be secondary to parvovirus, rickettsial, and *Dirofilaria* spp. infection. Most of these disorders have associated systemic or laboratory abnormalities. Patients who appear healthy apart from the head tilt/nystagmus could have an arteriovenous malformation. If a brain scan and a CSF tap are done soon after the development of clinical signs, a diagnosis of cerebrovascular accident may be made.

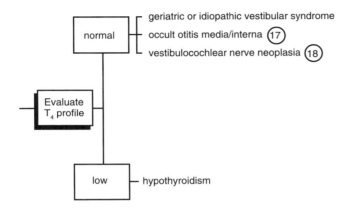

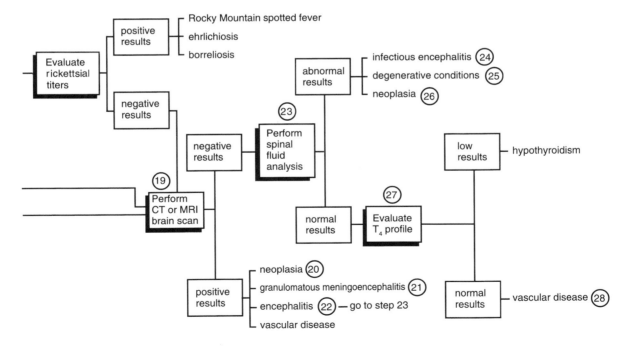

1 Ataxia is a sign of sensory dysfunction, producing "wobbliness" or incoordination of the limbs, head, or trunk. CNS disorders commonly produce ataxia, but systemic illness, endocrinopathies, cardiovascular disturbance, and metabolic disorders also can cause ataxia for poorly defined reasons. Ataxia is divided into three types: sensory (proprioceptive), vestibular, and cerebellar. All three types produce changes in limb coordination, but vestibular and cerebellar ataxia also cause changes in head and neck coordination.

2 The history should establish the possibility of trauma, exposure to toxins or drugs, and the presence of preexisting disease or other clinical signs. If cardiac or respiratory compromise is evident, the ataxia could be due to reduced CNS oxygenation. Physical examination findings including fever, weight loss, cardiac murmurs or arrhythmias, alopecia, or pale mucous membranes suggest a nonneurological cause of ataxia. Head tremors or bobbing, whole body tremors, hypermetria, nystagmus, or a head tilt suggest a neurological cause of ataxia.

3 Otitis externa is a relatively common finding on physical examination and can be unrelated to the ataxia. However, otitis externa also can extend into the middle and inner ear and cause vestibular ataxia.

4 The client should be questioned about any possibility of toxin exposure. Potential toxins include flea control products, lead, and ethylene glycol. Other systemic or neurological signs often are present. Note that ataxia, seizures, or depression can be the first sign of ethylene glycol intoxification.

5 Preexisting diseases that can cause ataxia include congestive heart failure, hepatic encephalopathy, and hypoglycemia due to an insulinoma or fasting in toy-breed dogs.

6 Sedatives, tranquilizers, and anticonvulsants can cause ataxia. Metronidazole can cause vestibular signs, rear limb weakness, and seizures. If drugs are discontinued, ataxia usually resolves.

7 If neurological signs are present, proceed with the neurological examination to determine if the ataxia is cerebellar, vestibular, spinal, or neuromuscular in origin. If the findings are normal or suggestive of systemic disease, if only ataxia or tremors are found, exclude metabolic disorders with a hemogram and chemistry screen (including CK).

8 Signs of cerebellar ataxia include tremors of the head and/or body, hypermetric gait, intention tremors, and positional nystagmus or an absent menace response. Although a CT scan of this area can yield positive results, an MRI scan will define the area better and without artifacts.

9 Cerebellar hypoplasia is a congenital maldevelopment of the cerebellum. The signs are seen in kittens and puppies as they begin to ambulate and do not progress over time. Underlying causes include exposure to panleukopenia virus in kittens in utero.

10 Animals with cerebellar abiotrophy or lysosomal storage diseases usually are normal initially but develop cerebellar signs over time. No treatment is available.

11 Infectious diseases that affect the cerebellum include CDV, FIP virus, toxoplasmosis, and rickettsial and fungal organisms. Brain scans and CSF analysis can make the diagnosis.

12 GME is an inflammatory disease of unknown etiology producing diffuse or focal cerebral and brainstem changes.

13 Neoplasia, fungal granulomas, GME, and abscesses cause the appearance of cerebral masses.

14 Swaying, leaning, or tilting to one side, head tilt, and nystagmus most often characterize vestibular ataxia (see the algorithm for head tilt).

15 Muscle weakness can cause an ataxic gait. Spinal reflexes can be reduced and muscle atrophy can be present. If such signs are found in all limbs, then a generalized muscle or nerve disorder should be suspected and testing should include serum CK and serum thyroid concentrations.

16 If serum CK is elevated, infectious and immunological disorders should be pursued. Test for infectious diseases present in the region. Immunological tests that might be worthwhile include ANA titers.

17 Hypothyroidism can cause ataxia by producing muscle weakness or vestibular signs.

18 Hyperthyroidism in cats can cause muscle weakness, although the mechanism is not fully understood. Ataxia and ventroflexion of the neck are common.

19 If muscle or nerve disease is suspected, consider muscle biopsy or a referral to a specialist for further electrodiagnostic testing, such as electromyography (EMG) or nerve conduction studies (NCS).

20 If muscle atrophy and ataxia are localized to the pelvic limbs, the lower lumbar spinal cord or lumbar nerve roots/peripheral nerves are likely to be affected. Testing would begin with spinal radiographs of this area. Potential problems include disc herniation, trauma, neoplasia, discospondylitis, and LS spondylosis.

21 If spinal radiographs are normal and only ataxia is present, have the patient rest and perform serial neurological examinations. If the signs are progressive, pursue appropriate diagnostic testing by referring to the appropriate algorithm (e.g., paraparesis). If signs are nonprogressive, likely possibilities include disc herniation, trauma, and fibrocartilaginous embolism.

22 Some patients with portosystemic shunts have intermittent ataxia as the primary presenting complaint. If intermittent ataxia occurs in a dog or cat less than 1 year of age or if the BUN or albumin is low, evaluate liver function tests (e.g., bile acids) to assess for liver disease.

23 Ataxia in an adult dog with increased serum cholesterol or triglycerides suggests the need to exclude hypothyroidism.

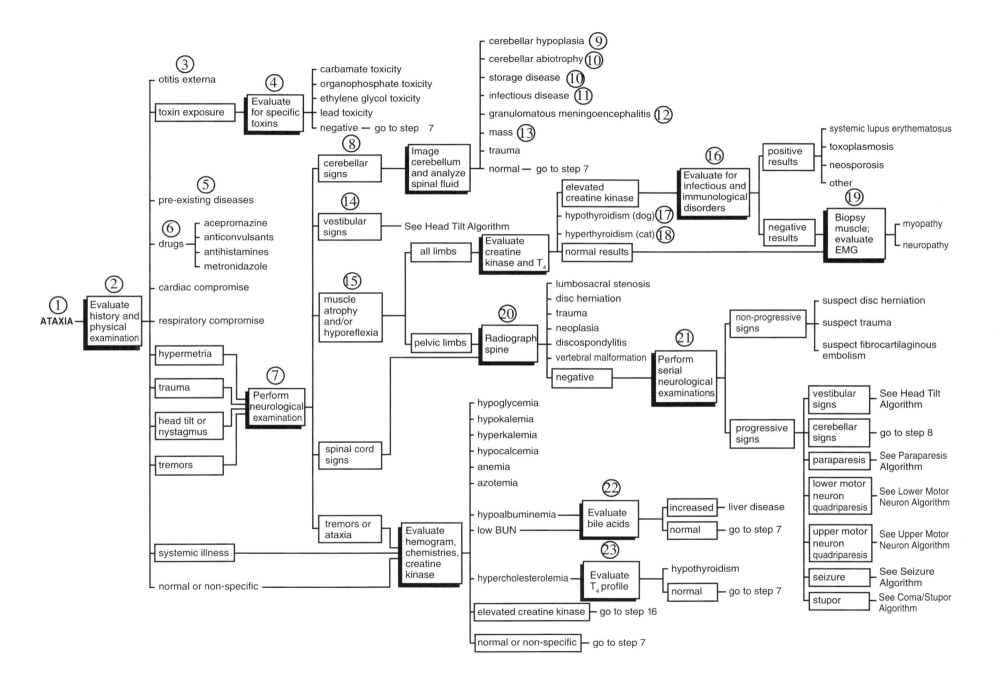

1 Upper motor neuron (UMN) quadriparesis or quadriplegia is weakness or complete lack of voluntary motor activity, respectively, in all limbs. Quadriparetic patients can be ambulatory. Severely affected ones are not. Quadriparesis due to a UMN lesion can be differentiated from that due to a lower motor neuron (LMN) lesion by the presence of exaggerated spinal reflexes and normal muscle tone in the former. Occasionally brain rather than spinal lesions cause UMN quadriparesis (step 15).

2 Slowly compressive lesions (type II disc herniation, cervical vertebral malformation, some neoplasms) cause slow-onset of weakness. Trauma, type I disc herniation, fibrocartilaginous embolism (FCE), and some neoplasms cause acute-onset signs.

3 Neurological examination localizes weakness to the cervical area if spinal reflexes are intact or exaggerated and there is no sign of primary brain disease. Depressed or absent spinal reflexes suggests LMN quadriparesis. A history of seizures or other cerebral signs (dementia, pacing, getting lost in corners, inappropriate behavior) suggests cerebral disease. Weakness usually is mild with cerebral disease. Cranial nerve abnormalities (head tilt, facial paralysis, pupil dilation, tongue atrophy) suggest brainstem lesions. Severe depression, stupor, or coma often is present.

4 If a cervical lesion is suspected, spinal radiographs are the next step. Sedation or general anesthesia is needed for positioning. Survey radiographs show discospondylitis, bony neoplasia, atlantoaxial subluxation, spinal fractures, and luxations. Disc mineralization and sometimes disc material can be seen in the spinal canal.

5 Atlantoaxial subluxations most commonly occur in small dogs and result from malformation/fracture of the dens of the axis. Neck pain, hypermetria, proprioceptive deficits, and weakness are common. Avoid manipulation of the neck in these patients to reduce the chance of further injury.

6 The most common cervical malformation in large-breed dogs (especially Doberman pinschers and Great Danes) is cervical vertebral malformation/malarticulation ("wobbler," cervical stenosis) syndrome. Signs are chronic and progressive or acute. Acute signs usually are associated with intervertebral disc herniation that occurs as part of the syndrome. Survey radiographs may show dorsal tipping of the cranial portion of caudal cervical vertebrae, articular facet proliferation, and vertebral canal narrowing. However, myelography is needed to define the location of the lesion and the type and extent of compression.

7 Discospondylitis is a bacterial (rarely fungal) infection of the intervertebral disc and adjacent vertebral endplates. It may be associated with spinal pain, fever, weight loss, and hyporexia. Radiographic signs lag clinical signs by weeks to months. All affected dogs should be checked for *Brucella canis*, but *Staphylococcus* and *Streptococcus* spp. are most commonly isolated.

8 Myelitis is spinal cord inflammation due to a variety of agents (commonly CDV in dogs and FIP virus in cats). It is diagnosed by a combination of spinal fluid analysis, serum/spinal fluid titers, and cultures.

9 Spinal fluid cytology occasionally shows lymphoma.

10 If spinal radiographs and CSF analysis are negative, the next step is spinal imaging (myelography, CT/MRI scans).

11 FCE causes weakness/paralysis of sudden onset that does not worsen over time. Signs often are asymmetrical. Cervical pain is absent or minimal. Spinal cord swelling resolves/is minimal within a day or two. If deep pain perception remains intact, most patients improve over time, although their gait may never be normal. The causes of FCE are unknown, but material found ob-structing the spinal cord's blood supply has characteristics of disc material.

12 Cervical neoplasia affects bone, spinal cord, nerve roots, or any soft tissue structures in the area. Signs are progressive. Unless bone is affected, spinal imaging is needed to define a mass.

13 Normal spinal imaging leaves two possibilities: brainstem/cerebral lesions or problems within the parenchyma of the spinal cord. To investigate the first, a CT/MRI scan is needed (step 15). For parenchymal lesions in the cord, if onset is acute, trauma and FCE should be considered. If onset is slow and progressive, a degenerative spinal cord abnormality should be suspected.

14 Degenerative myelopathy of the cervical region is uncommon and requires spinal cord histopathology for diagnosis. It often is breed specific (e.g., rottweiler encephalomalacia, miniature poodle demyelinating myelopathy).

15 If a cerebral disorder is suspected (cranial nerve abnormalities, seizures, or behavioral changes), then a brain CT/MRI scan is needed. Many diseases affecting the brain result in asymmetrical weakness on neurological examination.

16 Congenital hydrocephalus causes gait deficits, hypermetria, ataxia, and mild weakness.

17 Intracranial arachnoid cysts are fluid-filled cavities lined with an arachnoid-like membrane. They occur in many areas of the brain but may be incidental findings.

18 Degenerative brain diseases include lysosomal storage disorders and cognitive dysfunction syndrome. These are relatively uncommon causes of quadriparesis, and most cause CNS signs that are more obvious than gait changes.

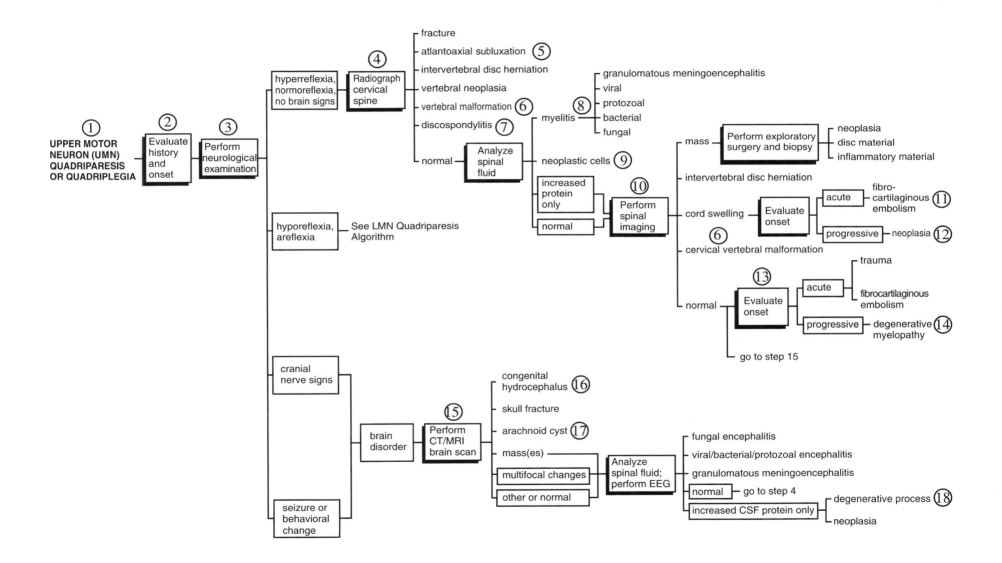

1 UMNs initiate voluntary movement. However, they can affect that movement only via LMNs and their axons. When LMNs, their axons, or receptors (i.e., muscle) are injured, patients exhibit weakness and decreased strength. Additionally, spinal reflexes are diminished to absent, and muscle tone is reduced because the effector side of the reflex arc does not function properly. These clinical manifestations are referred to as *LMN signs.*

2 Neurological weakness due to LMN disease must be distinguished from systemic disease causing weakness. The history and physical and neurological examinations should help make the differentiation. Causes of LMN quadriparesis differ in immature and mature animals. Congenital or inherited muscle and nerve disorders manifest most commonly in immature animals, while metabolic and endocrine disorders occur mostly in mature animals. PU, PD, hair loss, weight loss, coughing, vomiting, diarrhea, lymphadenopathy, fever, or abdominal masses may be found if systemic illness (neoplasia, endocrine, or inflammatory disease) is contributing to quadriparesis.

3 Neurological examination allows LMN and UMN weakness to be distinguished on the basis of spinal reflexes and muscle tone.

4 LMN weakness should be suspected if spinal reflexes and muscle tone are reduced. Since causes of acute LMN quadriparesis are different from those of chronic or progressive LMN quadriparesis, the rate of onset of clinical signs should be determined.

5 If LMN weakness develops rapidly, the differential diagnosis includes myasthenia gravis, tick paralysis, botulism, *Toxoplasma* spp. myoneuritis, and acute polyradiculoneuritis.

6 Mature animals with chronic, progressive LMN signs need routine laboratory work to investigate the possibility of systemic or generalized illness. Investigation begins with a hemogram, chemistry profile, and CK determination. The patient's environment also should be examined for toxins since many of these cause chronic polyneuropathies.

7 If the patient has had a history of intermittent, exercise-induced weakness that resolves with rest, myasthenia gravis is a potential cause. Serum can be evaluated for circulating antibodies to acetylcholine receptors in muscle. Tensilon testing (using intravenous edrophonium chloride) also can be performed. Some patients with polymyositis improve with edrophonium, so do not base the diagnosis only on a positive response to the drug.

8 Carefully examine the patient for engorged female ticks (*Dermacentor* spp.) that can cause tick paralysis. In the United States, clinical signs improve within hours and patients are normal once ticks are removed (manually or with insecticidal sprays or dips). This is not the case in other parts of the world (e.g., Australia) where ticks that cause tick paralysis (e.g., *Ixodes* spp.) frequently cause progressive, severe clinical signs and death.

9 Question clients carefully about the possibility of exposure to carrion or spoiled foodstuffs that could contain toxins produced by *Clostridium botulinum.* The toxin blocks acetylcholine release at the neuromuscular junction. Clinical signs can include mydriasis, urinary and fecal retention, and weakness of facial, esophageal, and pharyngeal musculature.

10 If muscle pain, fever, or gastrointestinal signs are present, ask about potential exposure to *Toxoplasma gondii* via ingestion of cat feces, rodents, or uncooked meat. Cats may be asymptomatic.

11 If the patient is a hunting dog and was bitten by/exposed to a raccoon 1 to 2 weeks prior to the onset of acute LMN signs, polyradiculoneuritis or coonhound paralysis is likely. Weakness typically begins in the pelvic limbs and progresses forward. Most dogs retain the ability to wag the tail voluntarily, urinate, and defecate. They may be unusually sensitive to touch. Immune-mediated demyelination and axonopathy is the most likely cause, but the triggering element is unknown. Clinical cases do appear to occur in dogs that have not been exposed to raccoons, so there are likely to be other sources of antigenic stimulation. Clinical signs usually improve within 6 to 8 weeks, but full recovery may take months.

12 Needle EMG, motor nerve conduction velocity (MNCV), and decremental response (DR) testing of nerve and muscle function can be performed at teaching hospitals or specialty clinics.

13 Diabetes mellitus–induced polyneuropathy affects cats more often than dogs. Pelvic limbs are most commonly affected, often producing "dropped hocks."

14 If signalment (e.g., a mature dog of a medium to large breed), history (e.g., lethargy, heat seeking, weight gain), physical examination (e.g., symmetrical hair loss, thin haircoat, obesity), or laboratory findings (e.g., hypercholesterolemia) suggest hypothyroidism, the thyroid hormone concentration should be evaluated. If this is lower than normal, investigate the possibility of hypothyroidism with other thyroid function tests prior to trial therapy with replacement hormone.

15 If weakness is gradual and progressive and accompanied by elevations in ALP, assess for hyperadrenocorticism (pot-bellied appearance, alopecia, PU, PD, polyphagia). An ACTH response test or other screening tests can be used to diagnose this condition. Needle EMG may show myotonic discharges.

16 Exposure to *T. gondii* is frequently based on titer results. If clinical signs are due to active infection a good response to treatment is expected within several days.

17 If the patient is middle-aged or older, consider paraneoplastic neuropathy/myopathy. Thoracic radiographs and abdominal ultrasonography can be beneficial in detecting masses.

18 If the patient is young, congenital, inherited, or inflammatory muscle or nerve disorders are possible.

19 Muscle and nerve disorders often can be confirmed and defined via electrodiagnostics and biopsy of nerve and/or muscle.

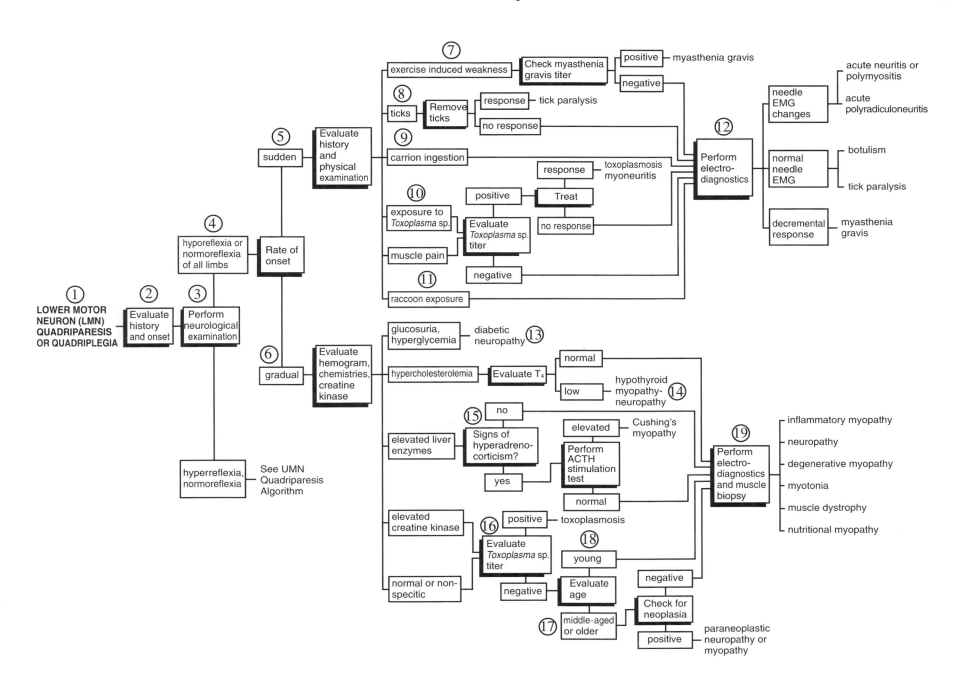

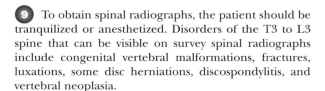
1 Paraparesis is weakness in and paraplegia is lack of pelvic limb movement. Paraparetic patients can be ambulatory but have weak voluntary movements. More severely affected patients are nonambulatory but still have the ability to move the rear limbs voluntarily. Even more severely affected patients lack voluntary movement; voluntary urination is also absent. Most severe cases of paraparesis/paraplegia are neurological in origin (spinal cord or peripheral nerve disorders). Metabolic, muscle, and cardiovascular diseases can cause mild paraparesis.

2 Knowing the speed of onset and progression of clinical signs aids the differential diagnosis. In general, weakness of sudden onset is caused by traumatic, vascular, or neoplastic disease. Gradual onset and progressive signs suggest inflammatory, infectious, degenerative, and neoplastic causes. Age also is a consideration since inflammatory and infectious diseases of the nervous system occur most commonly in younger patients, while neoplastic disorders are found in middle-aged to older patients. Intervertebral disc herniation is a common cause of paraparesis and paraplegia in dogs over 3 years of age, and signs are acute (chondrodysplastic breeds) or gradual.

3 Physical examination can suggest cardiovascular, metabolic, or systemic diseases. Older dogs presenting with pelvic limb weakness and pale mucous membranes may have acute internal hemorrhage from a ruptured abdominal hemangiosarcoma. Finding petechiation in a paraparetic patient should make the clinician suspect vasculitis (Rocky Mountain spotted fever, ehrlichiosis) or a coagulopathy (DIC). Patients with hypoglycemia and hypocalcemia can present with pelvic limb tremors and/or weakness. For these reasons, routine laboratory tests for paraparetic patients should be evaluated. Femoral pulses should be assessed in any cat presenting with pelvic limb weakness since aortic thromboembolism is a common cause of paraparesis and paraplegia in cats. The problem occurs rarely in dogs.

4 Results of the hemogram and serum chemistry profile (including CK) can eliminate or verify most metabolic causes of paraparesis. Such disorders rarely cause paraplegia.

5 If there is a possibility of exposure to protozoal agents or if CK is elevated, evaluate blood titers for toxoplasmosis and neosporosis. If these are strongly suspected, begin treatment while awaiting test results.

6 In the nonambulatory or paralyzed patient, a complete neurological examination is needed to localize the site of dysfunction. If thoracic limbs are normal and pelvic limbs are paralyzed, the lesion is located below the T2 vertebra. If the pelvic limbs are weak but the patient is still ambulatory, the lesion can be located anywhere along the spinal cord or possibly is associated with muscle or peripheral nerves.

7 If a patient with paraparesis or paralysis shows evidence of mentation changes, cranial nerve signs, or seizure activity, then a diffuse CNS disorder is possible. Potential causes include infection (CDV, fungal or protozoal encephalomyelitis, FIP, rickettsial vasculitis), degenerative processes (lysosomal storage disorders), toxins (lead, organophosphates), and diffuse neoplasia (lymphoma).

8 To localize problems to a specific area of the spinal cord or peripheral nervous system, evaluate spinal reflexes. The patient must be relaxed to obtain reflexes that can be assessed accurately. While evaluating spinal reflexes, assess the muscle tone and mass. If the pelvic limb muscles are normal in size and have normal tone, then the lesion is likely to be a UMN lesion located from T3 to L3 (provided that thoracic limbs are normal). Additionally if pelvic limbs have exaggerated spinal reflexes, a positive crossed extensor reflex, or a positive Babinski sign, then a UMN lesion from T3 to L3 is most likely. Severe pelvic limb muscle atrophy or absent to depressed spinal reflexes is suggestive of LMN disease. Pelvic limb LMN signs can be due to disease of the lower lumbar spinal cord, peripheral nerves of the pelvic limbs, or pelvic limb muscles. In practice, it is usually easier to evaluate the lower lumbar spinal cord and vertebrae radiographically (step 10) than to evaluate muscles and nerves. Normal pelvic limb reflexes are compatible with either a UMN or an LMN lesion, and radiographs should be obtained of the T3 to L3 area as well as the L4 region and distally.

9 To obtain spinal radiographs, the patient should be tranquilized or anesthetized. Disorders of the T3 to L3 spine that can be visible on survey spinal radiographs include congenital vertebral malformations, fractures, luxations, some disc herniations, discospondylitis, and vertebral neoplasia.

10 Disorders of the lower lumbar spine visible on survey spinal radiographs include those listed in step 9 and lumbosacral stenosis.

11 If a T3 to L3 spinal cord lesion is suspected and survey radiographs are normal, further spinal imaging is indicated in paralyzed patients and recommended in paraparetic patients. However, before performing contrast spinal radiographic studies or a CT/MRI scan, CSF should be analyzed to exclude meningitis, myelitis, and some types of neoplasia (e.g., lymphoma). Nonspecific increases in CSF protein in conjunction with normal cell counts occur with many compressive, traumatic, degenerative, and inflammatory processes.

12 Myelography is best for evaluating spinal cord compression by intervertebral disc herniation or a mass. Spinal CT or MRI scans provide more information about the spinal cord parenchyma or nerve roots.

13 Signs of lumbosacral stenosis include paraparesis, atrophy of muscles innervated by the sciatic nerve, fecal or urinary incontinence, weak tail movements, weak perineal reflexes, and pain on dorsiflexion of the tail or palpation of the lumbosacral area. Such signs warrant spinal imaging via CT/MRI scans or epidurography. If these tests are not available and the evidence is sufficient, then exploratory laminectomy can yield a diagnosis and treat the problem at the same time.

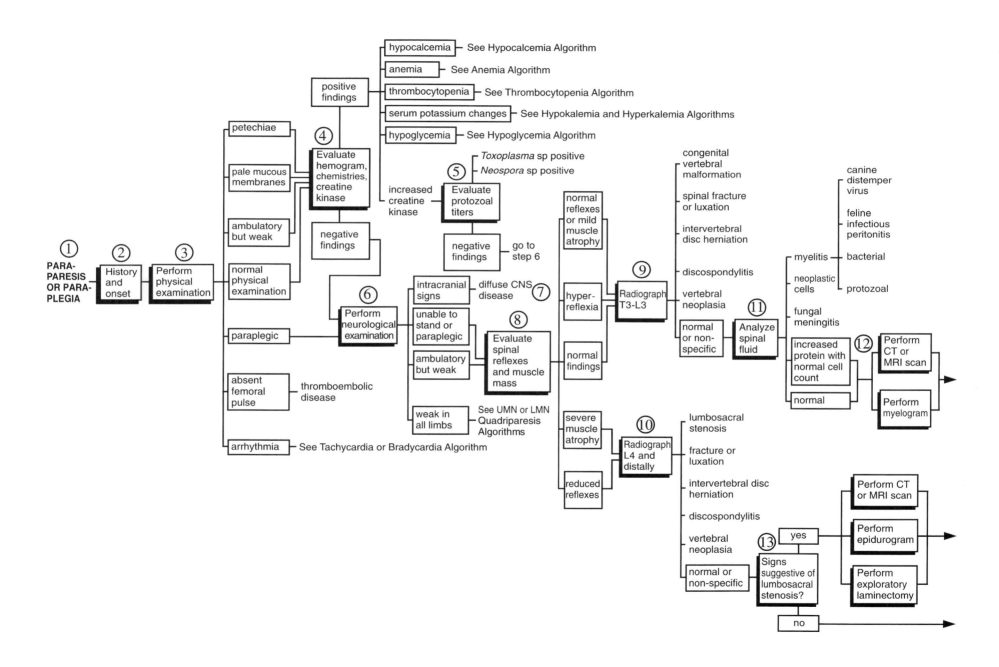

14 If a mass effect is seen on spinal imaging, exploratory surgery is recommended to biopsy the mass for histopathological evaluation, to remove as much of the mass as possible, or to decompress the area and relieve the clinical signs.

15 GME is a nonsuppurative meningoencephalomyelitis of unknown cause. It is uncommon in the spinal cord or nerve roots. It occurs mostly in smaller breeds of dogs (miniature poodles, terriers). The cause is unknown. The only way to obtain a positive diagnosis is via tissue biopsy or necropsy.

16 Spinal cord neoplasia can be primary or metastatic. Primary neural tumors include astrocytoma, glioma, ependymoma, neuroepithelioma, malignant nerve sheath neoplasia, meningioma, and lymphoma. The spinal cord also can be compressed by extradural tumors originating from surrounding structures (bone, cartilage, and vertebral bone). Lymphoma is the most commonly seen spinal tumor in cats.

17 FCE occurs acutely and results in ischemic myelopathy. The emboli occlude arteries and/or veins in the spinal cord. Predisposing factors are unknown. Patients commonly are large to giant-breed dogs of any age. Patients often are severely paraparetic but nonpainful, and signs are nonprogressive after the first 12 hours. Clinical signs depend on the location of the lesion. Diagnosis is made by excluding other causes of myelopathy. Spinal radiographs and CSF analysis usually are normal or nonspecific. Mild spinal cord swelling may be seen on a myelogram.

18 Slowly progressive ataxia, pelvic limb paresis, and conscious proprioceptive deficits characterize degenerative myelopathy. There is demyelination of the entire white matter of the spinal cord, especially in the thoracic segments. Neurological examination indicates a myelopathy between T3 and L3. The underlying causes are unknown. The increased incidence in German shepherds suggests a genetic predisposition. Diagnosis is based on the clinical findings, age of the dog, and breed. Spinal radiographs are normal, and significant myelographic abnormalities are not found. No effective treatment has been reported.

19 If imaging of the lower lumbar area does not yield a diagnosis of stenosis, a mass, or disc herniation, the next step is to analyze spinal fluid. Spinal fluid analysis can be done after CT or MRI imaging; however, it is best to perform CSF analysis before an epidurogram in case some of the contrast medium reaches the subarachnoid space.

20 If CSF analysis does not yield a diagnosis of myelitis, neoplasia, or fungal meningitis, needle EMG can be used to determine that the disease process is more generalized than was originally thought or that it is localized to the lower lumbar spine. If needle EMG does not show changes in the pelvic limb muscles, then consider the possibility that the disease process is cranial to L4. Myelography or CT/MRI scans are used to image the spinal cord above L4.

21 Hydromyelia (dilation of the central canal of the spinal cord) and syringomyelia (spinal cord cavitation) may occur together or separately, may be associated with congenital conditions, or may be acquired. Clinical findings of paraparesis usually are progressive but may be acute initially.

22 If the tests performed up to this point do not yield a specific diagnosis, then reevaluate the onset of clinical signs. Fibrocartilaginous emboli are sudden in onset, but clients may misinterpret subsequent muscle wasting as a sign of progressive disease. Some clients may also attribute slowly progressive pelvic limb weakness to hip dysplasia and may misinterpret progression. Degenerative myelopathy can affect spinal nerve roots and present as LMN signs. Finally, if test results do not yield an answer, consider myelitis that may not show up on CSF analysis because it is either mild or may produce only subtle CSF changes.

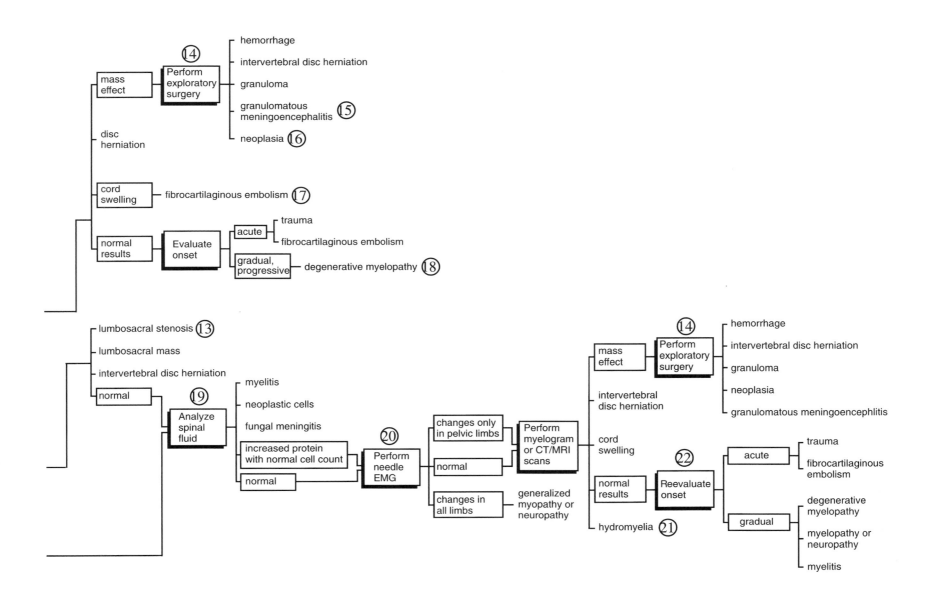

1 Urinary incontinence is loss of voluntary control of urination. It has both neurogenic and nonneurogenic causes. With neurogenic causes there usually are historical or neurological findings (ataxia or a weak gait, dropped tail, fecal incontinence) that point to neurological problems. Nonneurogenic disorders are anatomical or physiological abnormalities of the lower urinary tract (e.g., ectopic ureters, cystitis, neoplasia, urolithiasis, or prostatic disease).

2 Do not decide that a patient is incontinent until a thorough description of the problem is obtained. Clients can confuse both PU and stranguria with incontinence. Inquire about increased water intake; if it is increased, suspect PD causing PU and "urge incontinence." If the animal's water consumption is unknown, have the client measure it over 24 hours. In cats, suspect feline lower urinary tract disease (FLUTD), a condition that is far more common in cats than incontinence. Cats with FLUTD often urinate in inappropriate places. Large volumes of urine found in the house are more suggestive of PU or inappropriate urination than of incontinence. Signs of incontinence include dribbling urine when walking or sleeping. Dribbling of urine usually occurs without the patient posturing to urinate.

3 Palpate the urinary bladder to evaluate its size, tone, and wall thickness, as well as for the presence of uroliths. Try to express the bladder manually. If the bladder has poor tone and is easily expressed, a neurological abnormality should be suspected. If the bladder cannot be expressed, the pet could be normal or have reflex dyssynergia or urethral obstruction. Palpate the prostate gland in all male dogs.

4 Detailed neurological examination determines if nerve dysfunction is causing incontinence. Cerebral, cerebellar, or spinal cord abnormalities can result in neurogenic incontinence. Incontinence caused by cerebral or cerebellar abnormalities is unusual and is not generally the main presenting sign. Spinal cord diseases, particularly at L4 to S3, are common causes of urinary incontinence. Finding a weak perineal reflex, decreased anal/tail tone, lumbosacral hyperpathia, proprioceptive deficits, or fecal incontinence suggests an L4 to S3 lesion.

5 If the neurological examination is normal, pursuit of a lower urinary tract problem causing incontinence is warranted. Start with analysis of a urine sample collected by cystocentesis.

6 The presence of glucose and/or ketones in urine suggests PU caused by diabetes mellitus.

7 The presence of bacteriuria or pyuria suggests a urinary tract infection (UTI), but it can be difficult to determine if this is the primary reason for urinary incontinence or if it is a secondary complication (the most common problem resulting from urinary incontinence is the development of a UTI). Urine can be cultured or the patient treated empirically with an antibiotic that achieves high concentrations in the urinary tract. If there is no response to the antibiotic, urine culture definitely is warranted. If there is a response to the antibiotic but clinical signs recur, then the UTI is probably a complication of an underlying disease process.

8 A positive urine culture indicates either primary or secondary infection of the urinary tract. Primary infections are not associated with underlying disease. Secondary infections are associated with structural abnormalities such as uroliths (kidney or bladder), neoplasia, bladder diverticulae, or urethral/ureteral strictures. There is no way of knowing if structural abnormalities are present without performing imaging studies. These studies are not indicated unless clinical signs do not resolve with appropriate therapy or recur after treatment.

9 If the urinalysis is normal, PD has been excluded, and the patient is a spayed female dog, there is a good chance that the condition is hormone-responsive urinary incontinence. If there is no response to appropriate medical management (phenylpropanolamine or low-dose estrogen), imaging of the lower urinary tract is required to exclude structural disorders.

10 Intermittent dribbling of urine during rest has been observed in FeLV-positive cats. The significance of this association is not known.

11 In patients with signs of spinal cord disease, spinal radiographs often confirm vertebral trauma, disc herniation, lumbosacral stenosis, discospondylitis, vertebral neoplasia, or sacrocaudal dysgenesis. However, some spinal cord disorders are difficult to diagnose on survey radiographs, making myelography or CT/MRI scanning necessary.

12 FCE may cause sudden urinary incontinence. Patients do not have pain, other neurological deficits are present, and often signs are asymmetrical. Myelography and MRI/CT scans may be normal or may show cord swelling, especially if evaluation occurs within a few days of the onset of clinical signs. Neurological signs do not progress and may improve.

13 Cats can get their tails caught under car tires, in doors, or in other objects. When the cat pulls away, stretching or trauma to the nerves of the tail, anus, and bladder results in paralysis of these areas. If deep pain perception to the anal area is not present within 2 weeks post injury, the prognosis for return of urinary continence is guarded.

14 Dysautonomia is an idiopathic sympathetic and parasympathetic (autonomic nervous system) polyneuropathy that may present as urinary or fecal incontinence. The bladder is easily expressed manually. Dry mucous membranes, dilated pupils, and megaesophagus are other features of the condition.

15 If urine culture results are negative or if the animal has recurrent UTIs, abdominal radiographs or ultrasound are indicated. Uroliths and soft tissue masses of the bladder or caudal abdomen can cause urinary incontinence.

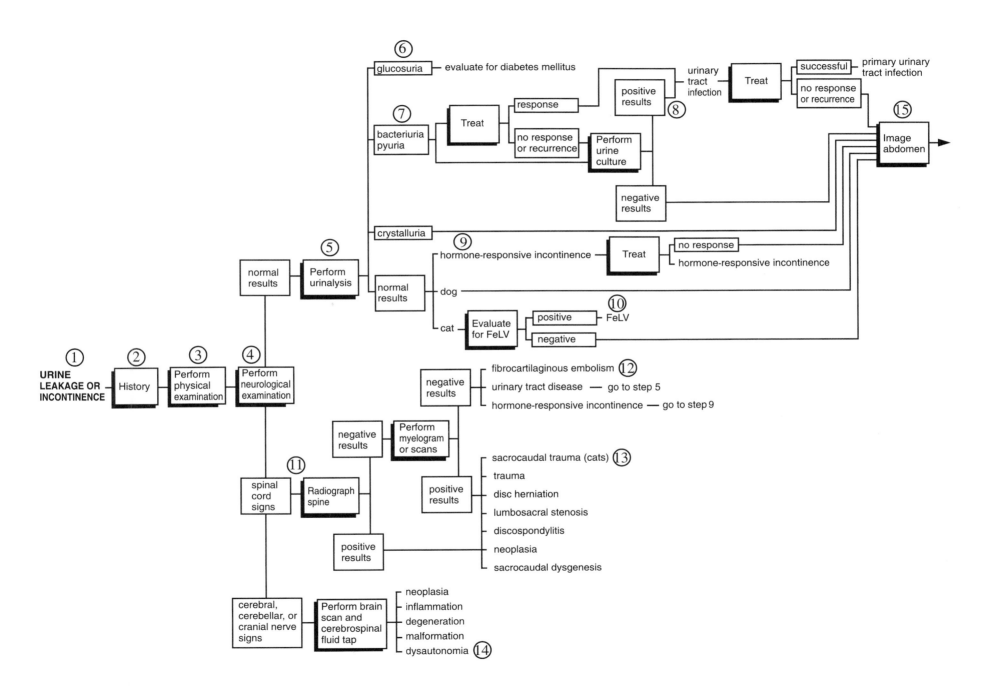

16 If initial abdominal imaging findings are normal or inconclusive, contrast radiographic studies become necessary. Radiographic imaging of the renal pelvis and ureters (areas unlikely to be associated with urinary incontinence unless there is abnormal implantation of the ureters into the urethra) is accomplished via excretory urography. To evaluate the urethra and bladder, positive-contrast cystourethrography or vaginourethrography and double-contrast cystography are used. Urethrocystography detects uroliths, bladder diverticulae, bladder or urethral neoplasia, and urethral strictures. Many of these disorders cause dysuria or stranguria, but some of them (most notably ectopic ureters and urethral calculi) cause urinary incontinence.

17 If contrast studies yield negative results, repeat the neurological examination to determine if a progressive disorder of the nervous system is causing clinical signs.

Other neurological deficits could develop and be detected on a later examination.

18 If the second neurological examination is normal, the patient probably has urethral incompetence. This is the most common micturation disorder in dogs and is characterized by intermittent resting urinary incontinence. It has been associated with prostatic disease, urethral inflammation or infiltrative disease, and congenital anatomical anomalies (e.g., ectopic ureters and vaginal strictures or bands), many of which should have been detected on physical examination or via imaging of the urinary tract prior to this stage of the algorithm. The last disorder associated with urethral incompetence and urinary incontinence is hormone-responsive incontinence, a disorder recognized in both neutered female and male dogs. The incidence of this problem in spayed female dogs is quite high (up to 20%). Variables that contribute to an increased incidence of this problem include body size, obesity, genetic factors, urethral length, urinary bladder position, and concurrent vaginal anomalies. Urethral incompetence can be confirmed via urethral pressure profilometry, but this test is not widely available outside of teaching hospitals. Pharmacological management using alpha-adrenergic agents or reproductive hormone replacement therapy usually controls the clinical signs.

19 Urodynamic studies evaluate the micturation reflex and bladder storage capacity. These tests measure pressure, volume, and flow in the urinary bladder and urethra. Tests include cystometrography and urethral pressure profilometry. Urethral pressure profilometry confirms urethral incompetence (see step 18).

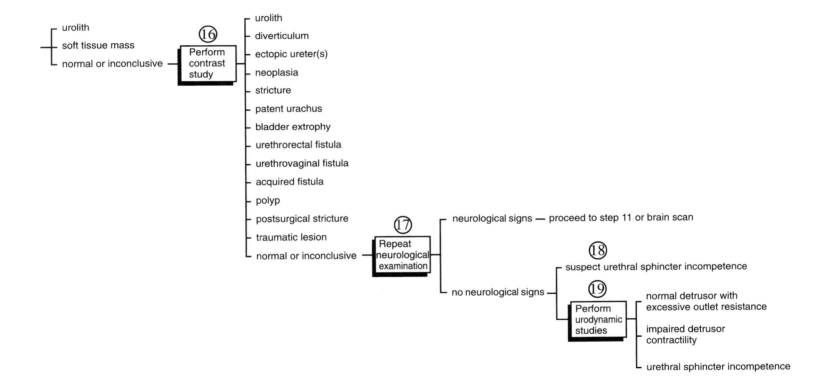

urolith
soft tissue mass
normal or inconclusive ——

⑯ Perform contrast study

urolith
diverticulum
ectopic ureter(s)
neoplasia
stricture
patent urachus
bladder extrophy
urethrorectal fistula
urethrovaginal fistula
acquired fistula
polyp
postsurgical stricture
traumatic lesion
normal or inconclusive ——

⑰ Repeat neurological examination

neurological signs — proceed to step 11 or brain scan

no neurological signs ——

⑱ suspect urethral sphincter incompetence

⑲ Perform urodynamic studies

normal detrusor with excessive outlet resistance
impaired detrusor contractility
urethral sphincter incompetence

SECTION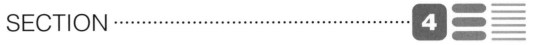

Hematological Disorders

1 Bleeding that occurs spontaneously or for a prolonged period following trauma or surgery indicates a problem with hemostasis resulting from coagulation factor deficiencies, blood vessel wall problems, or platelet problems.

2 A thorough history and physical examination can help to determine whether the problem involves formation of the primary or secondary hemostatic plug.

3 Problems with formation of the primary hemostatic plug include platelet dysfunction (quantitative/qualitative), von Willebrand's disease (vWD), and some vascular disorders. Conditions cause spontaneous bleeding of short duration from the gums, nose, gastrointestinal tract, or urinary tract. Petechiae/ecchymoses also can be seen. The platelet count and buccal mucosal bleeding time (BMBT) are used to evaluate these problems.

4 Problems with formation of the secondary hemostatic plug (coagulopathies) are acquired/congenital coagulation factor deficiencies. Signs include spontaneous, delayed-onset bleeding of long duration, hematoma formation, hemarthrosis, and hemorrhage into body cavities or deep tissues. Evaluation of a platelet count, activated partial thromboplastin time (PTT), and one-stage prothrombin time (PT) can classify the defect as involving the intrinsic, extrinsic, or common coagulation pathways.

5 If the platelet count, PT, and PTT are normal, evaluate BMBT for platelet function. Perform this test only if platelet counts are normal, since thrombocytopenic animals are expected to have a prolonged BMBT. The test has low sensitivity, meaning that a normal BMBT does not eliminate the possibility of a platelet function defect. Buccal mucosa is a common site for testing. Normal BMBT for dogs is 2.62 ± 0.49 minutes, and for cats it is 1.9 ± 0.5 minutes.

6 Prolonged BMBT indicates platelet dysfunction or a vascular wall defect. A hemogram and serum chemistry profile can suggest underlying systemic diseases (e.g., hyperadrenocorticism, sepsis, and vasculitis) as potential causes. If vWD is suspected, assay the patient's plasma for the concentration of von Willebrand factor antigen (vWF:Ag).

7 In general, an abnormal coagulogram suggests specific factor deficiencies, DIC, or anticoagulant rodenticide intoxication.

8 Decreased platelets with normal PT and PTT can indicate early DIC or thrombocytopenia alone. Thrombocytopenia with prolonged PT and/or PTT suggests DIC or platelet consumption secondary to bleeding. If bleeding is severe, more than expected for thrombocytopenia alone, or if there is systemic illness, testing for fibrinogen degradation products (FDPs) can establish a diagnosis of DIC. False FDP elevations occur with heparin administration or dysfibrinogenemia.

9 If only PT is prolonged, a defect in the extrinsic coagulation pathway is likely, specifically factor VII deficiency. Factor VII has a short half-life and is thus sensitive to vitamin K deficiency or antagonism (e.g., anticoagulant rodenticide intoxication). Laboratories can test for anticoagulant rodenticide exposure (proteins induced by vitamin K antagonism testing).

10 Factor VII deficiency is inherited in beagles and Alaskan malamutes. It causes mild bleeding problems, especially when there is additional stress on the hemostatic system (e.g., surgery, trauma).

11 Dietary deficiency of vitamin K is not a problem in dogs and cats on commercial diets. However, patients with chronic malabsorption (abnormal fat assimilation or lymphatic transport) or biliary obstruction may develop vitamin K deficiency, particularly if bacterial synthesis of vitamin K is also inhibited by oral antibiotics.

12 Prolongation of PTT suggests abnormalities of the intrinsic coagulation pathway (factors VIII, IX, XI, and XII). The activated clotting time (ACT) also evaluates the intrinsic coagulation pathway. This test can be performed quickly in the hospital as an initial evaluation.

13 vWD is inherited autosomally, with incomplete dominance of the gene. Bleeding can be mild to severe.

PT is normal, and PTT is normal or prolonged. The BMBT usually is prolonged. The concentration of vWF:Ag in plasma can be assayed to confirm vWD.

14 Factor VIII deficiency is inherited as an X-linked recessive trait in many dog and cat breeds and in mongrels. The BMBT is normal, but the plug formed may not hold and rebleeding occurs.

15 Factor IX deficiency is inherited as an X-linked recessive trait in dogs and cats. Acquired factor IX deficiency is associated with nephrotic syndrome in human beings.

16 Factor XI deficiency is documented in springer spaniels and Great Pyrenees. The BMBT is normal, but rebleeding may occur since the initial plug may not hold.

17 Factor XII deficiency, in cats and poodles is usually subclinical.

18 If the platelet count is normal but the PT and PTT are prolonged, a common coagulation pathway abnormality involving factors I, II, V, and X is likely.

19 From 3 to 4 days after exposure to an anticoagulant rodenticide, the PT becomes prolonged. Bleeding problems become more frequent later as deficiencies of factors IX, X, and II develop. Platelet counts usually are normal or only slightly decreased.

20 Severe acute hepatopathies (infectious hepatitis, lipidosis) prolong the PT and PTT. Chronic, partially compensated hepatopathies cause slight prolongation of the PTT; the PT is normal. Most patients do not bleed unless challenged (surgery, trauma) or until quantitative/qualitative platelet function is affected.

21 DIC is excessive stimulation of hemostasis leading to consumption of platelets and coagulation factor. Typically, patients have thrombocytopenia and, later, prolongation of PT and PTT, with elevations in FDPs.

22 Hemoptysis is "spitting up" blood or blood-stained sputum, but the term is often used to describe coughing up of blood.

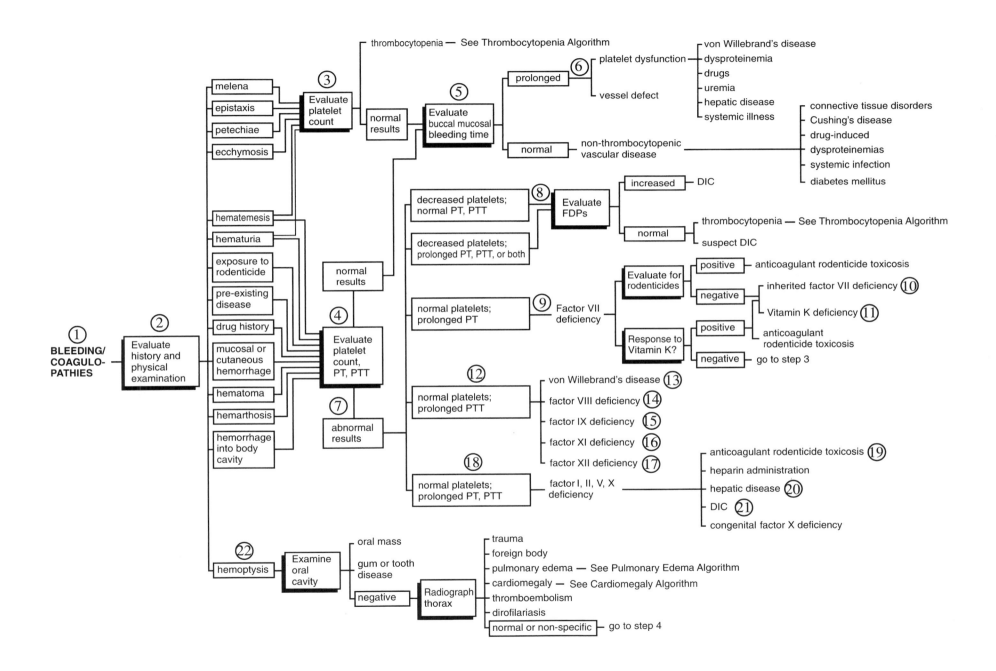

1 Lymphadenopathy is focal or diffuse enlargement of peripheral or internal lymph nodes. Enlarged lymph nodes are the result of proliferation of normal cells (reactive lymphadenopathy) or infiltration by inflammatory cells (lymphadenitis) or neoplastic cells (primary lymphoid neoplasia or metastatic neoplasia). The condition may be benign or malignant.

2 Certain infectious diseases (e.g., leishmaniasis, salmon poisoning, plague, some systemic mycoses) have defined geographic distributions; therefore, a travel history is important. Additionally, some diseases that manifest with lymphadenopathy have seasonal distributions (e.g., Rocky Mountain spotted fever). Some cats and dogs develop generalized reactive lymphadenopathy shortly after vaccination. Dermatitis or localized infections (abscesses, periodontal disease, paronychia) cause reactive lymph node hyperplasia. If the patient is a puppy with draining purulent material from lymph nodes, especially of the head and neck, lymphadenitis (*puppy strangles*) should be suspected. This is a steroid-responsive condition that is suspected to be immune mediated. The presence of severe clinical signs in association with lymphadenopathy is more suggestive of systemic infections than of lymphoma.

3 Palpation of all external lymph nodes allows characterization of lymphadenopathy as local, regional, or generalized. With regional or local lymphadenopathy, the primary lesion will probably be in the area drained by the affected node(s). Patients with deep (intra-abdominal or intrathoracic) solitary or regional lymphadenopathy generally have metastatic neoplasia or systemic infectious disease. Most dogs and cats with generalized lymphadenopathy have systemic fungal or rickettsial infection, hematopoietic neoplasia, or idiopathic lymph node hyperplasia. Marked lymphadenopathy (lymph nodes 5 to 10 times the normal size) occurs almost exclusively with lymphadenitis and lymphoma.

With lymphadenitis the node may be soft, tender, and warm and may adhere to surrounding structures, resulting in fixed lymphadenopathy.

4 Fine-needle aspiration of an enlarged node or nodes is the first step toward establishing a diagnosis. Superficial lymph nodes can be aspirated with minimal difficulty. Aspiration of intrathoracic or intra-abdominal lymph nodes requires a surgical preparation and adequate patient restraint (usually sedation). Ultrasound guidance is generally recommended. A 22- to 25-gauge needle is used, and the needle is redirected within the node several times when aspiration is performed. Withdraw the needle from the lymph node, making sure that there is no suction left in the syringe. Detach the needle from the syringe, draw 6–8 ml air into the syringe, reattach the needle, and force the cells out onto a clean glass slide by pushing the air out of the syringe. Slides are then air-dried and stained for cytological evaluation to distinguish reactive, inflammatory, and neoplastic lymphadenopathy. Note that administration of glucocorticoids before aspiration can make the diagnosis of lymphoma more difficult.

5 If nondiagnostic samples are obtained on the first aspiration, repeat the aspiration or move on to step 6.

6 A hemogram and a serum chemistry profile can be evaluated for signs of inflammatory or neoplastic diseases, especially in patients with generalized lymphadenopathy. Some changes on the hemogram that may suggest systemic inflammation include neutrophilic leukocytosis, a left shift, and monocytosis. Circulating blast cells, marked lymphocytosis, or thrombocytosis suggest underlying neoplasia. Occasionally, infectious organisms may be found on a blood or buffy coat smear (*Histoplasma* spp., *Trypanosoma* spp., *Babesia* spp.). Hypercalcemia in conjunction with lymphadenopathy leads to consideration of lymphoma or very rarely multiple myeloma, be-

nign parathyroid tumors, and blastomycosis in dogs and lymphoma, squamous cell carcinoma, fibrosarcoma, or very rarely myeloma and benign parathyroid tumors in cats. If hyperglobulinemia is present on the serum chemistry screen, determine whether it is monoclonal or polyclonal. If it is monoclonal, consider multiple myeloma, chronic lymphocytic leukemia, lymphoma, ehrlichiosis (dogs), and leishmaniasis. If the hyperglobulinemia is polyclonal, systemic mycoses, FIP, ehrlichiosis, and lymphoma are possibilities. Cats with lymphadenopathy should have their FeLV and FIV status evaluated as part of the minimum database.

7 A syndrome of idiopathic lymphadenopathy (or distinctive peripheral lymph node hyperplasia) has been described in some FeLV- and FIV-positive cats. Some cats are clinically normal except for the lymphadenopathy, while others have a variety of clinical signs. Signs may resolve but often recur later, and lymphoma may develop.

8 If the hemogram and chemistry results are normal, are nonspecific, or show only mild anemia or thrombocytopenia, evaluate the patient for infectious diseases endemic to the area. These include ehrlichiosis, Rocky Mountain spotted fever, blastomycosis, coccidioidomycosis, histoplasmosis, and cryptococcosis. Serology may be useful in some instances. Histopathology, cytology, and specialized cultures are important for some conditions.

9 If evaluation for infectious disease is nonproductive or if hypercalcemia, hyperglobulinemia, or lymphocytosis is present, obtain a lymph node biopsy specimen (step 12) and/or bone marrow aspirate to look for hematopoietic neoplasia or systemic infectious diseases (e.g., ehrlichiosis). Choose between lymph node biopsy and bone marrow aspiration based on the patient's clinical signs. In some dogs bone marrow aspiration can be performed under sedation and with local anesthesia.

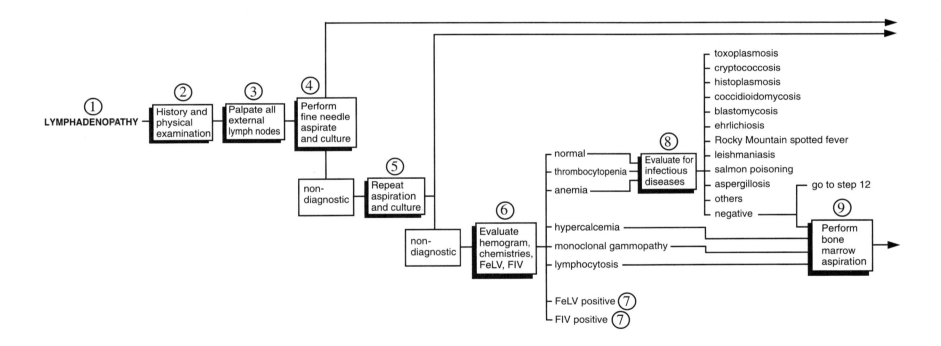

① **LYMPHADENOPATHY**

② History and physical examination

③ Palpate all external lymph nodes

④ Perform fine needle aspirate and culture

non-diagnostic

⑤ Repeat aspiration and culture

non-diagnostic

⑥ Evaluate hemogram, chemistries, FeLV, FIV

- normal
- thrombocytopenia
- anemia

⑧ Evaluate for infectious diseases

- toxoplasmosis
- cryptococcosis
- histoplasmosis
- coccidioidomycosis
- blastomycosis
- ehrlichiosis
- Rocky Mountain spotted fever
- leishmaniasis
- salmon poisoning
- aspergillosis
- others
- negative

- hypercalcemia
- monoclonal gammopathy
- lymphocytosis

- FeLV positive ⑦
- FIV positive ⑦

go to step 12

⑨ Perform bone marrow aspiration

10 Hematopoietic neoplasms that can be diagnosed on bone marrow aspiration cytology or lymph node biopsy include leukemias, lymphoma, multiple myeloma, malignant histiocytosis, and systemic mast cell tumor spread.

11 If the bone marrow aspirate or lymph node biopsy specimen suggests an infectious process rather than hematopoietic neoplasia, evaluate for infectious diseases common in the local area or in regions to which the patient has traveled. Evaluation may involve serology (best for coccidioidomycosis, cryptococcosis, ehrlichiosis, Rocky Mountain spotted fever, babesiosis, and toxoplasmosis), lymph node histopathology, special tissue stains for specific organisms (e.g., atypical mycobacteria, *Nocardia* spp., *Actinomyces* spp.), and specialized culture techniques.

12 If bone marrow aspiration cytology and tests for infectious diseases are done first and are negative, the next step is lymph node biopsy. Excision of an affected node is preferable to core or needle biopsy because lymph node architecture is preserved. If there is generalized lymphadenopathy, a popliteal lymph node usually is excised since these nodes are easily accessible.

13 Viral causes of lymphadenopathy in the dog are uncommon but include canine infectious hepatitis, herpes virus, and viral enteritides. In the cat, FIP, FIV, and FeLV have been known to cause lymphadenopathy.

14 Localized bacterial infections (e.g., cellulitis) often cause localized lymphadenopathy that resolves when the infection is treated appropriately. Bacterial infections can also cause generalized lymphadenopathy (e.g., strangles). Other bacterial agents that cause lymphadenopathy include *Corynebacterium* spp., *Brucella* spp., *Mycobacteria* spp., *Actinomyces* spp., *Nocardia* spp., *Yersinia pestis* (cats), and *Francisella tularensis* (cats).

15 Plexiform vascularization is an uncommon disorder characterized by solitary cervical or inguinal lymphadenopathy in cats aged 3 to 14 years. Cats are usually asymptomatic except for the enlarged nodes. Histologically, lymph nodes are characterized by replacement of interfollicular tissues with plexiform proliferation of small capillary-sized vascular channels and lymphoid atrophy.

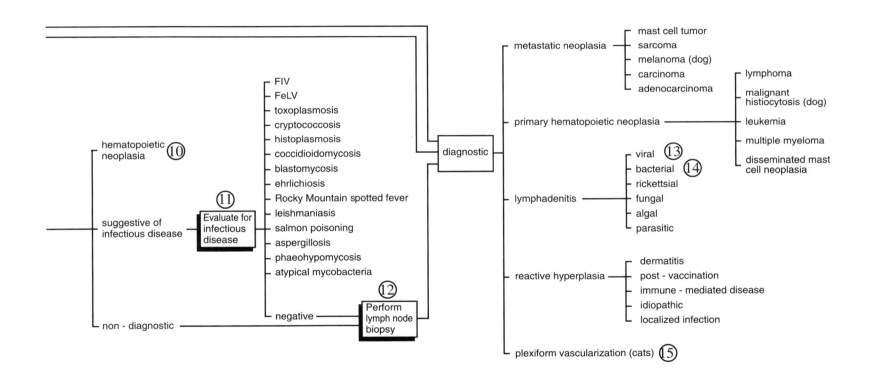

hematopoietic neoplasia ⑩

suggestive of infectious disease

Evaluate for infectious disease ⑪
- FIV
- FeLV
- toxoplasmosis
- cryptococcosis
- histoplasmosis
- coccidioidomycosis
- blastomycosis
- ehrlichiosis
- Rocky Mountain spotted fever
- leishmaniasis
- salmon poisoning
- aspergillosis
- phaeohypomycosis
- atypical mycobacteria

non - diagnostic — negative — **Perform lymph node biopsy** ⑫

diagnostic

metastatic neoplasia
- mast cell tumor
- sarcoma
- melanoma (dog)
- carcinoma
- adenocarcinoma

primary hematopoietic neoplasia
- lymphoma
- malignant histiocytosis (dog)
- leukemia
- multiple myeloma
- disseminated mast cell neoplasia

lymphadenitis
- viral ⑬
- bacterial ⑭
- rickettsial
- fungal
- algal
- parasitic

reactive hyperplasia
- dermatitis
- post - vaccination
- immune - mediated disease
- idiopathic
- localized infection

plexiform vascularization (cats) ⑮

1 Splenomegaly is enlargement of the spleen, which may be focal (e.g., a mass within the spleen) or diffuse (e.g., enlargement due to extramedullary hematopoiesis). Focal splenomegaly (usually a mass lesion) is more common in dogs, whereas cats tend to present more frequently with diffuse disease. Splenomegaly may be the result of many disease processes but also may be normal for an individual. Certain species (e.g., ferrets) and dog breeds (e.g., basset hounds) may have prominent spleens. It is unusual for splenomegaly to be the presenting complaint, although occasionally the spleen is so large that abdominal distention or a mass effect is felt through the body wall.

2 Patients that have splenomegaly on physical examination or imaging of the abdomen tend to present with nonspecific signs such as lethargy, weakness, anorexia, PU, PD, and diarrhea. This is true with both primary splenic disease (e.g., a mass or torsion) and splenic enlargement secondary to systemic problems (e.g., autoimmune hemolytic anemia, septicemia, leukemia, pyometra). With systemic disease causing splenomegaly, clinical signs are probably related to the underlying condition. Review of the patient's history can reveal pharmacological agents likely to cause splenomegaly because they cause splenic vein dilation and splenic congestion.

3 Drugs causing splenomegaly include barbiturates used in anesthesia (e.g., thiopental) and as anticonvulsants (e.g., phenobarbital), as well as sedatives (e.g., phenothiazine). All these agents cause splenic vascular dilation and blood pooling.

4 Review of the history can reveal preexisting diseases that cause or are associated with splenomegaly (e.g., autoimmune hemolytic anemia, endocarditis, red blood cell parasitism, and leukemia).

5 Physical examination often detects splenomegaly and allows the clinician to distinguish focal and diffuse enlargement. This is not the case in every patient (e.g., obese animals and very deep-chested dogs, in which much of the spleen is mainly located within the rib cage). It also allows detection of abdominal fluid, which may suggest that a splenic mass has ruptured. This is important because if diagnostic facilities or client finances are limited, palpating a mass is a good indication that surgical exploration is needed following laboratory work and thoracic radiographs. Physical examination also can suggest more systemic problems resulting in splenomegaly (e.g., white or icteric mucous membranes with autoimmune hemolytic anemia and red blood cell parasitism, fever with a variety of infectious conditions, back pain with discospondylitis, and heart murmurs with bacterial endocarditis).

6 Diffuse splenomegaly requires more extensive evaluation for underlying disease via laboratory work, ultrasound, or other imaging techniques, possibly followed by splenic aspiration for cytology.

7 A minimum database (hemogram, chemistry profile, and FeLV/FIV tests for cats) should be obtained at this point to assess the patient's general health, involvement of other body systems, and suitability for any surgery. Often, the information obtained will not contribute directly to the diagnosis. Occasionally, however, the hemogram can provide the diagnosis (e.g., if neoplastic cells or red blood cell [RBC] parasites are found on the peripheral blood smear). Note that patients can have more than one problem causing splenomegaly (e.g., FeLV-positive cats can have neoplastic or hematopoietic infiltrates in the spleen as well as *Haemobartonella felis* in their RBCs as a result of immunosuppression). The chemistry profile also can provide further information about the underlying cause of splenomegaly. For example, hyperbilirubinemia and bilirubinuria, with or without anemia, suggest immune-mediated hemolytic anemia, other causes of RBC breakdown, and splenic masses or splenic torsion as potential underlying causes of splenomegaly. In such cases, radiographs or abdominal ultrasound are indicated.

8 Imaging the abdomen allows determination of whether splenic enlargement is focal or diffuse, whether there is abdominal fluid, and whether there are other problems (e.g., masses elsewhere, concurrent gastric torsion). Radiographs often distinguish diffuse splenic enlargement and focal masses, as well as splenic torsion. Ultrasound is needed to evaluate the parenchyma of the spleen (e.g., for masses within the spleen that do not distort the outer capsule, diffuse enlargement with alterations in the echogenicity of the spleen that suggest infiltrative disease). Abdominal ultrasound also is useful for determining whether other structures in the abdomen are affected (e.g., metastatic lesions in the liver from a splenic mass, lymphadenopathy, and small amounts of abdominal fluid). Abdominal ultrasound can be more sensitive than radiographs in identifying total or partial splenic torsion.

9 Splenic torsion can be difficult to diagnose both radiographically and with ultrasound. Clinically, it may be associated with very nonspecific signs, and there is a risk of sudden death associated with the problem. Therefore, if patient signalment is appropriate (e.g., a large or giant breed of dog) and if other causes of splenomegaly have been excluded, surgical exploration of the abdomen is recommended above other diagnostic tests.

10 Splenectomy and histopathological evaluation of tissue are recommended above needle aspiration for cytology when there is a focal mass lesion. Excisional biopsy is more likely to provide a definitive diagnosis (e.g., of a benign lesion such as a hematoma, granuloma, or abscess or a malignant lesion such as a hemangiosarcoma, fibrosarcoma, or leiomyosarcoma) since splenic masses often do not exfoliate well. It also reduces the risks of shedding neoplastic cells within the abdominal cavity during aspiration, leading to metastasis.

11 If free fluid is present in the abdomen, abdominocentesis should be performed. If blood is found, ruptured hemangiosarcoma or other malignant splenic masses must be considered. Exploratory laparotomy is in order.

12 Fine-needle aspiration of the spleen may require ultrasound guidance to allow aspiration of focally abnormal areas or just to ensure that the spleen is the tissue being aspirated. Needle aspiration of the spleen has few contraindications, especially where splenic enlargement is diffuse and there is no obvious mass or cavitation. Caution is needed in patients with thrombocytopenia and an obvious tendency to bleed. A small (22- or 25-gauge) needle is recommended.

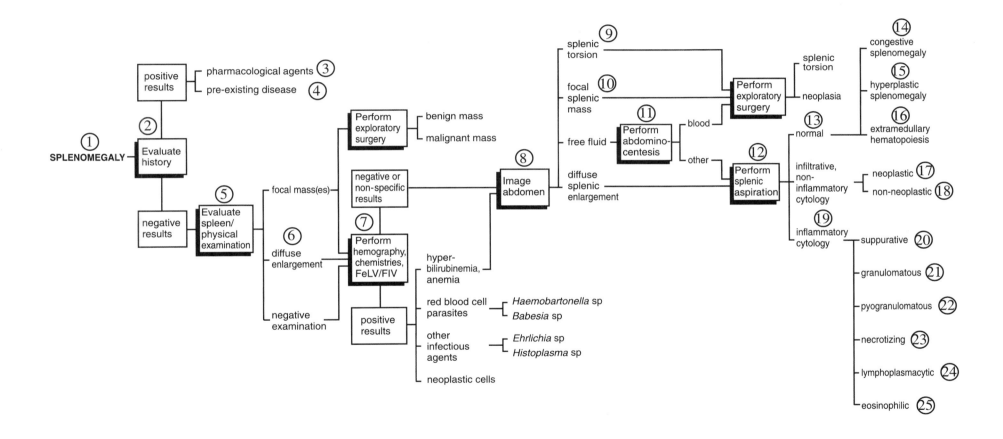

SPLENOMEGALY ① — ② Evaluate history

positive results — pharmacological agents ③
positive results — pre-existing disease ④

negative results — ⑤ Evaluate spleen/physical examination

⑤ Evaluate spleen/physical examination:
- focal mass(es)
- ⑥ diffuse enlargement
- negative examination

Perform exploratory surgery:
- benign mass
- malignant mass

negative or non-specific results — ⑧ Image abdomen

⑦ Perform hemography, chemistries, FeLV/FIV

positive results:
- hyper-bilirubinemia, anemia
- red blood cell parasites — Haemobartonella sp / Babesia sp
- other infectious agents — Ehrlichia sp / Histoplasma sp
- neoplastic cells

⑧ Image abdomen:
- splenic torsion ⑨
- focal splenic mass ⑩
- free fluid
- diffuse splenic enlargement

⑪ Perform abdomino-centesis:
- blood
- other

Perform exploratory surgery:
- splenic torsion
- neoplasia

⑫ Perform splenic aspiration:
- ⑬ normal
- infiltrative, non-inflammatory cytology
- ⑲ inflammatory cytology

normal ⑬:
- congestive splenomegaly ⑭
- hyperplastic splenomegaly ⑮
- extramedullary hematopoiesis ⑯

infiltrative, non-inflammatory cytology:
- neoplastic ⑰
- non-neoplastic ⑱

inflammatory cytology ⑲:
- suppurative ⑳
- granulomatous ㉑
- pyogranulomatous ㉒
- necrotizing ㉓
- lymphoplasmacytic ㉔
- eosinophilic ㉕

13 Where cytology of a splenic aspirate indicates a normal or hyperplastic population of cellular elements, splenic enlargement is likely to be due to accumulation of blood within the spleen (congestion), hyperplasia, or extramedullary hematopoiesis.

14 Splenic congestion can be caused by drugs, splenic torsion, portal hypertension (e.g., secondary to acquired hepatic cirrhosis or due to congenital hepatic shunts), splenic vein thrombosis, or heart failure.

15 Splenic hyperplasia is thought to occur as a reaction to blood-borne antigens and antigen-antibody complex formation in the circulation (e.g., with chronic endocarditis, discospondylitis, brucellosis, hemolysis, or SLE). Antigens and antibody-antigen complexes stimulate increased splenic activity, including phagocytosis of cells with foreign material within them or with antigens on the cell surface. Under some circumstances, RBCs phagocytosed by splenic macrophages may be seen on splenic aspirates. It is more usual to see increased lymphoid elements and cells of the reticuloendothelial system on aspirates.

16 Extramedullary hematopoiesis occurs where the residual hematopoietic function of the spleen is reactivated, due either to excessive demand for RBC production or to failure of bone marrow function, and the spleen starts to make RBCs, white blood cells (WBCs), and platelets. Extramedullary hematopoiesis is more common in dogs than in cats.

17 Neoplastic infiltrative disease is more common than nonneoplastic splenic infiltrates in both dogs and cats. It is one of the most common causes of diffuse splenomegaly in both species. Neoplastic infiltrative disease is due either to a primary neoplasm or to infiltration with a more systemic neoplasm (e.g., mastocytosis, plasma cell myeloma, malignant histiocytosis, acute and chronic leukemia, and lymphoma). The spleen is rarely a site for metastatic neoplasia.

18 Nonneoplastic splenic infiltrates include those seen with lymphomatoid granulomatosis (in dogs), hypereosinophilic syndrome (in cats), and amyloidosis.

19 Inflammatory infiltrates also can result in diffuse splenic enlargement, except in the rare case of a focal abscess or granuloma. Conditions causing inflammatory infiltrates generally are either infectious or granulomatous. Conditions may be classified according to either the duration of the problem (acute, subacute, or chronic) or the main cellular infiltrate seen.

20 Suppurative infiltrates are neutrophilic and usually represent acute disease. Common causes of suppurative splenic infiltrates are systemic infectious conditions and include septicemia, bacterial endocarditis, acute canine adenovirus infection (infectious canine hepatitis), toxoplasmosis, and foreign bodies in or direct wounds to the spleen.

21 Granulomatous splenic infiltrates have macrophages, lymphocytes, and multinucleated giant cells on splenic cytology and most commonly represent chronic inflammation. Causes include histoplasmosis, mycobacterial infection, and leishmaniasis.

22 Pyogranulomatous splenic infiltrates have a combination of neutrophilic and granulomatous inflammation on cytology and can be seen with blastomycosis, sporotrichosis, and FIP infections.

23 Predominantly necrotic tissue and cellular debris on splenic cytology are compatible with underlying conditions such as splenic torsion, large splenic neoplasms with necrotic centers, acute canine adenovirus infection, and salmonellosis.

24 Lymphocytes and plasma cells are associated with chronic canine adenovirus infection, chronic ehrlichiosis, pyometra, brucellosis, and hemobartonellosis.

25 Eosinophilic infiltrates are seen with eosinophilic gastroenteritis/hepatitis and hypereosinophilic syndrome (in cats).

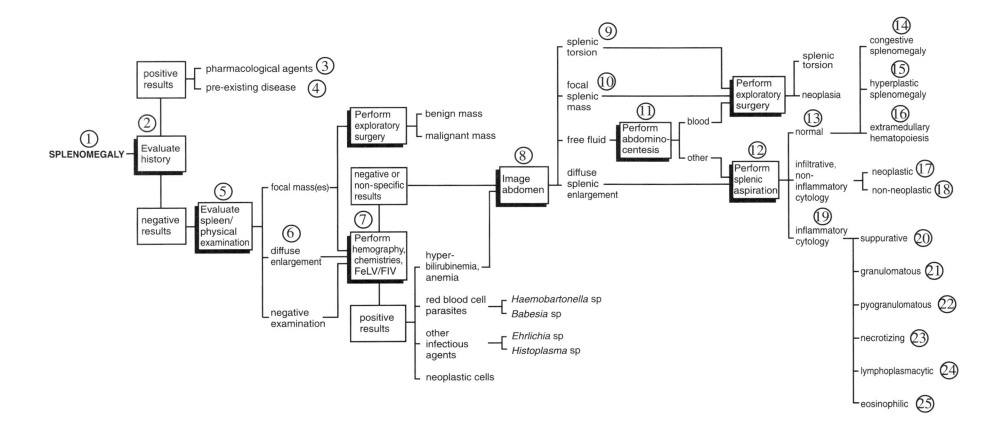

SPLENOMEGALY ① — Evaluate history ②

positive results
— pharmacological agents ③
— pre-existing disease ④

negative results

Evaluate spleen/ physical examination ⑤

focal mass(es)

Perform exploratory surgery
— benign mass
— malignant mass

negative or non-specific results

diffuse enlargement

Perform hemography, chemistries, FeLV/FIV ⑦

negative examination

positive results
— hyper-bilirubinemia, anemia
— red blood cell parasites
 — *Haemobartonella* sp
 — *Babesia* sp
— other infectious agents
 — *Ehrlichia* sp
 — *Histoplasma* sp
— neoplastic cells

Image abdomen ⑧

splenic torsion ⑨

focal splenic mass ⑩

free fluid

Perform abdomino-centesis ⑪
— blood
— other

diffuse splenic enlargement

Perform exploratory surgery
— splenic torsion
— neoplasia

Perform splenic aspiration ⑫

normal ⑬
— congestive splenomegaly ⑭
— hyperplastic splenomegaly ⑮
— extramedullary hematopoiesis ⑯

infiltrative, non-inflammatory cytology
— neoplastic ⑰
— non-neoplastic ⑱

inflammatory cytology ⑲
— suppurative ⑳
— granulomatous ㉑
— pyogranulomatous ㉒
— necrotizing ㉓
— lymphoplasmacytic ㉔
— eosinophilic ㉕

1 Anemia is characterized by a reduced packed cell volume (PCV), RBC count, and hemoglobin (Hb) concentration. It reduces the oxygen-carrying capacity of blood. The first step is to determine if anemia is regenerative or nonregenerative by calculating the corrected reticulocyte count and the reticulocyte production index (RPI) and evaluating RBC morphology.

2 Regenerative anemia (RA) is characterized by reticulocyte counts of 60,000–500,000/μl. The reticulocyte percentage can be converted to a count by multiplying it by the RBC count. Normal patients have reticulocyte percentages of 1% of total RBCs. This percentage increases in RA and must be corrected if the patient is anemic. Correction is based on the RPI and on reticulocyte maturation and release time from the bone marrow. The RPI equals the reticulocyte percentage multiplied by the patient's PCV (Hb) divided by the average PCV (or Hb). This result is then divided by a correction factor:

PCV of 45% = correction factor
PCV of 35–44% = correction factor of 1.5
PCV of 25–34% = correction factor of 2
PCV of 15–24% = correction factor of 2.5

An RPI greater than 2.5 is considered regenerative in dogs. Values are lower in cats (RPI of 1–1.5). Less reliable signs of regeneration include polychromasia, increased mean corpuscular volume (MCV), and decreased mean corpuscular hemoglobin concentration.

3 Nonregenerative anemia has reticulocyte counts less than 60,000/μl or an RPI less than 2.5. Nonregenerative anemia indicates failure of bone marrow to produce RBCs at an adequate rate. Other cell lines (platelets, neutrophils) also can be affected.

4 If the anemia is regenerative, then the cause is either blood loss (hemorrhage) or hemolysis. Evaluation of the plasma protein concentration is the next step. With hemolytic disease, there is selective destruction of RBCs and the plasma protein concentration is normal. When blood is lost from the vascular space, fluid replacement occurs over several hours as the body attempts to restore the circulating volume. Thus, plasma proteins will be diluted. External hemorrhage often results in more severe hypoproteinemia than internal hemorrhage.

5 Severe hypophosphatemia (<2 mg/dl) can cause intravascular hemolysis. Hypophosphatemia is rare but is associated with treatment of ketoacidotic diabetes mellitus, total parental nutrition, and excessive use of phosphate binders.

6 Destruction of RBCs can cause hemoglobinemia (usually intravascular hemolysis), hemoglobinuria, and hyperbilirubinemia. Hyperbilirubinemia can occur with both hemolysis and internal hemorrhage, and occurs when the rate of hemoglobin catabolism exceeds the ability of the liver to process heme pigment. Hemoglobin catabolism is usually greater with hemolytic disease than with internal hemorrhage; thus, hemolysis is more likely to cause hyperbilirubinemia.

7 When hemolysis is present, evaluate RBC morphology for spherocytes, Heinz bodies, anisocytosis, and so on.

8 Massive oxidation of heme iron causes methemoglobin production and prevents/reduces RBC transportation of oxygen. Affected patients have cyanotic/muddy gums and severe dyspnea, and their blood is brown after exposure to air (oxygen). Benzocaine-containing creams and sprays, acetaminophen (Tylenol), and phenazopyridine (a urinary tract analgesic) cause severe methemoglobinemia in cats within minutes to hours of exposure.

9 Fragmented erythrocytes or schistocytes often are associated with microangiopathic disease (e.g., hemangiosarcoma, hypersplenism, and DIC). Intravascular hemolysis causes RBC shearing destruction.

10 RBC parasites shorten cellular survival times. Parasites may be seen on a blood smear. Examining RBCs in or just below the buffy coat or smearing blood collected from a capillary bed increases the chance of seeing organisms.

11 Spherocytes and RBC agglutination suggest immune-mediated hemolytic anemia (IMHA). Spherocytes result from partial phagocytosis or lysis of RBCs. These are spherical RBCs that are microcytic, with no central pallor. Seeing many spherocytes suggests IMHA in dogs, although smaller numbers can be seen in other diseases (hypophosphatemia, zinc toxicity, microangiopathic hemolysis). Spherocytes are difficult to identify in cats because their RBCs normally are small and lack central pallor. Autoagglutination may be seen when blood is placed in an EDTA tube or occurs as small clumps of RBCs on a stained blood smear or in a saline wet mount. Clumping is different from rouleaux formation (where RBCs are stacked up on top of each other). Rouleaux formation is normal in cats.

12 The majority of drugs and toxins that cause hemolytic anemia in dogs and cats are "oxidants" that injure cell membranes, denature hemoglobin (causing Heinz body formation), or oxidize heme iron (causing methemoglobin production). Causes of Heinz body hemolytic anemia include onions, methylene blue, D,L-methionine, and vitamin K.

13 Ingestion of zinc-containing nuts and bolts, U.S. pennies, and zinc oxide-containing ointments can cause hemolytic anemia. Zinc-containing objects can be seen on radiographs or serum zinc concentrations can be measured.

14 If RA is present without signs of external blood loss or hemolysis, consider internal blood loss (e.g., due to ruptured hemangiosarcoma). Careful abdominal palpation followed by abdominal imaging is warranted. Patients usually are middle-aged and older dogs, especially Labradors, golden retrievers, and German shepherds. Bleeding into the thoracic cavity also can occur, but dyspnea is the most likely presenting complaint.

15 If hemolysis and internal or obvious external blood loss are not found, look for hookworms or other parasites. These can cause severe anemia, usually RA, in young animals.

16 Ensure that the blood loss is not coming from the urinary tract by evaluating a urine sample.

17 After eliminating sources of blood loss, reevaluate RBC morphology and indices via another hemogram.

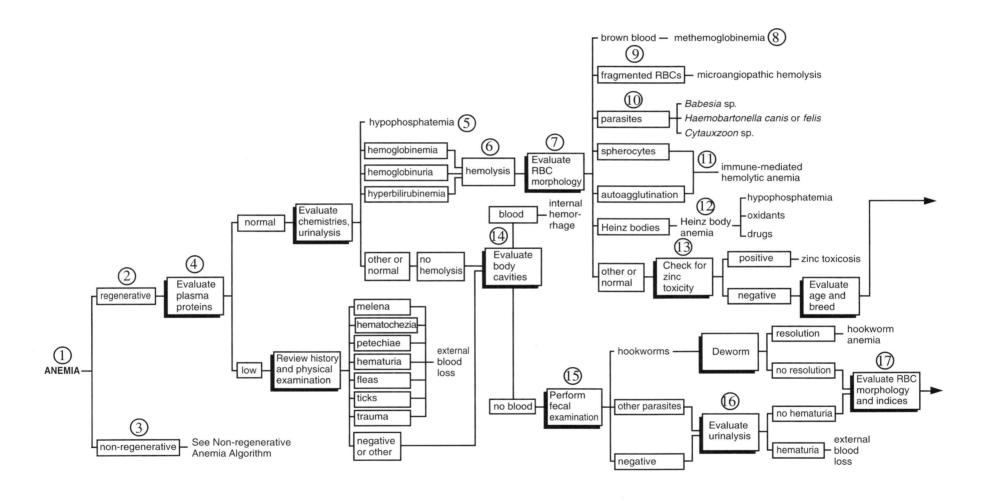

18 Copper toxicity causes severe intravascular hemolysis and some methemoglobinemia. It has been associated with fulminant hepatic failure caused by copper storage disease in Bedlington terriers.

19 Pyruvate kinase deficiency has been documented in several dog breeds and in cats. It causes hemolytic anemia with massive regeneration. It is inherited as an autosomal recessive trait. Polychromasia often is present and PCVs range from 10 to 33%, with marked increases in MCV and reticulocyte counts as high as 20–60%. Bone marrow cytology/biopsy terminally shows myelofibrosis and osteosclerosis. Radiographs of long bones show osteosclerosis.

20 Phosphofructokinase deficiency is inherited as an autosomal recessive disorder in springer spaniels and American cocker spaniels. It has also been reported in mixed-breed dogs. Clinical features include inducible hemolytic crises, mild myopathy, and pigmenturia. Exercise and tachypnea cause metabolic acidosis and induce hemolysis.

21 Hereditary nonspherocytic hemolytic anemia of poodles is an uncommon, autosomally inherited, macrocytic, hypochromic anemia.

22 *H. felis* infection should be considered in any cat with hemolytic anemia, even if the organism is not found on peripheral blood smears. The organism will not be seen if blood samples are placed in EDTA tubes or if the patient has already started therapy. If a response is seen to appropriate treatment for hemobartonellosis, then the algorithm can end. A polymerase chain reaction (PCR) exists for detection of *H. felis* infection.

23 Congenital porphyria has been diagnosed in a few Siamese and domestic shorthaired cats. This is an autosomal dominant condition causing anemia and dental discoloration.

24 Erythrocyte alloantibodies (isoantibodies) are antibodies directed against normal RBC antigens that determine the blood type within a species. Alloantibodies occur naturally in cats. In dogs they are mostly produced after sensitization via mismatched blood transfusions. Therefore, neonatal isoerythrolysis (NI) is not a clinical problem in dogs unless the bitch has previously received an incompatible blood product. However, NI is a problem in type A and AB kittens born to primiparous type B queens.

25 The direct Coombs' test detects antibodies and/or complement on the canine RBC surface when anti-RBC antibody strength or concentration is too low to cause spontaneous autoagglutination. It is not necessary to perform this test if reasonable numbers of spherocytes are seen on a blood smear since this can provide a definitive diagnosis of IMHA. The direct Coombs' test does not discriminate between primary and secondary (associated with drugs or underlying disease) IMHA.

26 Dogs with a negative Coombs' test should be reevaluated for other causes of hemolytic anemia.

27 Severe iron deficiency anemia is characterized by hypochromic, microcytic anemia. This is due to decreased synthesis of Hb, delayed cell maturation, and extra mitotic steps occurring in bone marrow. It can be associated with mild to moderate reticulocytosis. The serum iron concentration is low, ranging from 5 to 60 $\mu g/dl$ compared to the normal range of 60 to 230 $\mu g/dl$. The serum iron concentration is affected by many variables including hemolysis, recent transfusion, and iron supplementation, so care needs to be taken when interpreting the values obtained.

28 Fragmented RBCs are seen with iron deficiency anemia (Step 27), DIC, and following blood transfusion. A coagulogram is needed to establish a diagnosis of DIC. Decreased platelet numbers with normal PT and PTT val-

ues can indicate early DIC, so clinical signs and the coagulogram should be monitored closely. Thrombocytopenia with prolonged PT and/or PTT suggests DIC or platelet consumption secondary to bleeding. The presence of FDPs strongly supports a diagnosis of DIC. False FDP elevations occur in patients receiving heparin or having dysfibrinogenemia.

29 Lead intoxication is usually associated with mild anemia. It is characterized morphologically by nucleated RBCs and basophilic stippling of RBCs. Most commercial laboratories can evaluate blood samples for lead concentrations. Exposure to lead usually is seen in dogs that chew wood containing old lead-based paint.

30 Severe hepatic disease/fibrosis and acquired or congenital portal systemic shunting lead to insufficient iron storage capability. This initially can manifest as microcytosis and hypochromia, with or without anemia. The liver should be assessed via ultrasonography, ultrasound-guided liver aspiration or biopsy, or liver function testing (pre- and postprandial bile acids, fasting serum ammonia concentrations, or BSP retention testing). Depending on the underlying liver problem, the anemia may be regenerative or nonregenerative (anemia of chronic disease).

31 If a diagnosis has not yet been made, repeat the basic tests and look again for clues on the hemogram as above.

32 If internal or external blood loss is suspected but not found, the next step is gastrointestinal endoscopy or exploratory surgery with biopsies to try to identify the source of internal or external blood loss.

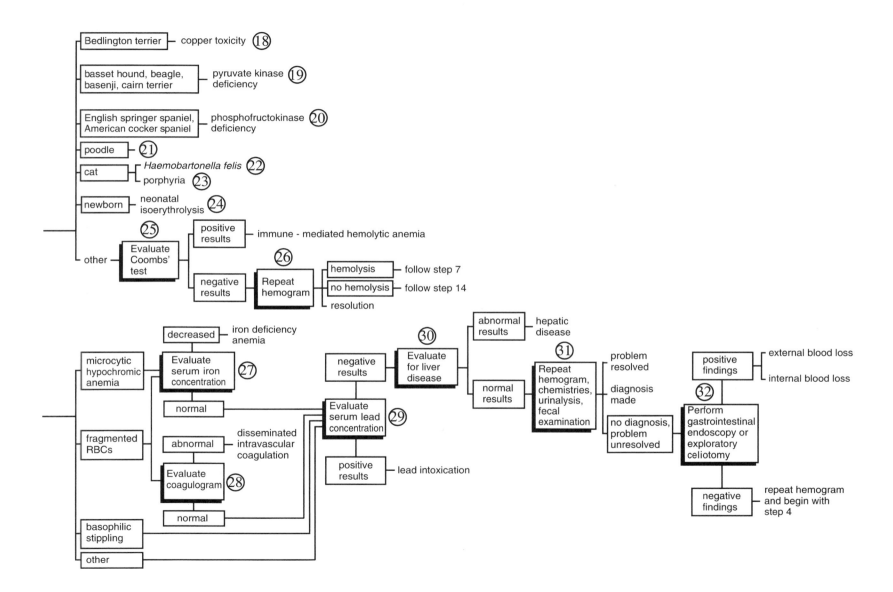

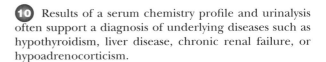

1 Anemia is characterized by a reduced PCV, RBC count, and Hb concentration. It reduces the oxygen-carrying capacity of blood. The first diagnostic step is to determine whether anemia is regenerative or nonregenerative. Nonregenerative anemia has a reticulocyte production index less than 2.5 (for dogs; values are lower for cats). Other findings that can help to make the distinction include RBC morphology and staining characteristics.

2 Nonregenerative anemia is usually normocytic and normochromic. Usually there are no changes in RBC morphology. Many nonregenerative anemias are mild to moderate and are complications of systemic diseases.

3 If a cause of the nonregenerative anemia is not immediately obvious, evaluate the history and physical examination findings carefully. Look at the patient's environment and travel history, drug or toxin exposure, and stool color, and check for external parasites and signs of systemic disease.

4 The most common cause of nonregenerative anemia in dogs and cats is "anemia of chronic disease." This accompanies infection, neoplasia, and other debilitating diseases, including hypothyroidism, chronic hepatic disease, and hypoadrenocorticism. This type of anemia is mild to moderate in severity and develops slowly over at least 2 to 3 weeks. The hematocrit seldom drops below 25%. Because cat RBCs have a shorter life span than those of dogs, the hematocrit can decrease more quickly and to a greater degree. Anemia is usually normocytic and normochromic but in some cases can be microcytic and hypochromic, causing confusion with iron deficiency anemia. Chronic renal failure produces mild to severe nonregenerative anemia, depending on the duration of the problem.

5 Elevated serum estrogen concentrations affect stem cell differentiation and cause aplastic anemia or pancytopenia. Hyperestrogenism is seen in male dogs with testicular tumors (usually Sertoli cell tumors but occasionally seminomas and interstitial cell tumors). Many affected male dogs show signs of feminization. Estrogen toxicity also can be seen in females given estradiol cyclopentylpropionate (ECP) to prevent pregnancy and diethylstilbestrol (DES) for urinary incontinence.

6 Very recent trauma with external blood loss causes apparent nonregenerative anemia. Regeneration, with increased reticulocyte counts, develops about 3 days after hemorrhage, with peak reticulocytosis occurring 5 days posthemorrhage.

7 A variety of drugs besides estrogen cause bone marrow dyscrasias and nonregenerative anemia. In dogs, drugs include quinidine, sulfonamides, phenylbutazone, meclofenamic acid, chloramphenicol, cephalosporins, phenobarbital, primidone, phenytoin, various chemotherapeutic agents, thiacetarsamide, and phenothiazines. In cats, drugs include chemotherapeutic agents, chloramphenicol, griseofulvin, propylthiouracil, albendazole, fenbendazole, and methimazole.

8 Fleas cause chronic external blood loss. The resulting anemia usually is regenerative unless the animal is young and nursing (milk is very low in iron), in which case iron deficiency anemia can develop and the anemia becomes nonregenerative.

9 Fecal examination (mainly looking for hookworm eggs) and fecal occult blood testing (for dogs only) should be performed next. Hookworms ingest blood and also cause point source bleeding from the intestinal wall leading to chronic blood loss anemia (initially regenerative, then becoming nonregenerative). Other causes of chronic gastrointestinal blood loss include gastrointestinal neoplasia and ulcerogenic drugs (glucocorticoids, salicylates, and nonsteroidal anti-inflammatory agents). Melena may be present in such cases but may not be obvious with low-grade blood loss. Blood can be found via occult fecal blood testing, but the value of this test is controversial. If the patient has not been on a meat-free diet for 3–4 days prior to collection of feces, a false-positive result could be obtained. A false-negative result could be obtained if the blood is not homogeneously distributed throughout feces or if the patient has received vitamin C supplementation.

10 Results of a serum chemistry profile and urinalysis often support a diagnosis of underlying diseases such as hypothyroidism, liver disease, chronic renal failure, or hypoadrenocorticism.

11 Cats should be checked for FeLV infection in peripheral blood. This virus can cause severe, usually nonregenerative, anemia. The virus also causes RBC dysplasias. Whenever macrocytic anemia occurs without reticulocytosis in a cat, FeLV infection should be suspected.

12 The peritubular endothelial cells in the renal cortex are the main production sites of erythropoietin. This hormone is the principal stimulus for erythropoiesis. Not only is there decreased production of erythropoietin in chronic renal failure due to loss of normal renal tissue, but the RBCs have shortened life spans. Thus, anemia is a major problem in chronic renal failure. Anemia usually is normocytic and normochromic, with few or no reticulocytes. Patients are azotemic, with fixed urine specific gravities.

13 Nonregenerative anemia is a common finding in liver disease. In most instances it is normocytic and normochromic. Target cells and poikilocytes also are found in liver disease and are most likely due to inefficient utilization of systemic iron stores.

14 Nonregenerative anemia commonly is present in dogs with chronic ehrlichiosis unless anemia is associated with hemorrhage from severe thrombocytopenia or hemolysis.

15 Hemobartonellosis in cats is generally associated with RA. Occasionally nonregenerative anemia is present when the organism is an opportunistic infection in an immunosuppressed or debilitated animal. Such patients should be tested for FeLV.

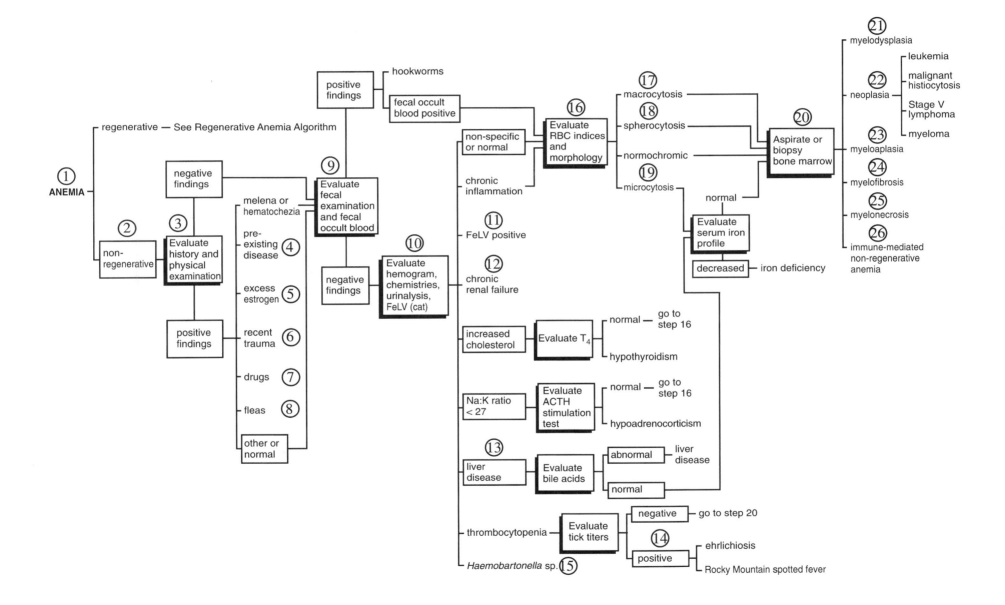

16 Nonregenerative anemia is typically normocytic and normochromic. However, there are times when RBC indices suggest that cells are either larger or smaller than normal.

17 Macrocytosis often is associated with bone marrow abnormalities (myelodysplasia). In cats, macrocytic nonregenerative anemia may occur with FIV and FeLV infections, and the anemia tends to be nonregenerative. In rare cases, macrocytic, normochromic RBCs indicate folate or cobalamin deficiency (e.g., due to malabsorption).

18 Spherocytosis with nonregenerative anemia may indicate acute hemolytic anemia when insufficient time has elapsed for reticulocytosis to develop. Signs of regeneration should be present within 3–4 days. If reticulocytosis does not develop, consider the possibility of immune-mediated anemia in which RBC precursors are destroyed in the marrow.

19 Microcytic anemia usually is associated with iron deficiency. While some cases of iron deficiency anemia are regenerative, chronic blood loss can lead to iron depletion and lack of regeneration, especially if the diet is inadequate for replacement of iron or if the patient is young and nursing. Most patients with iron deficiency anemia have microcytic, hypochromic indices, mild reticulocytosis (1–5%), thrombocytosis, low serum iron concentrations, low transferrin and low serum ferritin concentrations, and low iron stores in bone marrow. Microcytic, nonregenerative anemia also is seen in some cases of hepatic disease, including congenital portal systemic shunts.

20 After extramedullary causes of nonregenerative anemia are excluded, bone marrow aspiration or biopsy usually is indicated to detect hypoproliferative anemias. These are secondary to neoplastic, inflammatory, or dysplastic bone marrow disorders. In such cases, there is either crowding out of the normal erythroid precursors in bone marrow by neoplastic or inflammatory cells (myelophthisis), ineffective erythropoiesis, or RBC maturation arrest.

21 Myelodysplasia is a preneoplastic bone marrow condition. The marrow is usually hypercellular because of maturation arrest in some cell lines. Abnormal cells generally die in the marrow without completing the maturation process. There may be increased stainable iron in marrow as a result. How far back in the cellular differentiation process maturation arrest occurs affects the number of cell lines involved. RBC megaloblastic changes are common. Myelodysplasia is relatively common in cats, probably associated with FeLV infection in bone marrow. It may progress to leukemia in time. Myelodysplasia is rare in dogs.

22 Neoplasia can invade bone marrow and crowd out normal erythroid precursors.

23 Myeloaplasia is diagnosed by retrieval of fat alone on bone marrow biopsy or aspiration. No stem cells are left in the marrow, and all cell lines usually are affected.

24 In myelofibrosis normal marrow tissue is replaced by fibrous tissue. This is probably a manifestation of end-stage marrow failure, and it may not be possible to identify the underlying cause. The condition is irreversible.

25 Myelonecrosis can occur secondary to severe systemic disease (e.g., sepsis or endotoxemia), drug-induced marrow damage, and viral infection. With supportive care and removal of the underlying cause, the condition can be reversed.

26 RBC precursors in the bone marrow can be destroyed by immune-mediated attack, just as they can be in the circulation. If there is an immune-mediated attack on RBC precursors in the marrow, anemia will be nonregenerative and a pure RBC aplasia will be seen. Sometimes spherocytes are found in the circulation and the Coombs' test may be positive.

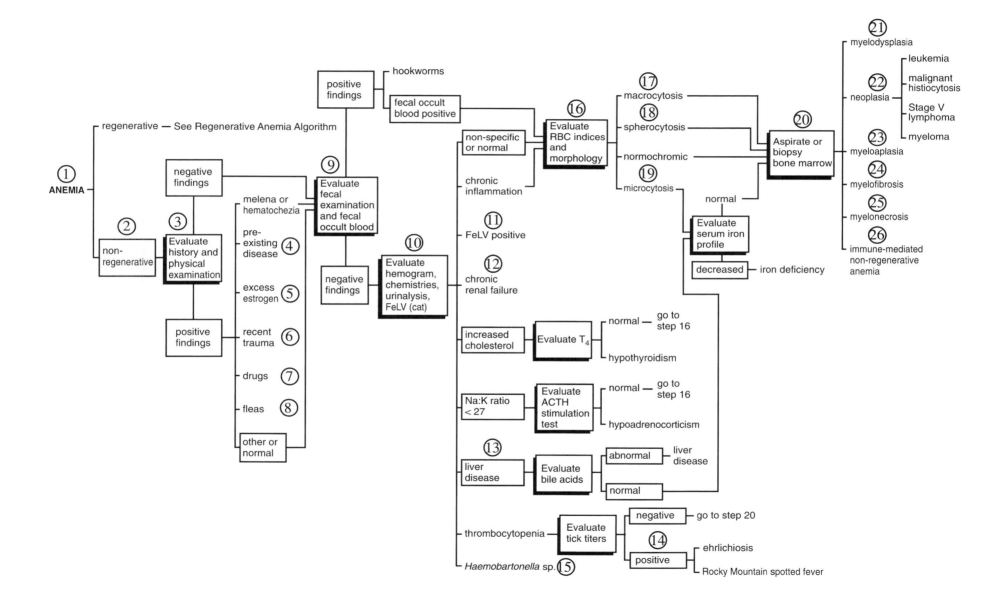

1 Polycythemia is an increase in the number of RBCs in the circulation. The underlying causes may be physiological (dehydration, splenic contracture, hypoxia) or pathological (secondary to erythropoietin-producing kidney tumors, bone marrow dyscrasias). Polycythemia that results from a decrease in serum plasma volume relative to RBCs is known as *relative polycythemia*. Polycythemia that does not result from dehydration or splenic contracture is known as *absolute polycythemia*. Absolute polycythemia may be primary (polycythemia vera, a rare bone marrow disorder) or secondary (the result of conditions such as hypoxia or renal disease, which increase erythropoietin production). Patients present with clinical signs of underlying disease (e.g., vomiting and diarrhea leading to dehydration, dyspnea due to pulmonary disease) or effects of excessive RBC numbers (PD, PU, mental confusion, injected/bright red mucous membranes).

2 The first step is to confirm the presence of polycythemia. PCVs greater than 65% are suspicious for polycythemia. Generally, there will be a related increase in the RBC count and the circulating Hb concentration. Patients with relative polycythemia have lower PCVs (60–75%) than those with absolute polycythemia (75–82%). However, there is considerable overlap between the PCVs in each condition, so counts alone cannot be used to diagnose the problem.

3 Evaluate the historical and physical examination findings. Drugs such as erythropoietin, androgens, and glucocorticoids may cause mild polycythemia. Patients living at very high altitudes and those with right-to-left cardiac shunts (e.g., reversed patent ductus arteriosus), severe pulmonary disease, or gross obesity have secondary absolute polycythemia because tissue hypoxia stimulates overproduction of erythropoietin. In these patients, hypoxia must be confirmed via arterial blood gas analysis prior to making this diagnosis, but a more detailed evaluation of the condition is probably not needed. Patients with gastrointestinal signs (vomiting, diarrhea) or a history of hyperthermia (due either to excessive heat exposure or to fever), or who appear clinically dehydrated (e.g., dry oral mucous membranes, sunken eyes, skin tenting in response to pinching), may be assumed initially to have relative polycythemia due to dehydration. Patients suspected of being dehydrated and those with no remarkable findings on the history and physical examination should have a serum chemistry profile evaluated, and their response to rehydration should be assessed prior to pursuing further diagnostic testing.

4 A serum chemistry profile (including electrolytes) and urinalysis may be used to confirm dehydration. Patients have elevated concentrations of serum protein and albumin, sodium and chloride, azotemia, and concentrated urine (urine specific gravity greater than 1.035 in dogs and 1.045 in cats). It is particularly important to assess the urinalysis because some underlying causes of secondary absolute polycythemia (renal neoplasia and pyelonephritis) may cause polycythemia but reduce the urine-concentrating ability. Other conditions detectable on laboratory tests also may lead to dehydration (e.g., diabetes mellitus, hepatic disease, renal failure) and hemoconcentration.

5 In patients presenting with polycythemia, fluid diuresis is both therapeutic and a useful diagnostic test. Care should be taken in rehydrating patients with underlying heart disease who may be predisposed to congestive heart failure, hyperosmolar ketoacidotic diabetics, patients with potential anuric renal failure, and hypertensive patients. However, there are very few absolute contraindications to rehydration, and the speed with which rehydration is performed should depend on the patient's condition and additional medical problems.

6 In patients in which polycythemia resolves with fluid therapy and findings suggest dehydration as the underlying problem, the diagnosis is relative polycythemia. Diagnostic evaluation and therapy should be directed toward the underlying cause.

7 Patients that do not show an appropriate decrease in PCV and RBC counts after rehydration have absolute polycythemia. Further screening tests are needed to distinguish between primary and secondary polycythemia. Patients with known or suspected cardiovascular disease causing right-to-left shunting of blood (e.g., reversed patent ductus arteriosus or tetralogy of Fallot), gross obesity, or chronic respiratory disease are likely to have secondary polycythemia. The underlying condition needs to be documented and the presence of hypoxia confirmed by arterial blood gas measurement. Other cases may prove more challenging to diagnose.

8 Depending on the facilities available to the clinician, the next step is to evaluate for low partial pressures of oxygen (PaO_2) in arterial blood. Arterial PaO_2 may be assessed indirectly using a pulse oximeter to assess the percentage of oxygen saturation of blood. A more accurate measurement may be made by measuring the arterial blood gas oxygen content, which will provide the actual PaO_2 value. When the PaO_2 is low, the kidneys are stimulated to produce erythropoietin, so that the bone marrow generates more RBCs in an attempt to improve the body's oxygen-carrying capacity. If the underlying cause of hypoxia is not immediately obvious (e.g., being obese or living on top of a high mountain), it may be sought via thoracic radiographs, echocardiography, and measurement of pulmonary artery wedge pressures. It also may be necessary to measure the serum erythropoietin concentration (step 12) to assess whether this is elevated. The serum erythropoietin concentration should be elevated when hypoxia is the underlying stimulus for polycythemia.

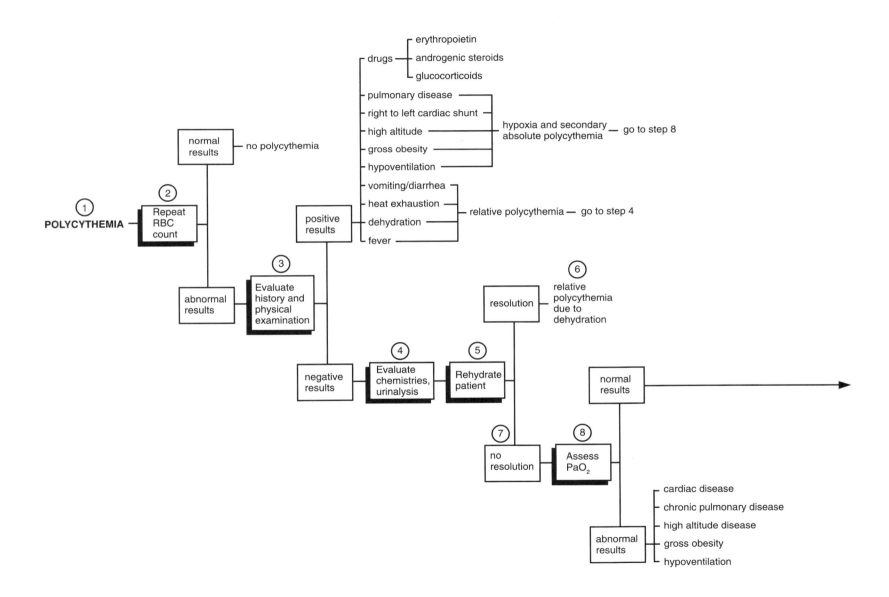

9 When PaO_2 is normal, other underlying causes of polycythemia must be sought. The next most common cause of absolute polycythemia is renal disease, particularly renal tumors (e.g., carcinoma, lymphoma). These lead to inappropriate overproduction of erythropoietin. In human beings, tumors elsewhere in the body also have been reported to produce erythropoietin and erythropoietin-like substances. Rarely, other renal conditions such as pyelonephritis also have been reported to cause polycythemia. The next most useful diagnostic test at this point is probably some type of abdominal imaging. Plain abdominal radiographs may indicate an abnormally shaped or enlarged kidney, a mineralized adrenal lesion (hyperadrenocorticism may cause mild elevations in RBC counts through a variety of mechanisms), or other abdominal masses. However, abdominal ultrasound, CT scan, or MRI scan is more likely to provide information about abnormalities within the kidneys and other organs. These techniques will highlight small masses, dilation of either renal pelvis that might suggest pyelonephritis, and adrenal gland enlargement/masses. A skilled ultrasonographer may also be able to assess for rarer causes of polycythemia, such as renal artery stenosis; however, this is more likely to require a selective contrast study for documentation. Renal imaging should be combined with a urinalysis, mainly for infection, although in rare cases neoplastic cells may be seen in the sediment.

10 Hyperadrenocorticism due to both endogenous and exogenous glucocorticoids and androgens may result in polycythemia. In general, elevation of RBC counts caused by the relatively mild stimulating effect of these hormones on the bone marrow is not great, and they rarely fall into the category of true polycythemias. However, adrenal enlargement found on an ultrasound scan or a patient with PU, PD, polyphagia, and other classical presenting signs of hyperadrenocorticism accompanying mild to moderate polycythemia justifies pursuit of the problem. A good clinical history should bring to light exogenous glucocorticoid or androgen administration early on (step 3). Serum erythropoietin concentrations are normal or low in these patients since they directly stimulate bone marrow to produce RBCs.

11 If the kidneys appear normal but another abdominal mass lesion is identified, this should be pursued by means of cytological evaluation and incisional or excisional biopsy to determine the lesion type. Exploratory surgery has the benefit of allowing removal of some mass lesions, thus permitting determination of whether polycythemia subsequently resolves. It also may be worth while to measure serum erythropoietin concentrations (step 12).

12 In patients with confusing clinical signs, an indefinite diagnosis, or absolute polycythemia with no obvious underlying cause, serum erythropoietin concentrations should be measured. Elevated concentrations suggest an underlying cause of absolute (secondary) polycythemia that has not yet been discovered. This may suggest a need for more invasive testing (e.g., Swan-Ganz cardiac catheterization to determine whether a patient has pulmonary hypertension, arteriography to look for renal artery stenosis, or pursuit of other lesions previously thought to be unrelated to the polycythemia).

13 If serum erythropoietin concentrations are normal or low, this suggests primary polycythemia or polycythemia vera. The latter is a rare bone marrow dyscrasia that causes unregulated production of RBCs independent of erythropoietin. Although the condition is not neoplastic, later transformation to erythroleukemia or development of RBC aplasia or myelophthisis may occur. Bone marrow examination in these patients shows hyperplasia of erythroid cell lines. Patients may have hepatosplenomegaly, neurological signs (e.g., dementia, altered behavior, seizures), or evidence of hyperviscosity (dilated and tortuous retinal vessels, congestive heart failure). While polycythemia vera is the most likely diagnosis at this point in the algorithm, production of erythropoietin-like factors (generally by neoplastic tissues) that do not react with the test to measure serum erythropoietin concentrations cannot be excluded from the diagnosis completely.

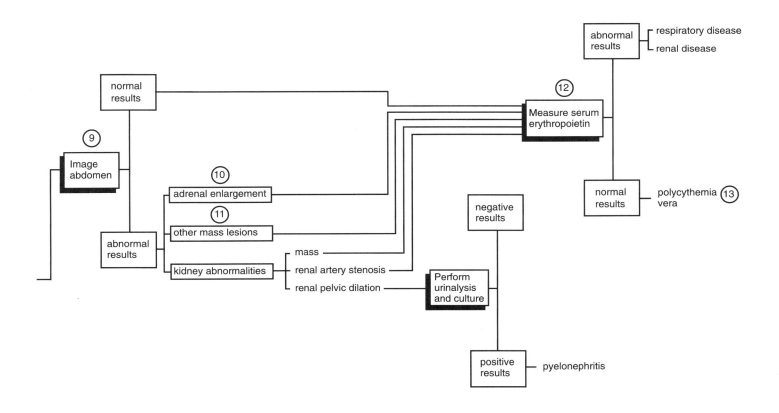

1 Pancytopenia is defined as a decrease in all cell lines (red and white cells and platelets) in peripheral blood. The algorithm applies to bicytopenia and some monocytopenias as well, since many conditions that affect cells in peripheral blood do not affect all cell lines or do not affect them at the same rate. For example, RBCs have the longest life span, meaning that acute conditions affect neutrophils and platelets before causing anemia. Pancytopenia always reflects underlying bone marrow disease, and marrow examination is indicated in most cases. Clinical signs include petechial/ecchymotic hemorrhages or epistaxis due to thrombocytopenia, weakness, collapse, and pallor due to anemia, as well as fever because of infection due to neutropenia.

2 Patients with pan/bicytopenias should have a complete CBC and differential repeated 3 to 4 days later to establish that low cell counts persist. A reticulocyte count determines whether anemia is regenerative or nonregenerative. Nonregenerative anemia is common with pancytopenia because of failure of bone marrow stem cell activity. Rarely, anemia is regenerative if the marrow problem is immune-mediated.

3 Signs of blood cell destruction and regeneration (reticulocytes, spherocytes, giant platelets, RBC autoagglutination) suggest an immune-mediated cause of pancytopenia or at least of thrombocytopenia or anemia and the possibility of a response to immunosuppressive therapy. A Coombs' test may be appropriate for antibodies against RBCs; this is unnecessary if spherocytosis is seen. Some patients with immune-mediated disease have antibodies against marrow stem cells and no regeneration, but spherocytosis or autoagglutination is seen.

4 Neutropenic patients and those immunosuppressed for other reasons may acquire *H. felis/canis* or *Babesia* spp. infection and develop RA. A blood smear should be reviewed for intracellular organisms, and titers for *H. felis* and *Babesia* spp. can be obtained.

5 Any drug can affect marrow stem cells idiosyncratically or induce immune-mediated disease. Drugs consistently associated with pancytopenia include chemotherapeutic agents (busulfan, cyclophosphamide, chlorambucil, melphalan, cytarabine, platinum-containing compounds,

doxorubicin, mitoxantrone, methotrexate), trimethoprim sulfa, chloramphenicol, cephalosporins, estrogens, phenobarbital, primidone, phenytoin, phenylbutazone, meclofenamic acid, quinidine, albendazole, fenbendazole, methimazole,* propylthiouracil,* griseofulvin,* thiacetarsamide). Those marked with an asterisk in particular cause pancytopenia in cats (griseofulvin especially in conjunction with retroviral infection). Chemotherapeutic drugs commonly cause neutropenia and/or thrombocytopenia 5 to 10 days after administration since most of them affect rapidly dividing cells. Nitrosoureas affect stem cells, with slow-onset neutropenia but prolonged effects and the risk of permanent bone marrow damage. In most instances, removal of a myelosuppressive agent will allow bone marrow recovery. This may not be the case with some chemotherapeutic agents and phenylbutazone. Phenylbutazone should not be used in dogs and cats.

6 Toxins include benzene derivatives (gasoline, solvents), phenol, organophosphates, organochlorides, and thallium.

7 Radiation exposure leading to pancytopenia is highly unlikely in any normal environment. However, it may occur with half-body irradiation for lymphoma.

8 In feline patients with pancytopenia, the retrovirus status should be tested. Being FeLV or FIV positive may not be the cause of pancytopenia, but it may affect the client's desire to pursue further testing. FeLV has been directly associated with marrow suppression (aplastic anemia, myelodysplasia, bone marrow neoplasia). Patients who are FeLV negative may not have been exposed to the virus or may have been exposed and mounted an adequate immune response to eradicate it. However, they also may have been exposed to FeLV and mounted a partial immune response, allowing virus sequestration in tissues. Marrow is a common site of virus sequestration. Immunofluorescence (IFA) of bone marrow for FeLV antigens is possible.

9 Young or poorly vaccinated cats or very old cats with pancytopenia and gastrointestinal signs may have feline panleukopenia virus (FePLV). No specific test exists for this virus.

10 Young or poorly vaccinated dogs and very old immunosuppressed dogs that present with pancytopenia and gastrointestinal signs may be infected with parvovirus or CDV. Canine parvovirus infection is confirmed by fecal antigen testing. False positives may be seen in patients that have been recently vaccinated against the virus. CDV infection is more difficult to confirm, although IFA on conjunctival scrapes is possible.

11 Older intact male dogs should have their testicles checked for masses. Sertoli cell tumors and occasionally seminomas and interstitial cell tumors may suppress bone marrow by producing estrogens. Tumors more commonly occur in intra-abdominal testicles. Elevated serum estrogen affects stem cell differentiation, causing marrow aplasia, pancytopenia, or aplastic anemia. Estrogen-induced anemia/pancytopenia often is irreversible. Most dogs show feminization (gynecomastia, attraction of intact males).

12 For neutered male dogs, the neutering history should be checked to see whether it was very recent or straightforward, or if only the descended testicle was removed in a cryptorchid patient.

13 Hyperestrogenism is rare in female patients, but older, intact females should be checked for ovarian masses. In rare cases, granulosa cell tumors and ovarian follicular cysts increase estrogen concentrations and suppress marrow production of cellular elements.

14 If the patient has a questionable neutering history or if hyperestrogenism is a concern, abdominal ultrasound is indicated to look for intra-abdominal masses, retained testicles, or abnormal ovarian tissue that might be a source of estrogen and marrow suppression.

15 Serum estrogen concentrations can be measured in patients suspected of having hyperestrogenism and in which no obvious source of estrogen has been identified. Such assays are not used as the first line of testing because it is usually easier to arrive at a diagnosis by another method and not all forms of estrogen are tested for in the assay. However, concentrations can be measured prior to more invasive testing, such as exploratory laparotomy.

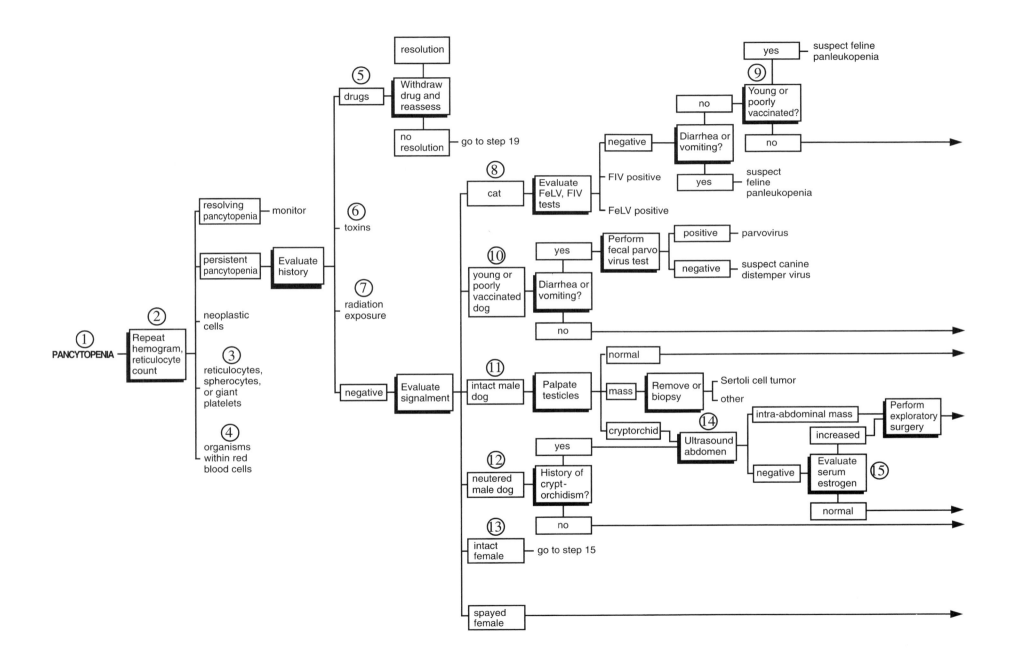

16 For canine patients in which hyperestrogenism appears to have been excluded from the differential diagnosis list, the next step is to obtain a tick exposure history and, if appropriate, titers for *Ehrlichia canis*. This is especially important in patients with hyperglobuline-mia, protein-losing nephropathy, and/or renal failure. However, it is important to note that other conditions that cause pancytopenia (e.g., immune-mediated disease and neoplasia) may cause similar problems. Chronic *E. canis* infection leads to pancytopenia or variable cytopenias via bone marrow suppression (only plasma cells in the marrow are hyperplastic). The condition is sometimes complicated by hemolytic anemia due to concurrent *Babesia* spp. infection or blood loss secondary to thrombocytopenia. Patients that are positive for *E. canis* should be treated appropriately. Eradication of the infection should lead to resolution of clinical signs and laboratory abnormalities in time.

17 In many patients with pancytopenia, physical examination findings are nonspecific (weight loss, poor body condition) or reflect bone marrow suppression (petechial or ecchymotic hemorrhages and epistaxis due to thrombocytopenia; weakness, collapse, tachycardia, and pale mucous membranes due to anemia; oral ulcers due to neutropenia). In some instances, physical examination may be helpful in determining the next diagnostic step.

18 Patients with lymphadenopathy can undergo fine-needle aspiration or biopsy of a lymph node for cytological evaluation/histopathology. These tests may reveal neoplasia, allowing the underlying cause of pancytopenia to be diagnosed and obviating the need for bone marrow aspiration except for further staging. Hepatosplenomegaly may be due to infiltration of tissues with neoplastic cells or may be a normal response of extramedullary hematopoietic tissues trying to produce sufficient peripheral blood cells in the face of bone marrow failure. Aspiration of liver and spleen will probably require ultrasound guidance (although not always in cats, in which the spleen is easily fixed through the body wall for aspiration). Aspiration should be performed with caution in thrombocytopenic patients. Bone marrow ex-

amination is still likely to be needed if neoplastic cells are not found on aspirates.

19 Bone marrow examination is the ultimate diagnostic test for any patient with persistent pancytopenia and for most patients with bicytopenias. It may be indicated earlier in the diagnostic process than suggested by this algorithm. Bone marrow examination in pancytopenic patients should consist of both aspiration for cytology and a core biopsy. This is the case because there may be so little marrow tissue left that a negative aspirate could indicate myelofibrosis/myelophthisis or could be the result of inadequate sampling. Analysis of the bone marrow core biopsy specimen can answer this question. Either sample, if adequate, should be able to diagnose bone marrow neoplasia (since to cause pancytopenia marrow neoplasia would have to be extensive), myelonecrosis, or myelodysplasia.

20 Myelodysplasia is a preneoplastic condition of bone marrow. Despite the presence of peripheral "cytopenias," the marrow is usually hypercellular because of maturation arrest in some cell lines. Abnormal cells die in the bone marrow without completing the maturation process. There also may be a buildup of stainable iron in marrow as a result of failure of RBC production. How far back in the differentiation process maturation arrest occurs determines the number of cell lines affected. Megaloblastic changes in RBCs are common. Myelodysplasia is relatively common in cats, probably associated with FeLV infection. It is rare in dogs. In both species it may progress to leukemia over time.

21 In myelofibrosis normal marrow tissue is replaced by fibrous tissue. This is probably a manifestation of end-stage marrow failure, and it may not be possible to identify an underlying cause. The condition is irreversible.

22 Myelonecrosis may occur secondary to severe systemic diseases such as sepsis and endotoxemia, drug-induced marrow toxicity, and viral infections. With supportive care and removal of the underlying cause, the condition may be reversible. Pancytopenia is seen only in severe, diffuse cases.

23 Osteosclerosis or increased bone thickness (extending into the marrow cavity) may be an end-stage, irreversible change with chronic conditions affecting bone marrow. Radiographically, osteosclerosis appears as increased bone density. Underlying causes include pyruvate kinase deficiency in dogs (which may be picked up earlier in the algorithm when assessing signalment and preexisting conditions). It is a condition known to affect several breeds of dogs, including basenjis, beagles, cairn terriers, West Highland white terriers, and a few other breeds. Patients generally are young to middle-aged and have a chronic history of marked RA. Although pyruvate kinase deficiency is also seen in some cat breeds, it does not lead to osteosclerosis. Osteosclerosis is seen as an end result of FeLV infection in cats.

24 Bone marrow neoplasia may result in pancytopenia if the marrow is filled with neoplastic cells. These cells may or may not be released into the circulation. Blast cells in the marrow undergo uncontrolled proliferation, abnormal differentiation, and failure of maturation. Another reason for pancytopenia is a soluble factor produced by blast cells that is known to inhibit hematopoietic progenitor cells. In fact, this inhibition may precede proliferation of the malignant clone. Pancytopenia is generally seen with acute leukemias of different cell lines. Circulating blast cells are a relatively common finding in such cases. Extramedullary neoplasms that may invade bone marrow and cause pancytopenias include lymphoma (stage V), plasma cell myeloma, and malignant histiocytosis.

25 Myeloaplasia or aplastic pancytopenia is diagnosed when only fat is retrieved on bone marrow biopsy. No stem cells are present, and there is no remaining marrow tissue. The condition is irreversible.

26 FeLV may be detected in bone marrow by IFA testing of cytology slides to detect the antigen. Positivity for FeLV in marrow is not an actual diagnosis but it may result in a number of conditions in cats, including myelodysplasia or aplasia, neoplasia, and aplastic anemia.

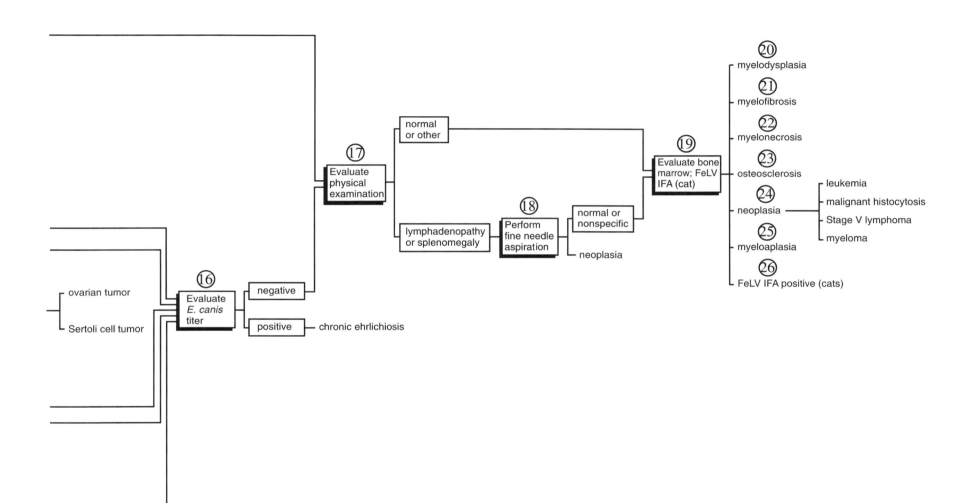

1 Neutropenia is defined as a low granulocytic cell count in the peripheral circulation (the term includes eosinophils, basophils, and neutrophils). The neutrophil is the main granulocytic cell. Neutrophils in blood form two distinct populations, the circulating pool (cells actually measured on the hemogram) and the marginated pool (cells associated with blood vessel walls which exchange into tissue pools of neutrophils). Circulating and marginated pools are approximately equal in size in dogs, whereas in cats the marginated pool is two to three times larger than the circulating pool. Patients do not present with neutropenia per se but with its consequences (e.g., signs of local/disseminated infection due to failure of neutrophil defense responses) or signs of the diseases underlying neutropenia. Many patients are not clinically affected, and neutropenia is an incidental finding when a hemogram is evaluated. Neutrophils are an intrinsic part of the immune system, responding acutely to infection and other conditions causing tissue inflammation. Low peripheral neutrophil counts can result from problems with neutrophil production, failure of neutrophil release into the peripheral circulation from marrow (bone marrow dysplasia or maturation defect), neutrophil sequestration, increased neutrophil margination, or an increased demand for neutrophils in tissues.

2 In any patient with neutropenia, counts should be rechecked in 24 to 48 hours, then 7 to 10 days later. Neutrophils have approximately a 7-hour half-life in the circulation. Proliferation and differentiation from the initial stem cell take 6 to 7 days in the dog. Patients with persistent neutropenia should be investigated further.

3 A number of drugs are associated with bone marrow problems, including suppression. Problems range from neutropenia to pancytopenia. The majority are reversible, provided that the problem is detected and drug administration is stopped. However, neutropenia or pancytopenia due to phenylbutazone and estrogen administration may be irreversible. Phenylbutazone should not be used in cats and dogs, and patients receiving estrogens and other potentially myelosuppressive agents should be closely monitored while they are receiving the drugs. Drugs associated with neutropenia include estrogens (stilbestrol, estradiol), chloramphenicol, nonsteroidal anti-inflammatory agents (NSAIDs) (phenylbutazone, meclofenamic acid), phenobarbital, trimethoprim-sulfadiazine, quinidine, antineoplastic agents, thiacetarsamide (dogs), methimazole (cats), and griseofulvin (cats). Neutropenia is a problem especially if griseofulvin is given to cats with FIV, and the FIV status should be known in all feline patients prior to griseofulvin administration. In some instances, the problem is one of immune-mediated attack on bone marrow stem cells; in others, there appears to be a direct suppressive effect on the marrow.

4 Very few causes of neutropenia are specifically breed related. However, cyclic neutropenia (also known as *cyclic hematopoiesis*) is an autosomal recessive condition in gray (i.e., color-dilute) collies. These animals have gray rather than black noses. Cyclic neutropenia and associated fever recur at 10- to 12-day intervals. Neutropenia is the most severe abnormality, but there also may be thrombocytopenia and anemia with low reticulocyte counts. The neutropenia is followed by neutrophilia and then recurrent neutropenia. Multiple hemograms may be needed to document the phenomenon. Patients are highly susceptible to infections as a result of recurrent neutropenia. Another consequence of recurrent infection and immune system overstimulation is immune complex diseases (e.g., amyloidosis). Very few patients survive beyond 1 year of age.

5 In any feline patient, of any age, with chronic neutropenia, the FeLV and FIV status should be checked. Cats may sequestrate FeLV in the bone marrow, leading to marrow suppression or dysplasia in the absence of circulating viremia.

6 Feline patients with neutropenia, especially those with bi- or pancytopenias, and clinical illness which includes fever, vomiting, and diarrhea, may have FePLV infection. This condition frequently is fatal in young kittens. Older patients often survive. Kittens exposed in utero may develop cerebellar hypoplasia, but they are not neutropenic. Vaccination against the virus is included in standard vaccination protocols. No specific test exists for the viral infection, but feces may be examined electron microscopically for the virus, and canine parvovirus enzyme-linked immunosorbent assay (ELISA) tests appear to detect the virus (not an approved method of diagnosis). Diagnosis generally is based on clinical signs and the vaccination history.

7 Young dogs are highly susceptible to a variety of viral diseases that directly affect bone marrow. This is especially the case in those with a poor or incomplete vaccination status.

8 In canine patients with neutropenia, especially those with vomiting and diarrhea, a fecal sample should be tested for parvovirus infection (an ELISA test). Note that patients that have been vaccinated recently can be positive on a fecal ELISA test due to virus shedding in the absence of clinical disease. Neutropenia due to parvoviral infection results from destruction of neutrophilic precursors in bone marrow. There also may be anemia and thrombocytopenia. If these patients receive supportive care, they should develop a regenerative response in the neutrophil cell line.

9 CDV also suppresses bone marrow, causing neutropenia in the acute phase of the disease. Again, patients generally are young and poorly vaccinated. Associated signs of distemper include oculonasal discharge, signs of upper and lower respiratory tract disease, diarrhea, and seizures. Diagnosis in acute cases is by IFA to identify the virus in conjunctival scrapes.

10 Historical evaluation looks for known causes of bone marrow suppression other than drug therapy (e.g., prior radiation exposure). Physical examination should include evaluation of descended and inguinal testicles in males for mass lesions, abdominal palpation, and fundic examination for vessel dilation/tortuosity (due to hyperviscosity and hyperglobulinemia). There should be evaluation of oral mucous membranes for pallor, suggesting anemia, and evaluation of skin and mucous membranes for bruising, ecchymoses, and petechiation, suggesting thrombocytopenia or vasculitis. Individual bones should be palpated for pain due to bone marrow or primary bone lesions. General patient health should be evaluated, looking for fever, dehydration, and other signs of severe systemic disease.

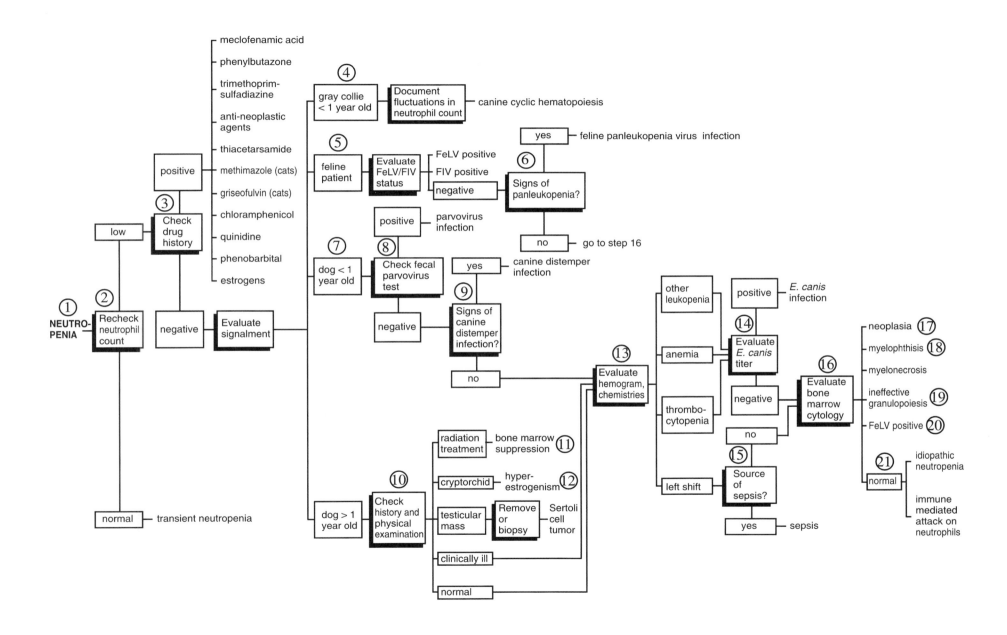

meclofenamic acid

phenylbutazone

trimethoprim-sulfadiazine

anti-neoplastic agents

thiacetarsamide

methimazole (cats)

griseofulvin (cats)

chloramphenicol

quinidine

phenobarbital

estrogens

① NEUTRO-PENIA

② Recheck neutrophil count

low

normal — transient neutropenia

③ Check drug history

positive

negative

Evaluate signalment

④ gray collie < 1 year old — Document fluctuations in neutrophil count — canine cyclic hematopoiesis

⑤ feline patient — Evaluate FeLV/FIV status — FeLV positive / FIV positive / negative

⑥ Signs of panleukopenia? — yes — feline panleukopenia virus infection — no — go to step 16

⑦ dog < 1 year old

⑧ Check fecal parvovirus test — positive — parvovirus infection — negative

⑨ Signs of canine distemper infection? — yes — canine distemper infection — no

⑩ dog > 1 year old — Check history and physical examination

radiation treatment — bone marrow suppression ⑪

cryptorchid — hyper-estrogenism ⑫

testicular mass — Remove or biopsy — Sertoli cell tumor

clinically ill

normal

⑬ Evaluate hemogram, chemistries

other leukopenia

anemia

thrombo-cytopenia

left shift

⑭ Evaluate E. canis titer — positive — E. canis infection — negative

⑮ Source of sepsis? — no — yes — sepsis

⑯ Evaluate bone marrow cytology

neoplasia ⑰

myelophthisis ⑱

myelonecrosis

ineffective granulopoiesis ⑲

FeLV positive ⑳

normal — ㉑ idiopathic neutropenia / immune mediated attack on neutrophils

11 In patients that have undergone radiation therapy bone marrow suppression may develop, especially where the radiation field has been extensive (e.g., half-body irradiation for lymphoma).

12 Male patients that were cryptorchid when neutered, those that have not been neutered, and/or those that are cryptorchid may have estrogen-producing testicular tumors (usually Sertoli cell tumors). Rarely, female patients have hyperestrogenemia and bone marrow suppression. Often, bone marrow suppression is extensive with hyperestrogenemia and also results in nonregenerative anemia and abnormalities in other cell lines.

13 Review the hemogram and serum chemistry profile to check for signs of severe systemic disease (e.g., chronic *E. canis* infection or septicemia), persistent neutropenia, and involvement of other blood cell lines. Patients with neutropenia with a left shift, especially a degenerative left shift (total neutrophil count more than 10% band neutrophils), and toxic changes in the neutrophils are more likely to be suffering from increased neutrophil consumption than failure of neutrophil production.

14 Canine patients with persistent neutropenia, with or without nonregenerative anemia, thrombocytopenia, or other problems (e.g., chronic weight loss, anterior uveitis, hyperglobulinemia), should be evaluated for *E. canis* infection via serology prior to bone marrow examination.

15 Patients with a left shift, signs of disseminated illness suggesting bacteremia or septicemia on physical examination (fever, heart murmur, pulmonary disease, extensive cutaneous lesions), or laboratory test abnormalities suggestive of sepsis (hypoalbuminemia, hypoglycemia, elevated alkaline phosphatase, degenerative left shift and associated neutropenia) should be evaluated for a source of septicemia. Bacteria associated with septicemia are generally gram negative. Neutropenia is generally the result of overwhelming tissue demand and depletion of peripheral and bone marrow reserves of neutrophils. There may be associated involvement of other cell lines (e.g., thrombocytopenia with incipient DIC). Evaluation should consist of urine culture (patients commonly culture positive for bacteria from urine with more dissemi-

nated sepsis) and blood culture (three cultures, from different vessels, within a 24-hour period, best performed at times when the patient is febrile). Additional evaluation includes thoracic radiographs (for signs of pneumonia or pleural fluid suggesting pyothorax), abdominal ultrasound (for focal abscessation, pyelonephritis, or peritonitis), fecal culture in patients with diarrhea (for *Salmonella* spp.), and culture of any wound. If all results are negative but septicemia is still a consideration (e.g., in neutropenic patients with a degenerative left shift), trial therapy with broad-spectrum intravenous antimicrobials may be appropriate. Focal or diffuse tissue necrosis without actual infection also may result in an excessive tissue demand for neutrophils and neutropenia on the hemogram.

16 If patients are persistently neutropenic, no left shift is seen, and no source of sepsis or inflammation is discovered, the next step is bone marrow examination. Even in patients with evidence of local or widespread infection, it should be remembered that neutropenia may predispose patients to sepsis as well as resulting from severe systemic disease. Cytological examination of bone marrow (with or without a marrow core biopsy) is the ultimate step in the investigation of any persistently neutropenic patient with no known underlying cause. This is particularly the case in patients with evidence of involvement of other marrow cell lines or when neutropenia persists with no obvious site of neutrophil sequestration in the body. It also may be indicated when the underlying cause of the neutropenia is known (e.g., secondary to administration of antineoplastic agents) but there is a need to assess the regenerative capability of marrow (presence of stem cells). Bone marrow aspiration may be performed under either heavy sedation or general anesthesia. Ideally, a hemogram should be evaluated within 7 to 10 hours of marrow sampling to allow complete assessment of the underlying condition, to evaluate for the presence of bone marrow arrest or dysplasia, and to decide whether the marrow is mounting a regenerative response in any cell line.

17 Bone marrow neoplasia, if extensive enough to alter peripheral neutrophil counts, will probably affect other cell lines, leading to bi-/pancytopenias. Extensive marrow involvement is seen with diffuse bone marrow neo-

plasms such as leukemia, lymphoma, and plasma cell myeloma.

18 Myelophthisis is replacement of bone marrow stem cells with fibrous tissue. This may be a primary problem or secondary to bone marrow exhaustion (e.g., due to chronic chemotherapy). Like diffuse bone marrow neoplasia, it is expected to affect more cell lines than granulocytes/neutrophils. Marrow necrosis can occur prior to the development of fibrosis.

19 Ineffective granulopoiesis (failure of adequate granulocyte differentiation from stem cells or maturation arrest within the bone marrow) is seen when peripheral neutropenia is accompanied by normal to increased numbers of developing neutrophils/granulocytes in the bone marrow. Cells may be destroyed within the marrow (e.g., as in parvovirus infection and in some drug reactions) or may reach a certain stage of maturation and then go no further. An immune-mediated attack on granulocyte stem cells leading to failure of differentiation and neutrophil production is also postulated and occurs in human beings. It is poorly documented in dogs, but glucocorticoid-responsive neutropenias with apparent stem cell involvement have been described in both dogs and cats. Ineffective granulopoiesis would not be expected to affect other cell lines (e.g., RBCs, platelets, and monocytes).

20 In addition to cytological evaluation, IFA for FeLV may be performed on bone marrow aspirates in cats to search for sequestrated virus. This may be found in patients that are not persistently viremic. Occult FeLV infection of bone marrow can cause suppression of one or more cell lines.

21 Patients with apparently normal bone marrow production and release of neutrophils but persistent neutropenia may have an immune-mediated attack on neutrophils in the periphery (rare and poorly documented in dogs and cats). They also may have neutropenia of unknown cause, which may be more common in cats than in dogs (but see the potential explanation in step 20).

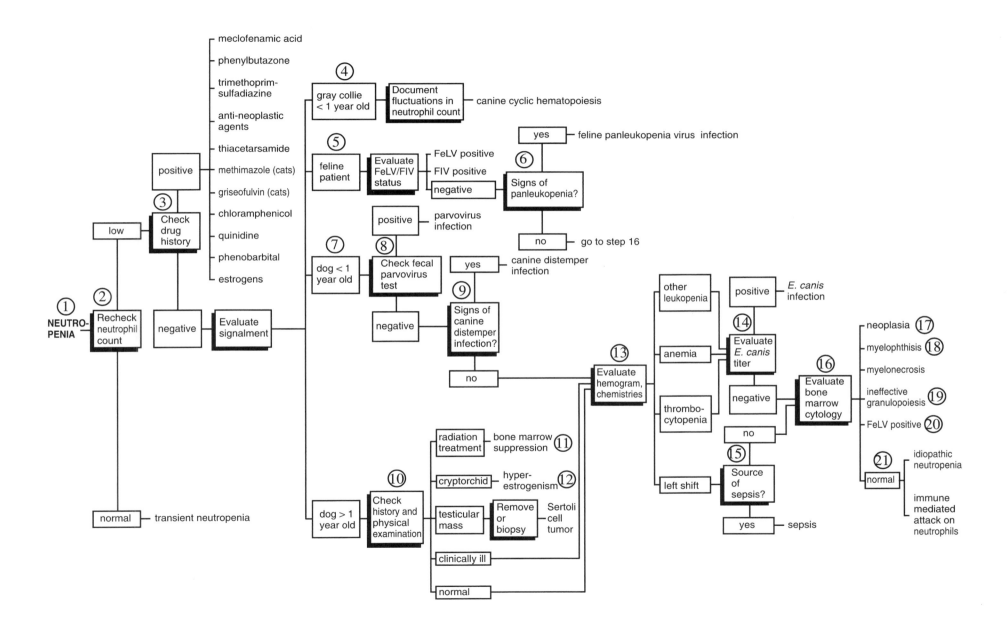

1 Thrombocytopenia is a platelet count below laboratory reference intervals. Reference intervals vary with the laboratory, but generally a platelet count less than 100,000/μl is considered low. Thrombocytopenia can be the result of platelet production failure (myeloproliferative disorders), excessive consumption of platelets (e.g., DIC, hemorrhage, rickettsial vasculitis, and immune-mediated disease causing vasculitis), platelet destruction (immune-mediated thrombocytopenia [IMT]), or platelet sequestration in liver or spleen. Sequestration and hemorrhage do not usually cause platelet counts to drop below 100,000/μl. Common findings associated with thrombocytopenia are petechial (pinpoint) hemorrhages and ecchymoses (larger hemorrhages) in the skin and mucous membranes, epistaxis, and gastrointestinal mucosal bleeding. Bleeding into body cavities is rare with thrombocytopenia. When thrombocytopenia is secondary to a systemic disease, other clinical signs of disease often are present.

2 The history should exclude drug therapy and recent vaccination as potential causes of immune-mediated thrombocytopenia and underlying neoplasia as a cause of increased platelet consumption or DIC.

3 The number of circulating platelets can be estimated from a blood smear. Six to seven platelets per oil immersion field (×1000) in the monolayer region of a smear correspond to about 100,000 platelets per microliter. Thus, fewer than three or four platelets per oil immersion field represents clinically significant thrombocytopenia. If the platelets are larger than normal (giant platelets), a regenerative response is probably present.

4 Results of the hemogram are useful for detecting concurrent cases of IMHA, anemia secondary to blood loss (concurrent reduction in serum proteins), or a bone marrow production problem (nonregenerative anemia).

5 If anticoagulant rodenticide exposure is suspected, a basic coagulogram (PT and PTT) should be obtained. FDPs should be added to facilitate the diagnosis of DIC.

6 Patients with DIC often have a prolonged PTT or PT and increased FDPs or some combination of these findings. Thrombocytopenia often is the first abnormality to develop. In cats, FIP virus infection can cause thrombocytopenia on its own or secondary to DIC.

7 Patients with anticoagulant rodenticide intoxication are likely to have normal or slightly reduced platelet counts, with marked prolongation of the PTT and PT. The PT may be prolonged before the PTT becomes abnormal.

8 Severe hemorrhage can reduce platelet numbers but seldom below 75,000/μl.

9 When IMHA is concurrent with thrombocytopenia, the hemogram may indicate RA, small RBCs, or spherocytes. Under these circumstances, thrombocytopenia is likely to be immune mediated.

10 A bone marrow production defect may affect WBCs (leukopenia) and RBCs (nonregenerative anemia) as well as platelets.

11 The most common infectious agents causing thrombocytopenia in dogs are *Rickettsia rickettsii*, *E. canis*, and *E. platys*. In the acute phase of *E. canis* infection, platelets are consumed or sequestered. In the chronic phase, platelet production is decreased due to bone marrow suppression. *E. platys* infection is characterized by 1- to 2-week parasitemic episodes during which morulae can be seen in platelets. These episodes are followed by periods of thrombocytopenia due to peripheral destruction of platelets. Other infectious agents in dogs that can cause thrombocytopenia include *H. canis*, *Leishmania* spp., *Babesia* spp., *Leptospira* spp., *Candida albicans*, *Histoplasma capsulatum*, adenovirus, herpes virus, and paramyxovirus infection. In cats, *H. felis* is an important cause of thrombocytopenia. Other causes include coronavirus (FIP), *Toxoplasma gondii*, and *Cytoxooan felis*. *Salmonella* spp. and *Dirofilaria immitis* can cause thrombocytopenia in both dogs and cats. Diseases common in or endemic to the patient's environment should be eliminated. Thrombocytopenic cats should be tested for FeLV and FIP (although the significance of a positive or negative coronavirus titer often is questionable).

12 Bone marrow aspiration and cytological examination are always indicated if the cause of persistent thrombocytopenia is uncertain or if other cell lines are involved (anemia and/or neutropenia).

13 With myeloproliferative or lymphoproliferative disorders, there may be accompanying changes on the hemogram (e.g., leukocytosis or leukopenia, abnormal blast cells). Bone marrow cytology will assist in determining the subclassification of the disorder.

14 The diagnosis of drug-induced thrombocytopenia may be based on a history of drug administration, otherwise unexplained thrombocytopenia, and a return of platelet counts toward normal in most instances when a drug is withdrawn (note that estrogen's toxic effects on marrow are irreversible). Drugs that cause thrombocytopenia include estrogens, chemotherapeutic agents, antithrombotic agents, and antimicrobial drugs such as trimethoprim-sulfa combinations and chloramphenicol. Propylthiouracil and methimazole cause thrombocytopenia in cats.

15 Antimegakaryocyte antibodies can be detected with direct IFA on bone marrow cytology samples and correlate quite well with IMT. Glucocorticoid therapy can result in a false-negative test.

16 Secondary IMT can be caused by a variety of inflammatory, infectious, autoimmune, and neoplastic disorders. Treatment must be directed at resolving the underlying disease as well as IMT.

17 With primary IMT, no underlying diseases can be found. Since platelets are being destroyed by the patient's own immune system, immunosuppressive therapy is administered. Once this point on the algorithm is reached response to immunosuppressive therapy is an appropriate diagnostic test.

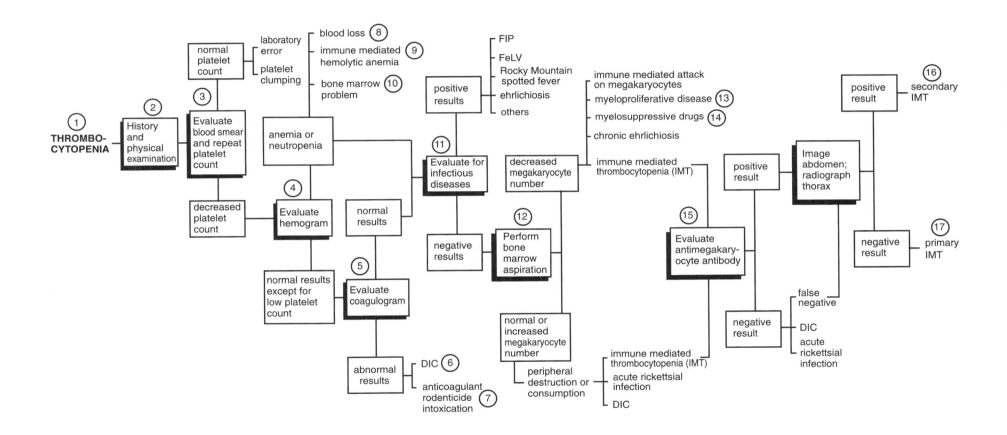

Metabolic/Electrolyte Disorders

1 Hypoalbuminemia is defined as a low concentration of albumin in serum. Low serum albumin develops due either to failure of production (severe liver disease or malnutrition leading to reduced protein manufacture) or increased loss from the body (renal, gastrointestinal, severe cutaneous injury, frank hemorrhage). Reference ranges for serum albumin concentrations vary among laboratories and species but, in general, serum albumin concentrations of less than 2.2–2.5 g/dl are considered low. Serum albumin concentrations of less than 1.6–1.8 g/dl may result in the formation of low-protein transudates in body cavities due to reduced plasma oncotic pressure. This is especially the case if there are other factors that concurrently impede venous return to the heart (either local or systemic), impede lymphatic drainage, or increase venous resistance (e.g., portal hypertension). Serum albumin concentrations below 1.0–1.2 g/dl are often associated with pitting edema of the extremities, formation of low-protein body cavity effusions, and reduced healing capacity. Other clinical signs vary with the underlying cause of the hypoalbuminemia. Patients with severe liver disease may be encephalopathic, anorexic, and nauseous. Patients with gastrointestinal protein losses often, although not always, have diarrhea and other gastrointestinal signs such as vomiting or anorexia. Patients with renal protein losses may or may not have clinical signs associated with renal failure, such as weight loss, anorexia, vomiting, and uremic ulceration of the oral mucosa. Patients with gastrointestinal and renal protein loss also may lose other small serum proteins such as antithrombin III (ATIII), which predisposes them to thromboembolic disease.

2 Signalment, history, and physical examination may suggest an initial route of diagnostic testing. Signalment is useful for identifying breeds predisposed to congenital, familial, or hereditary abnormalities that might result in hypoalbuminemia. For example, soft-coated wheaten terriers have familial protein-losing nephropathy, Yorkshire terriers and rottweilers are overrepresented among cases of intestinal lymphangiectasia, and young female Dobermans and some lines of American cocker spaniels are predisposed to chronic hepatitis/hepatopathy that eventually may progress to cirrhosis and liver failure. The history may determine a previously diagnosed condition that might result in hypoalbuminemia (e.g., gastrointestinal bleeding, inflammatory bowel disease,

exocrine pancreatic insufficiency) or inappropriate diet (severe malnourishment). The physical examination will detect severe burns or trauma wounds that might predispose to significant protein loss from the body. Physical examination also may reveal melena and hematochezia and suggest a primary gastrointestinal cause of the hypoalbuminemia. However, it must not be forgotten that severe renal and hepatic dysfunction also compromise gastrointestinal mucosal integrity and may lead to blood loss in the gastrointestinal tract.

3 A serum chemistry profile allows confirmation of low albumin. In combination with the urinalysis, it may pinpoint malfunction in a particular organ system that will direct the clinician toward investigation of that system as an underlying source of hypoalbuminemia (e.g., elevated liver enzymes or renal values).

4 Liver dysfunction must be very severe to result in failure of albumin production. Consequently, there may be little hepatic tissue remaining to produce liver enzymes such as ALT and ALP. Under those circumstances, liver enzymes may be normal in the face of severe hepatic dysfunction. If other substances normally produced by the liver (e.g., glucose, cholesterol, and BUN) are low in conjunction with hypoalbuminemia, severe liver dysfunction is suggested.

5 Panhypoproteinemia (low albumin and globulins) in the absence of burns, severe cutaneous abrasions, and obvious external hemorrhage strongly suggests gastrointestinal protein loss. Protein-losing nephropathy tends to result only in decreases in smaller protein molecules (albumin and ATIII) due to the size of the pores in the glomeruli. Liver failure leads to decreased production of albumin (and of coagulation factors which are not measured on a routine chemistry screen) because globulins are manufactured elsewhere in the body (by lymphocytes, etc.). However, protein loss from bowel commonly involves both low and high molecular weight proteins, especially in patients with lymphangiectasia, where lacteal rupture leads to loss of high-protein fluid into the lumen of the gut. Thus, panhypoproteinemia should lead the clinician to investigate the gastrointestinal tract as the source of the protein loss. In practice, it is usual to exclude hepatic dysfunction and renal protein losses as causes of hypoalbuminemia prior to anesthetizing pa-

tients for either endoscopic or full-thickness surgical bowel biopsies because such patients are often poor anesthetic and surgical candidates.

6 Patients with elevated renal values (BUN, creatinine, and phosphorus) and dilute urine have renal failure and should be evaluated for protein-losing nephropathy as a cause of hypoalbuminemia.

7 Liver function testing is useful in patients suspected of having hypoalbuminemia secondary to severe hepatic dysfunction, especially when there are no liver enzyme elevations and no significant decreases in other products of the liver (cholesterol, glucose, etc.). Which liver function test should be used depends on test availability, extent of the hypoalbuminemia, and alterations in body weight brought on by fluid accumulation. Measurement of fasting serum ammonia concentrations and BSP retention testing have somewhat restricted availability. Further, BSP retention testing may be affected both by decreased protein binding of BSP in hypoalbuminemic patients, leading to more rapid dye excretion, and by increased body weight compared to lean body mass in patients with ascites. Fasting serum ammonia concentrations may not be useful in patients who are anorexic, and ammonia challenge studies may decompensate hepatic encephalopathy. Pre- and postprandial bile acid measurement is difficult to perform in anorexic or vomiting patients, and there is considerable variation among laboratories as to the reliability of this test. Generally, more than one hepatic function test is advised to increase the accuracy of the diagnosis of liver dysfunction in veterinary patients. Liver function testing may be combined with radiographs, ultrasound, or other methods of imaging the liver in order to assess size, shape, outline, margins, and vascularity. Liver biopsy is the ultimate diagnostic test for patients suspected of having liver dysfunction.

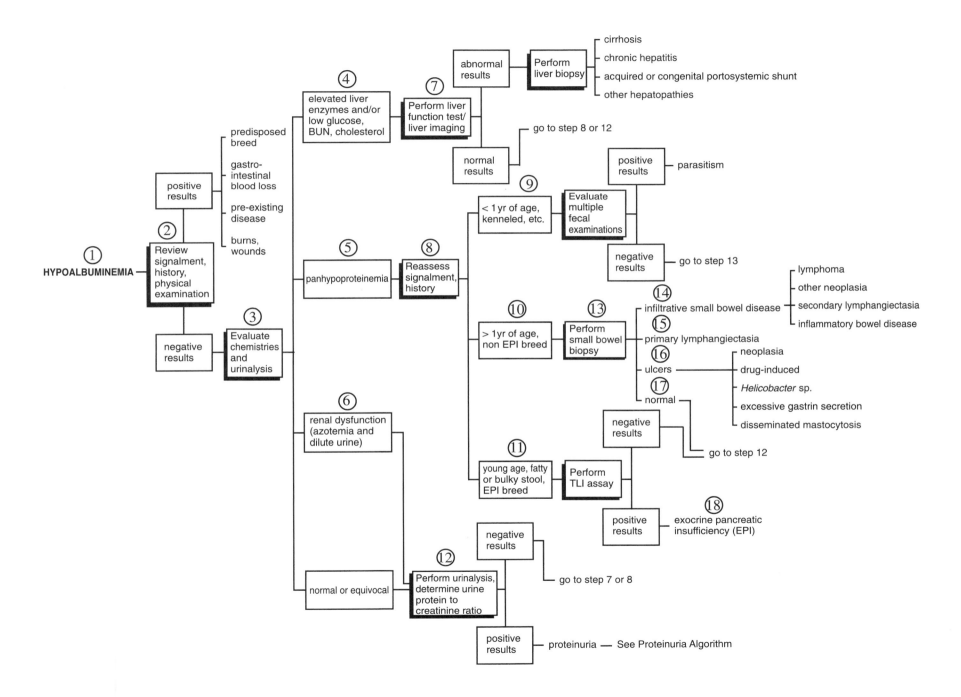

8 In patients suspected of having gastrointestinal protein losses, it is important to screen out the small minority of those in which the underlying condition can be diagnosed by less invasive methods than gastric and small intestinal biopsies.

9 Very young animals, particularly those kept in unclean surroundings or areas where there is potential for continuous reinfection with gastrointestinal parasites, and kenneled animals are predisposed to develop heavy parasite loads. Several fecal examinations and prophylactic deworming should be performed before considering intestinal biopsy.

10 For patients over 1 year of age, those that are kept in clean surroundings, and those that are not kenneled, it is necessary to progress to small intestinal biopsies to determine the underlying cause of the diarrhea. Patients that are not of a breed predisposed to develop exocrine pancreatic insufficiency and that do not have excessively bulky or fatty stools also need small intestinall biopsies.

11 Patients that have undergone drastic weight loss but that are otherwise bright and healthy, patients with very bulky or fatty stools, and those that appear to have undigested food in the stool should first have a fasted blood sample taken for a trypsin-like immunoreactivity (TLI) test. This test evaluates for failure of the pancreas to produce digestive enzymes, a condition known as *exocrine pancreatic insufficiency (EPI)*. Lack of these enzymes results in maldigestion and malabsorption of fat and protein. Although young German shepherd dogs are predisposed to EPI, the condition occurs idiosyncratically in all dog breeds and is seen occasionally in cats.

12 Urinalysis, preferably on a sample obtained by cystocentesis, is required to document failure of urine-concentrating ability in azotemic patients and to make the diagnosis of renal failure. A full urinalysis is also required to provide a rough measurement of urine protein losses and to assess the activity of the urine sediment. The urine protein/creatinine ratio should be measured on a urine sample with an inactive sediment in order to quantitate urine protein loss. A urine protein/creatinine ratio of more than 1.0 is definitely abnormal (a ratio above 0.5 may be indicative of protein loss) and suggests that the source of hypoalbuminemia is renal protein loss. A urine culture should always be performed where the urine protein/creatinine ratio is abnormal, even if the urine sediment does not reveal bacteria or pyuria, to exclude the possibility of occult infection as a cause of proteinuria. Dilute urine samples in hypoalbuminemic patients should have the protein/creatinine ratio determined even in the absence of obvious protein on the urine dipstick. Significant amounts of protein may be lost in dilute urine and show up as negative or trace proteinuria on a urine dipstick.

13 Gastric and small intestinal biopsies may be performed either endoscopically (mucosal biopsy) or at surgery (full-thickness biopsy). Upper endoscopy allows for direct examination of the mucosal surfaces of the stomach and proximal portions of the small intestine, and is a relatively fast, noninvasive way of obtaining biopsy specimens in a compromised patient. Endoscopic biopsies only sample mucosa and small amounts of submucosa and, in some circumstances, may not be diagnostic of the underlying condition. Surgery allows full-thickness biopsy specimens to be obtained and evaluation of the serosal surface of the intestine and lymphatic vessels in the mesentery (which may be important in patients with intestinal lymphangiectasia). It also allows evaluation of the whole length of the small intestine, which is important since lesions leading to protein loss may be regional and not within reach of the endoscope. However, hypoalbuminemic patients may have a reduced capacity to heal full-thickness intestinal biopsy sites, and those with ascites may have problems with fluid leakage and healing at the celiotomy site.

14 Small intestinal biopsy specimens may indicate cellular infiltrates into the intestine (inflammatory or neoplastic). These infiltrates may lead to protein-losing enteropathy or may result in secondary problems with lymphatic drainage and lymphangiectasia.

15 Primary intestinal lymphangiectasia develops in the absence of inflammatory infiltrates in the intestinal wall and may be the result of an acquired lymphatic problem (inflammatory, neoplastic, fibrotic) that leads to failure of gastrointestinal lymphatic drainage. It also may be the result of congenital lymphatic malformation in young animals. Before making the diagnosis of primary lymphangiectasia, more distant causes of lymphatic obstruction/increased lymphatic pressure (e.g., right-sided heart failure, intrathoracic conditions) need to be excluded.

16 Gastrointestinal ulceration may arise from a variety of causes (neoplasia, administration of glucocorticoids or NSAIDs), excessive gastrin secretion, *Helicobacter* spp. infection, etc.). Focal gastrointestinal ulceration must be severe and result in a great deal of protein exudation or blood loss to cause hypoalbuminemia.

17 Occasionally, patients suspected of having gastrointestinal protein loss have normal intestinal biopsy specimens. This may occur because incorrect areas of the bowel were sampled or because patients actually have severe glomerulopathy that results in loss of protein molecules of all sizes. Occasionally, patients have normal biopsy findings but underlying maldigestive/malabsorptive conditions (e.g., brush border enzyme deficiencies) that may prove very difficult to diagnose with the technology currently available in veterinary medicine.

18 Patients with EPI have a number of separate problems that cause maldigestion of dietary components and lead to malabsorption. If the condition is severe enough, it may result in hypoalbuminemia.

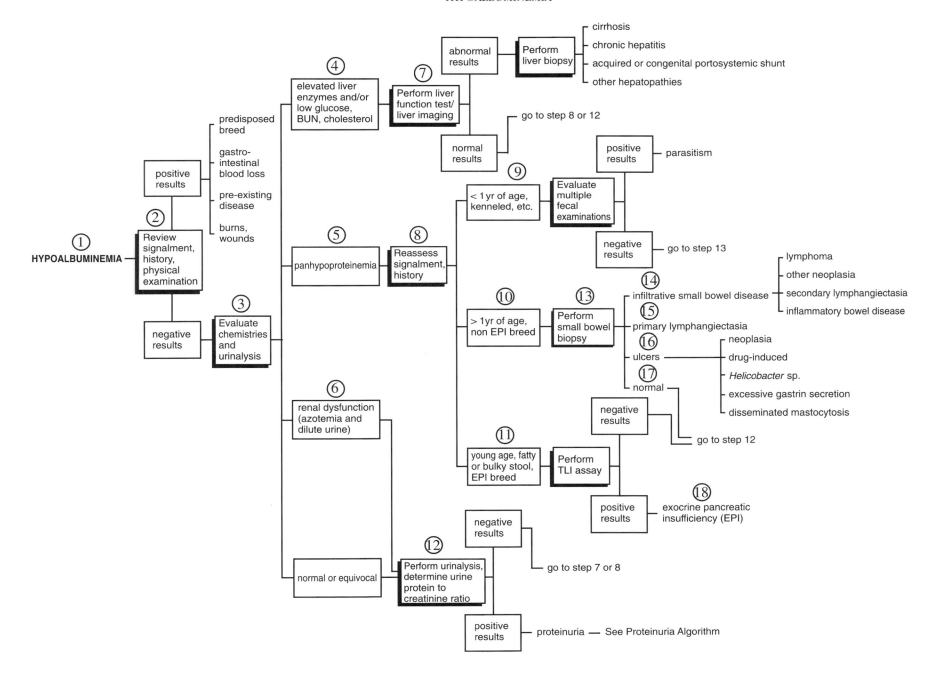

1 Hyperglobulinemia is an increased concentration of serum globulins. It may result from increases in non-immunoglobulins (acute phase proteins such as complement, fibrinogen, and alpha₂-macroglobulin, produced by the liver in systemic inflammation) or immunoglobulins (gamma globulins such as IgM and IgG, produced by lymphocytes in response to immune system exposure to antigens). Hyperglobulinemia results from inflammation, chronic stimulation of the immune system, or overproduction of one particular globulin group (generally by neoplastic cells). Patients with high serum globulin concentrations may be asymptomatic. However, severe hyperglobulinemia, especially due to IgM, causes signs of hyperviscosity, including reduced tissue oxygenation, coagulopathies, and interference with platelet function, resulting in bleeding problems including epistaxis. Patients may have neurological signs (seizures, depression, dementia), renal failure, congestive heart failure due to an increased cardiac workload, and retinal changes (dilated, tortuous vessels, retinal hemorrhage, retinal detachment). The normal range for serum globulins varies but is usually 2.8–3.8 g/dl. Elevations may be mild (4–5 g/dl), moderate (5–6 g/dl), or severe (>6 g/dl).

2 Patients presenting with increased serum globulin concentrations should be evaluated for dehydration (a history of vomiting, diarrhea, fever, water deprivation, or a finding of sunken eyes and dry oral mucous membranes). Dehydration reduces the water content of blood, causing relative increases in serum albumin, globulins, and RBCs.

3 Hyperglobulinemic patients should be checked for low serum albumin. Mild globulin increases maintain plasma oncotic pressure if albumin is low. However, globulin elevations also may cause compensatory decreases in albumin. Additionally, some hyperglobulinemic conditions are associated with reduced albumin synthesis (severe inflammatory liver disease) or loss (glomerulonephritis).

4 Drugs such as glucocorticoids may cause mild increases in serum globulin concentrations. Conditions such as neoplasia, dirofilariasis, and chronic inflammation due to immune-mediated disease and skin problems all can cause hyperglobulinemia.

5 An intact dog with hyperglobulinemia and suspected of having been bred should be evaluated for *Brucella canis*. Symptomatic patients may have uveitis, back pain, or bone pain, males may have deformed sperm, and females may have recurrent abortions. A rapid slide agglutination test (RSAT) is an immediate screening test. A negative RSAT has a high correlation with lack of infection. If the test is positive, it may be followed up by a tube agglutination test (TAT) or an agar gel immunodiffusion test (AGIDT) for confirmation. Intact females also should be checked for pyometra since this also may cause hyperglobulinemia.

6 Physical examination detects pyoderma, otitis externa, suspected immune-mediated skin disease, dental or gingival problems, and joint pain, all potentially resulting in hyperglobulinemia. It also detects lymphadenopathy, cutaneous/abdominal masses, heart murmurs, and thoracic or abdominal effusions that might need to be pursued prior to serum protein electrophoresis. Fundic examination is useful for hyperviscosity signs (tortuous retinal vessels, bleeding) and chorioretinitis (with some viral [FIP], fungal, and rickettsial [*Ehrlichia canis*] infections). Fever is an important physical examination finding but is nonspecific, since it may result from any infectious, neoplastic, or autoimmune source of immune system stimulation that increases cytokine activity and pyrogen release.

7 Enlarged lymph nodes and cutaneous, subcutaneous, or intra-abdominal masses should be evaluated cytologically or histopathologically. Lymphoma and reactive lymphadenopathy both may be associated with moderate to severe hyperglobulinemia. Patients with intra-abdominal masses or abdominal or thoracic fluid accumulation should have ultrasound or other imaging studies (radiographs, CT scans) to identify the tissues involved. Most tissues may be aspirated for cytology under ultrasound guidance. Biopsy usually requires a coagulation profile and general anesthesia, and it may not be possible to perform all biopsies under ultrasound guidance.

8 Dogs are primary reservoirs for a pathogenic flagellate protozoan *Leishmania* sp. Several different species exist, some indigenous to the Mediterranean region of Europe and some in the southern United States, Mexico, and South America. Clinical suspicion depends on the patient's location and travel history. Affected dogs show weight loss with a good appetite, cutaneous lesions, splenomegaly, gastrointestinal signs, and lymphadenopathy. Hyperglobulinemia usually is polyclonal, but monoclonal gammopathy has also been reported. Diagnosis requires the demonstration of amastigotes in tissues stained with Wright's or Giemsa stain. Cats are usually asymptomatic or subclinically affected.

9 Systemic fungal infections occur in both dogs and cats. Some are more common in one species (e.g., *Cryptococcus neoformans* and *Sporothrix schenckii* are seen more frequently in cats). Organisms are opportunistic pathogens, usually affecting only one animal in a group. Patients may present with skin lesions, upper respiratory tract, or systemic signs (pulmonary, bone, gastrointestinal tract). Rarely, systemic infections may be picked up on peripheral blood smears, bone marrow aspirates, or joint aspirates. Cultures of affected tissues may be needed for diagnosis.

10 Cats with abdominal effusions and elevated serum globulins should be evaluated for coronavirus infection (FIP), a very difficult condition to diagnose definitively. Cats are often young (<1 year old) or have had contact with other cats whose coronavirus status is unknown. They may be febrile and may have chorioretinitis, anterior uveitis, and neurological signs. Laboratory test abnormalities may include azotemia, elevated liver enzymes, anemia, thrombocytopenia, and neutropenia. Analysis of effusions often reveals high protein fluid levels (5–6 g/dl), with a yellow or straw-colored appearance and relatively low cellularity (nondegenerate neutrophils and lymphocytes). Positive serum titers only suggest exposure to coronavirus. To add to the confusion, some patients with FIP do not mount a good immune response to the coronavirus and have low or negative titers in the face of active disease. The only conclusive method of diagnosing FIP is by histopathological evaluation of affected tissues (liver, kidneys).

11 Patients with elevated globulins and fever or a heart murmur should be evaluated for endocarditis.

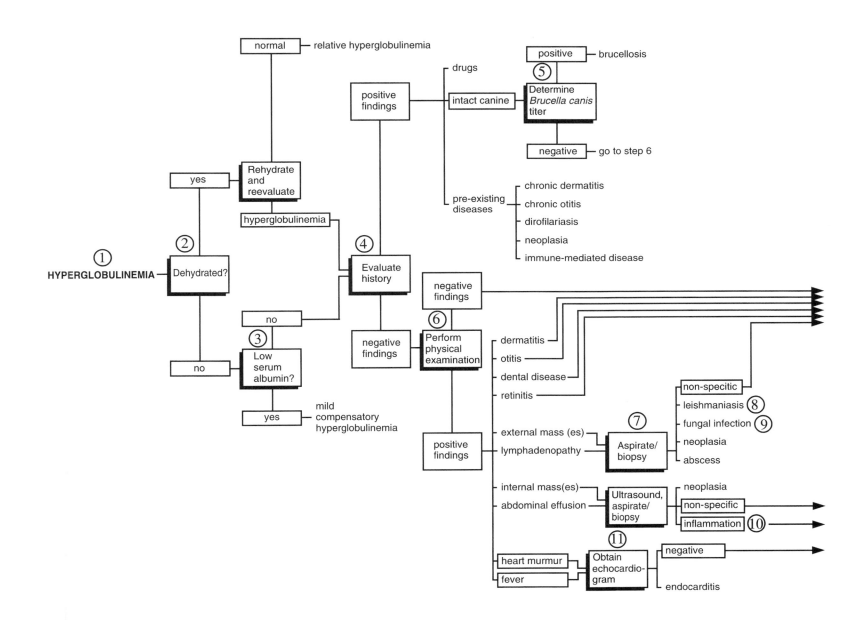

12 Serum protein electrophoresis determines the pattern of serum protein distribution. Results may take days to weeks, depending on the laboratory, so severely affected patients need other tests concurrently. Serum is mapped out on cellulose acetate gel to produce an electrophoretogram, with four regions corresponding to the four main protein types in serum (albumin and alpha, beta, and gamma globulins). Normal electrophoretograms have a tall, narrow spike in the region of albumin and low-level, broad-based spikes in the alpha, beta, and gamma globulin fractions. Patients with hyperglobulinemia frequently have increases in the gamma region (immunoglobulins) and, more rarely, in the alpha or beta regions (acute phase proteins associated with inflammation or liver disease). Occasional neoplastic monoclonal spikes have been reported in the beta globulin fraction. Elevations in the gamma fraction may be broad-based (polyclonal) or narrow-based and very tall (monoclonal).

13 Polyclonal gammopathy results from immune system stimulation by sterile inflammation or chronic bacterial, viral, fungal, parasitic, and *E. canis* infection. In dogs it commonly results from skin disease, dirofilariasis, and ehrlichiosis. In cats, FIP is a common cause.

14 Monoclonal gammopathy is excessive production of immunoglobulins or immunoglobulin light chains, usually by neoplastic cells. It is seen most commonly with multiple myeloma but has also been reported with lymphoma and extramedullary plasma cell tumors. Rarely, monoclonal gammopathy is associated with infections (FIP, *E. canis*, leishmaniasis) and skin disease (e.g., cutaneous amyloid).

15 Cats with marked polyclonal gammopathy commonly have FIP. Occasionally, monoclonal spikes occur. However these almost always occur on top of a broad-based elevation of globulins and acute phase proteins. Definitive diagnosis requires histopathology or tissue IFA to identify pyogranulomatous lesions and vasculitis. Coronavirus titers are difficult to interpret since a positive titer indicates only that the patient has been exposed, not that it has mounted the inappropriate immune response that underlies FIP. Negative titers do not mean freedom from clinical disease, especially in noneffusive FIP.

16 Although infection with either FeLV or FIV may cause broad-based gammopathy, infection is more likely to predispose patients to other infectious, neoplastic, or immune-mediated diseases, so a positive test is not necessarily the end of the algorithm.

17 Chronic or recurrent infections with several RBC parasites may lead to hyperglobulinemia due to chronic immune system stimulation. *E. canis* and some fungal organisms also may be detected in WBCs.

18 Immune-mediated diseases causing anemia may result in hyperglobulinemia. Many immune-mediated diseases do not have specific tests to diagnose the underlying condition. Most immune-mediated diseases cause only mild globulin elevations. However, when underlying conditions such as pyometra, otitis externa, and neoplasia trigger immune system overactivity, hyperglobulinemia may be more severe. ANA titers detect antibodies to cellular nuclear membranes. A positive ANA titer is helpful for diagnosing SLE, but it also may be seen with tissue necrosis or inflammation. Coombs' testing for anti-RBC antigens may be useful to confirm the presence of IMHA. However, spherocytosis and a positive in-saline autoagglutination test render Coombs' testing redundant.

19 Neoplastic cells on a blood smear are likely to be lymphocytes, thus making the diagnosis of lymphoblastic leukemia or stage V lymphoma (with bone marrow involvement). Rarely, leukemias originate in other cell lines and immunohistochemistry is required for diagnosis.

20 For undetermined causes of polyclonal gammopathy, where prior testing is negative or nonspecific, the next sequence of tests may be performed in any order. Thoracic radiographs are useful for screening. If they are positive, a variety of tests ranging from fine-needle aspiration and cytology of focal masses/lung tissue to bronchoscopy, thoracoscopy, and thoracotomy may be the next step. A variety of neoplasms, bacterial and fungal infections, and less specific "granulomatous" conditions such as lymphomatoid granulomatosis may be diagnosed this way.

21 Local fungal infections may not stimulate an antibody response, and patients with disseminated fungal infection may have such poor immune system function that fungal titers are not helpful. Currently available serum titers are most useful for *Cryptococcus* and *Coccidioidomycosis* spp.

22 Urine samples with inactive sediments and proteinuria can trace protein loss to the kidneys. Patients with monoclonal gammopathy have renal proteinuria due to loss of albumin (immune-mediated glomerulonephritis) or other proteins with severe glomerular damage or to excretion of immunoglobulin light chains from neoplastic cells (Bence Jones proteinuria). Bence Jones proteins will not be measured on urine dipstick evaluation but will be seen if a protein precipitation test is used. Bence Jones proteinuria is relatively uncommon in dogs and cats with multiple myeloma, but it is one of the criteria for making this diagnosis. Urine protein electrophoresis is also possible.

23 Patients with monoclonal gammopathy should be evaluated for bone pain, especially in the axial skeleton (pelvis, vertebrae). This determines the sites to radiograph to identify lytic lesions and guide bone marrow aspiration. Lytic lesions are another criterion for diagnosis of multiple myeloma. Bone scans may identify subtle lesions and increased bone turnover; however, myeloma lesions are often "cold" (i.e., negative). Although the majority of patients fulfilling these criteria have multiple myeloma, lymphoma and rarer conditions cannot be excluded without bone marrow aspiration.

24 If the bone marrow examination is negative, either the condition is neoplastic and isolated to certain bones or it is very rare (extramedullary plasmacytoma or idiopathic monoclonal gammopathy). Full skeletal radiographs or a bone scan may be performed to try to locate and aspirate a tumor site. If the findings are negative, exploratory surgery can be considered to try to locate extramedullary plasmacytoma (commonly bowel associated). Alternatively, the condition is considered idiopathic.

25 If the client is willing to have the patient treated and all potentially infectious causes of monoclonal gammopathy have been excluded, trial combination chemotherapy for round cell tumors could be considered and the diagnosis made by the response to therapy.

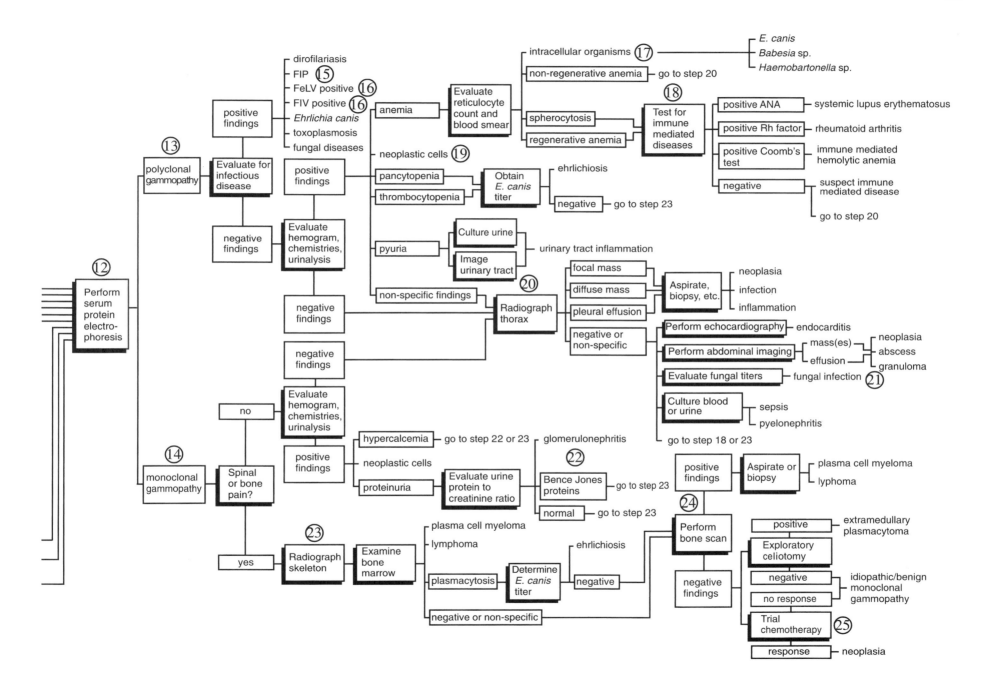

1 Hypoglycemia is a reduced blood glucose concentration, usually to below 50–60 mg/dl. The presence of clinical signs depends on how quickly glucose reduction occurred and how well the patient has adapted to reduced blood glucose concentrations. Clinical signs are not usually evident until blood glucose is less than 45 mg/dl. Nervousness, trembling, panting, and tachycardia can be followed by weakness, ataxia, mental dullness, collapse, stupor, coma, or seizures.

2 If serum or plasma is not separated from RBCs within 30–60 minutes after a blood sample is obtained, artifactual hypoglycemia can result due to glucose metabolism by RBCs. If it is not known whether RBCs were separated from serum or plasma appropriately, take another sample for glucose determination. Fasting samples are recommended to detect true hypoglycemia and avoid the effect of a recent meal temporarily boosting blood glucose. If the clinician suspects an insulinoma or intermittent hypoglycemia for other reasons, a 24- to 48-hour fast may be necessary to detect hypoglycemia with intermittent sampling of blood.

3 If artifactual hypoglycemia has been excluded by proper sample handling, assess the historical or physical examination findings that might explain hypoglycemia (e.g., toy breeds less than 1 year of age are likely to develop juvenile hypoglycemia due to inability to store glycogen).

4 Septic patients usually present with fever, collapse, shock, and poor appetite rather than hypoglycemia. An inflammatory leukogram is likely to be present. Appropriate cultures (blood, urine, and other body fluids) should identify the causative organism.

5 Vigorous exercise, especially in hunting dogs that have been fasted before a hunt, can cause low serum glucose and subsequent clinical signs. The diagnosis may be confirmed by measuring blood glucose while signs are present.

6 If the patient is less than 1 year of age, the differential diagnosis includes juvenile hypoglycemia, a heavy parasite burden, inadequate food intake, portosystemic shunt, or sepsis.

7 In patients less than 1 year of age, a heavy intestinal parasite load, especially hookworms, can result in hypoglycemia. Even if the fecal examination is negative (unlikely), deworming should be considered in such patients.

8 If a fecal examination is negative for parasites, obtain a hemogram and chemistry profile to evaluate for sepsis and liver disease. Normal young, growing dogs will probably have ALP elevation. Evidence of liver disease on routine laboratory tests includes microcytic, normochromic anemia, hypoalbuminemia, hypocholesterolemia, low BUN, and elevated liver enzymes.

9 To evaluate further for underlying liver disease in hypoglycemic patients, bile acid testing may be performed, along with measurement of fasting serum ammonia or ammonia challenge testing.

10 Transient juvenile hypoglycemia occurs predominantly in toy breeds of dogs between 6 weeks and 1 year of age. Precipitating events include inadequate nutrition, once or twice daily feedings, gastrointestinal parasites, and cold ambient temperature. Free choice feeding or feeding every 4 to 6 hours is recommended until such patients are mature.

11 In a young dog or cat, a congenital portosystemic shunt is more likely than acquired liver disease. If bile acid tests or other testing suggests liver dysfunction, abdominal ultrasound, CT scans, or MRI scans may be used to image the shunt. Plain abdominal radiographs show only microhepatica. Contrast portography may be needed to delineate abnormal vasculature.

12 If the patient is older than 1 year, and particularly if it is middle-aged or older, the differential diagnosis includes sepsis, hypoadrenocorticism (Addison's disease) in dogs, insulin-secreting tumors, and liver disease. Thus, a hemogram and chemistry profile are indicated.

13 Hypoadrenocorticism causes hyponatremia, hyperkalemia (Na:K ratio < 27:1), azotemia, and hypercalcemia in addition to hypoglycemia. Atypical Addison's disease is only a glucocorticoid deficiency; therefore, the patient will not have sodium and potassium abnormalities.

14 If the blood glucose concentration on a fasted sample is low, a concurrent serum insulin measurement should be obtained. The presence of an inappropriate serum insulin concentration (normal or high) in the face of hypoglycemia indicates a possible insulinoma. However, it does not differentiate an islet cell tumor from an insulin-producing tumor in other tissues.

15 If an insulin-secreting mass is suspected, abdominal ultrasound may image the lesion(s) or tumor metastasis. However, in dogs, insulin-producing pancreatic tumors often are very small and hard to detect via ultrasound. Exploratory celiotomy may be considered to find the lesion, to determine if the mass(es) can be removed, or to look for tumors outside of the pancreas (e.g., in small bowel) that rarely may cause hypoglycemia. Most insulin-secreting tumors of the pancreas are malignant carcinomas. If they cannot be surgically resected, medical management of hypoglycemia can be attempted with multiple small feedings of diets low in simple sugars, prednisone, or diazoxide.

16 If serum insulin concentrations are low in a hypoglycemic patient, consider the possibility of liver disease and perform liver function tests. Usually liver disease does not cause hypoglycemia until it is end-stage, and patients would be expected to be hypoalbuminemic and to have low cholesterol and BUN or coagulopathies as well.

17 An ACTH test can be obtained to exclude isolated glucocorticoid deficiency (atypical Addison's disease).

18 Occasional patients will have a low fasting blood glucose (55–65 mg/dl) for no apparent reason. If all other disease processes are eliminated, then one must consider this condition a variant of normal. However, occult neoplasia also should remain a consideration in such cases.

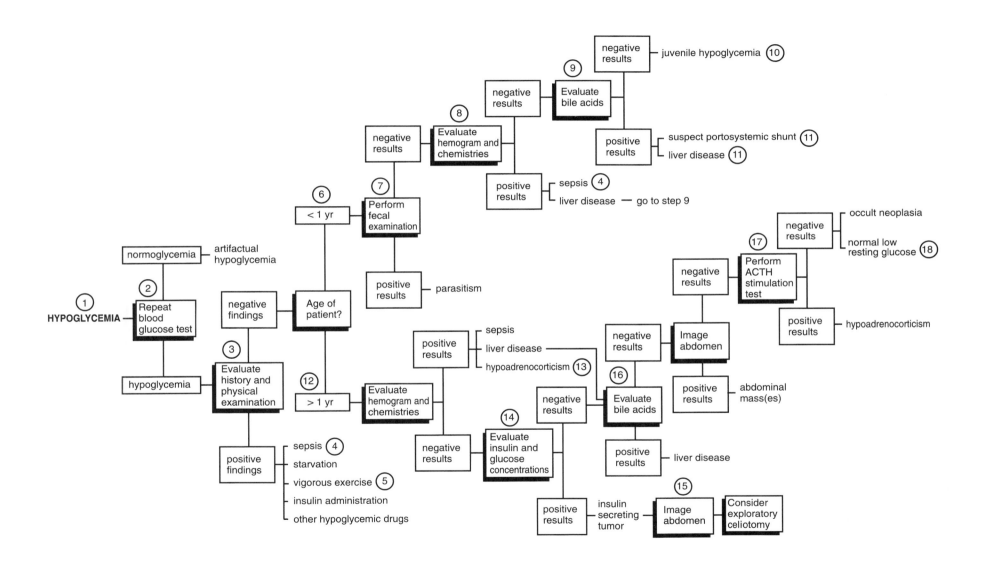

① **HYPOGLYCEMIA**

② Repeat blood glucose test
- normoglycemia — artifactual hypoglycemia
- hypoglycemia

③ Evaluate history and physical examination
- negative findings
- positive findings
  - sepsis ④
  - starvation
  - vigorous exercise ⑤
  - insulin administration
  - other hypoglycemic drugs

Age of patient?
- ⑥ < 1 yr
- ⑫ > 1 yr

⑦ Perform fecal examination
- negative results
- positive results — parasitism

⑧ Evaluate hemogram and chemistries
- negative results
- positive results
  - sepsis ④
  - liver disease — go to step 9

⑨ Evaluate bile acids
- negative results — juvenile hypoglycemia ⑩
- positive results
  - suspect portosystemic shunt ⑪
  - liver disease ⑪

⑫ Evaluate hemogram and chemistries
- positive results
  - sepsis
  - liver disease
  - hypoadrenocorticism ⑬
- negative results

⑭ Evaluate insulin and glucose concentrations
- negative results
- positive results — insulin secreting tumor

⑮ Image abdomen — Consider exploratory celiotomy

⑯ Evaluate bile acids
- negative results
- positive results — liver disease

Image abdomen
- negative results
- positive results — abdominal mass(es)

⑰ Perform ACTH stimulation test
- negative results
  - occult neoplasia
  - normal low resting glucose ⑱
- positive results — hypoadrenocorticism

1 Normal blood glucose values vary to some extent among laboratories. In general, values between 130 and 180 mg/dl are considered mild elevations. These may not be significant. However, if the patient presents with PU, PD, vomiting, pain, or other signs of illness, such values may be significant. Blood glucose values over 180 mg/dl are significant. Persistent fasting hyperglycemia results from relative insulin deficiency (in diabetes mellitus) or insulin resistance. If the blood glucose elevation is extreme (above 500–600 mg/dl), there may be CNS signs such as lethargy, stupor, and coma. The pathogenesis of impaired CNS function is not completely understood, but it may be due to hyperosmolality. As blood glucose concentrations exceed 180–200 mg/dl in the dog, the ability of renal tubular cells to reabsorb glucose from the glomerular ultrafiltrate is exceeded, resulting in glycosuria. The mean renal tubular threshold for normal cats is reportedly light (290 mg/dl). Glycosuria creates osmotic diuresis and PU. Compensatory PD prevents dehydration, but glycosuria causes caloric loss and hence weight loss.

2 Reasons for hyperglycemia may be found by reviewing the patient's history, drug history, and physical examination findings. The blood glucose concentration can be increased by a number of drugs such as glucocorticoids, thiazide diuretics, and megestrol acetate.

3 Although the mechanism is not understood, transient hyperglycemia has been observed in patients with severe head trauma or other insults to the brain.

4 Glucocorticoids raise the blood glucose concentration by increasing gluconeogenesis and antagonizing the effects of insulin. They induce synthesis of hepatic enzymes that promote glucose synthesis, and they promote hepatic glycogen synthesis.

5 Megestrol acetate induces oversecretion of growth hormone. This is a strongly diabetogenic hormone that causes insulin resistance in target tissues. Because of the risk of diabetes mellitus, patients with a history of megestrol acetate administration should have a urinalysis evaluated for glycosuria or ketonuria. This is true to a lesser extent of patients receiving glucocorticoids.

6 Mild hyperglycemia can occur up to 2 hours after feeding, especially if moist, soft food was consumed. Patients should be fasted and serum glucose concentrations reassessed.

7 *Stress* is a subjective term. The condition may not always be recognized and may evoke inconsistent responses in individual dogs and cats. Hyperglycemia (blood glucose elevations as high as 300–400 mg/dl) often can be stress-induced in cats in a hospital situation. However, concurrent glycosuria is rare because the transient nature of the increase in blood glucose prevents detectable concentrations of urine glucose from accumulating.

8 Evaluation of concurrent urine and blood glucose samples is helpful to distinguish stress-related hyperglycemia from diabetes mellitus.

9 The diagnosis of diabetes mellitus is based on finding glycosuria in conjunction with persistent hyperglycemia and other supporting clinical or historical signs (PU, PD, weight loss, polyphagia, increased susceptibility to infection).

10 Hyperglycemia in the cat, without concurrent glucosuria, is most likely due to stress. Possible causes of hyperglycemia, other than primary diabetes mellitus, in cats are acromegaly and pancreatitis. The last two conditions cause glycosuria because they cause hyperglycemia due to insulin antagonism.

11 Besides primary diabetes mellitus, hyperglycemia in the dog can be caused by pancreatitis, hyperadrenocorticism, and diestrus. These conditions cause insulin antagonism, diabetes mellitus, and glycosuria. Severe stress also can cause hyperglycemia.

12 In symptomatic patients, a full serum chemistry screen should be evaluated to look for underlying conditions that might lead to hyperglycemia, with or without the development of permanent diabetes mellitus.

13 Patients with necrotizing or other forms of pancreatitis may have hyperglycemia due to hyperglucagonemia and stress-related increases in catecholamine and cortisol concentrations. Hyperglycemia also may result from damage to insulin-producing beta cells in the pancreas. Some affected animals are diabetic following recovery from pancreatitis.

14 Progesterone secretion from the corpus luteum is greatest during diestrus. Progesterone induces growth hormone oversecretion. This can cause insulin resistance and subsequent hyperglycemia. Serum progesterone concentrations above 2 ng/ml are consistent with diestrus.

15 If the cause of hyperglycemia has not yet been determined, repeat serum glucose testing or evaluation to document persistent hyperglycemia. If this is found, it can be caused by early diabetes mellitus, exocrine pancreatic neoplasia, pheochromocytoma (in dogs), or acromegaly (in cats more than dogs).

16 Most acromegalic cats have concurrent diabetes mellitus due to insulin antagonism. Definitive diagnosis of acromegaly requires documentation of elevated growth hormone concentrations in serum, but a validated feline assay is not available. Pituitary scans (CT or MRI) can demonstrate a pituitary mass.

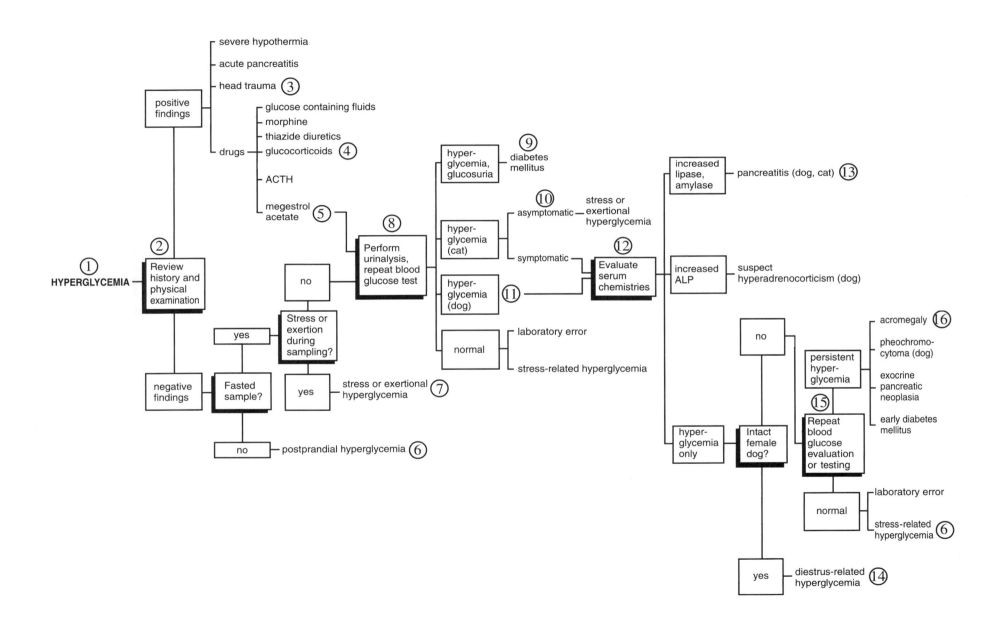

1 Hypokalemia is defined as a serum potassium (K^+) concentration less than 3.5 mEq/l. Causes include decreased dietary intake, gastrointestinal loss, transcellular shift, and renal loss. Most patients are asymptomatic until serum K^+ concentrations decrease to below 3 mEq/l. Then signs are primarily neuromuscular (muscle weakness, cervical ventroflexion) and cardiovascular (decreased cardiac output, arrhythmias). The signs or occurrence of hypokalemia are more common in cats than in dogs.

2 Review the patient's drug and dietary history. Many drugs and treatments can contribute to hypokalemia.

3 Iatrogenic hypokalemia is common in patients receiving intravenous fluids, especially replacement rather than maintenance fluids. Replacement fluids such as lactated Ringer's solution contain little or no K^+. Intravenous fluids containing glucose or bicarbonate also can cause transcellular shifts of K^+ (driving K^+ into cells).

4 Other causes of transcellular shifts of K^+ include administration of total or partial parenteral nutrition solutions, peritoneal dialysis with K^+-free dialysates, and administration of bicarbonate.

5 Administration of insulin to patients with diabetic ketoacidosis can drive K^+ into cells, causing hypokalemia. Patients usually have whole-body K^+ depletion due to osmotic diuresis, decreased intake, and gastrointestinal losses. Initial serum K^+ concentrations often are normal because of prerenal azotemia, insulin deficiency, and hyperosmolality. Only after insulin is administered does hypokalemia become a problem.

6 Loop and thiazide diuretics cause renal loss of K^+ by increasing flow to the distal convoluted tubules in nephrons.

7 Catecholamine release during acute illness and administration of B_2-agonists such as terbutaline can acutely decrease serum K^+ concentrations.

8 Diets deficient in K^+ and high in protein and acid have been associated with chronic tubulointerstitial nephritis and subsequent hypokalemic nephropathy in cats.

9 Another common cause of hypokalemia in dogs and cats is excessive K^+ loss with vomiting or diarrhea. Pyloric outflow obstruction and vomiting of gastric contents cause hypokalemia and metabolic acidosis. Hypochloridemia and hyponatremia further enhance urinary K^+ losses. Diarrhea also can cause hypokalemia.

10 Decreased oral intake of K^+ alone usually does not cause hypokalemia unless the patient is debilitated or severely anorexic.

11 If the patient has suffered urinary tract obstruction within the previous several days, hypokalemia is likely due to renal loss in postobstructive diuresis.

12 Hypokalemia has been reported in young Burmese cats with acute, recurrent episodes of weakness and increased serum CK concentrations. An intracellular shift of K^+ is suspected. The condition may be similar to hypokalemic periodic paralysis in human beings. There is a familial and inherited basis to the problem, with affected kittens produced in specific lines.

13 If an obvious cause for the hypokalemia has not yet been found, review the serum chemistry profile.

14 K^+ is excreted primarily by renal secretion. Large quantities of K^+ appear in the glomerular ultrafiltrate, but in normally functioning kidneys most K^+ is reabsorbed before reaching the distal tubules. Polyuric chronic renal failure (CRF) is a common cause of hypokalemia in cats and occasionally in dogs. Patients exhibit azotemia (elevated serum creatinine and BUN) in conjunction with a fixed, low urine specific gravity. In CRF patients, residual nephrons maintain K^+ balance by increasing the distal tubular secretion of K^+. Gastrointestinal secretion of K^+ also appears to be increased in CRF.

15 Alkalosis causes hypokalemia by shifting K^+ into cells.

16 Hypomagnesemia is not a common finding in small animals, but it causes enhanced aldosterone secretion, leading to hypokalemia. Hypokalemia may be severe and persistent until magnesium is replaced.

17 Finding hypernatremia, hypokalemia, and metabolic alkalosis should increase the suspicion of primary hyperaldosteronism (primary mineralocorticoid excess), which is often caused by an adrenal adenoma or adenocarcinoma. Abnormal zona glomerulosa tissue produces too much aldosterone. This leads to sodium retention, expansion of the extracellular fluid volume, and increased total body sodium content. K^+ depletion develops, contributing to metabolic alkalosis. The condition is rare but has been reported in both dogs and cats. Episodic weakness is a common presenting sign. Plasma aldosterone concentrations are increased but return to normal if the adrenal mass is removed.

18 Elevated liver enzymes in conjunction with historical signs (PU, PD, polyphagia) and physical examination findings (pendulous abdomen, thin skin, prominent ventral abdominal vessels, hepatomegaly) should alert the clinician to the possibility of hyperadrenocorticism. The mineralocorticoid effects of endogenous glucocorticoid overproduction can cause mild hypokalemia.

19 If acidosis or hyperchloremia is found, check the urine pH. If it is less than 6.0, suspect renal tubular acidosis, an uncommonly recognized renal disorder in veterinary medicine. Renal tubular acidosis is characterized by a hyperchloridemic metabolic acidosis due either to decreased bicarbonate reabsorption or to defective acid excretion in the presence of normal glomerular filtration rates.

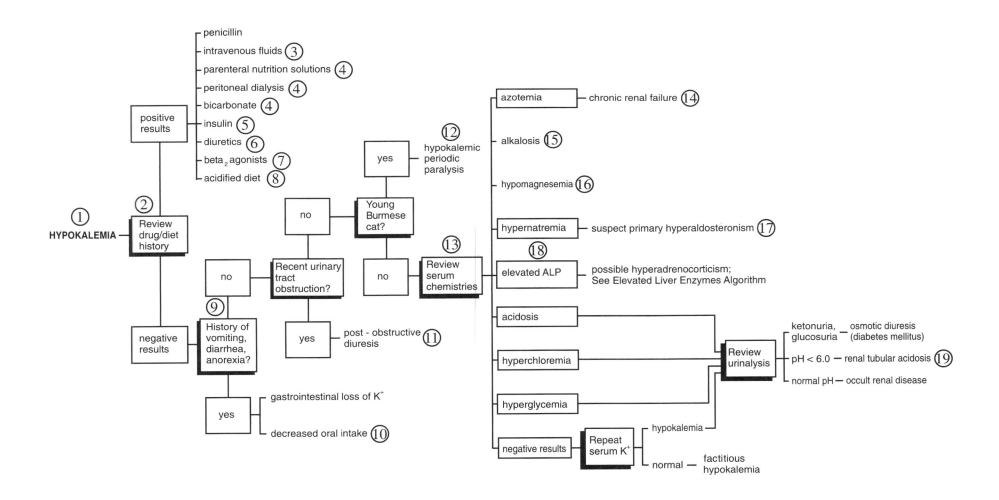

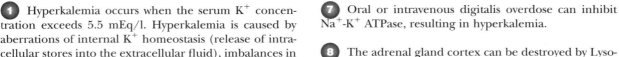

1 Hyperkalemia occurs when the serum K^+ concentration exceeds 5.5 mEq/l. Hyperkalemia is caused by aberrations of internal K^+ homeostasis (release of intracellular stores into the extracellular fluid), imbalances in external K^+ regulation (reduced excretion with or without increased intake), or a combination of both. Muscle weakness and cardiac abnormalities are the most common clinical signs, but nausea, vomiting, ileus, and abdominal pain also can occur. Mild increases in K^+ (5.6–7.0 mEq/l) cause lethargy and depression. If the K^+ concentration is 7.0 mEq/l or higher, muscular weakness and cardiac abnormalities (bradycardia, weak pulses) develop and can be life-threatening. When the serum K^+ concentration exceeds 8–9 mEq/l, impaired cardiac conduction results in heart block, idioventricular complexes, ventricular escape beats, and eventually ventricular fibrillation or asystole. Clinical signs of hyperkalemia are exacerbated by concurrent hyponatremia, hypocalcemia, and acidosis.

2 RBCs in the Akita have higher concentrations of K^+ than those in other breeds. If the blood sample is not analyzed or separated promptly, the serum K^+ concentration may be artificially elevated.

3 Concurrent medications can be an important cause of hyperkalemia. Drug-induced hyperkalemia often implies an underlying organ dysfunction because internal homeostatic mechanisms for K^+ are very effective. In normal patients, drugs usually do not cause K^+ to exceed 5.6 mEq/l unless renal or adrenal dysfunction is present.

4 Parental K^+, given at a more rapid rate than 0.5 mEq/kg/hr, increases the risk of cardiotoxicity. Any K^+ supplement can cause hyperkalemia if multiple forms of supplementation or other K^+-increasing drugs are given, or if occult renal or adrenal disease exists.

5 Massive transfusions using relatively aged blood result in RBC breakdown, which can release enough K^+ to cause hyperkalemia.

6 The K^+ salt of some drugs (e.g., potassium pencillin G) may cause hyperkalemia if given intravenously.

7 Oral or intravenous digitalis overdose can inhibit Na^+-K^+ ATPase, resulting in hyperkalemia.

8 The adrenal gland cortex can be destroyed by Lysodren (*o,p'*-DDD), creating hypoadrenocorticism and hyperkalemia.

9 NSAIDs inhibit aldosterone production by impairing renin secretion and decreasing urine flow.

10 K^+-sparing diuretics (spironolactone and triamterene) act by inhibiting the activity of aldosterone on distal tubular cells or by blocking the entry of Na^+ in the distal and collecting tubules. In normal animals, the plasma aldosterone concentration is relatively low. In dogs with heart failure, it is increased. Therefore, the effect of these diuretics on serum K^+ may be greater in such cases.

11 Prostaglandin inhibitors redistribute K^+.

12 β-blockers inhibit the β-adrenergic action of epinephrine. Epinephrine helps to lower the K^+ concentration.

13 Succinylcholine results in K^+ efflux from muscle cells, especially when repeated doses are given or when the drug is used in patients with intra-abdominal infection, burns, or UMN injuries.

14 Hyperkalemia is a potential complication with angiotensin-converting enzyme (ACE) inhibitors such as captopril and enalapril. It can result from severely reduced glomerular filtration and diminished release of aldosterone. Care should be taken if K^+-sparing diuretics are used in dogs receiving ACE-inhibiting drugs.

15 Massive cellular damage causes rapid release of intracellular K^+ into extracellular fluid. Potential causes of cellular damage include crush injuries, systemic arterial thromboembolism, widespread infections, heat stroke, tumor lysis syndrome, extensive surgery, and excessive seizure activity. With rhabdomyolysis, expect to find increased CK and/or myoglobinuria.

16 Since the kidney is the main route for K^+ excretion from the body, serum K^+ can increase with oliguria, anuria, or urinary outflow obstruction. Signs of urinary outflow obstruction include stranguria, dysuria, pollakiuria, and a large, distended urinary bladder. If the urinary bladder is small or normal, the possibility of renal failure should be eliminated by evaluation of serum chemistries and urinalysis.

17 Pseudohyperkalemia can occur with abnormal WBCs or RBCs in a blood sample (e.g., a hemolyzed blood sample or one with marked leukocytosis [$>100,000/mm^3$] or thrombocytosis [$>1,000,000/mm^3$]). Pseudohyperkalemia occurs as a result of increased release of K^+ from WBCs or RBCs during clotting. Both metabolic and respiratory acidosis can result in redistribution of K^+ and hyperkalemia. Renal failure, especially if acute, is a common cause of reduced K^+ excretion and hyperkalemia. If serum sodium (Na^+) is low in a hyperkalemic patient, hypoadrenocorticism should be suspected and evaluated via an ACTH stimulation test.

18 Hypoadrenocorticism typically causes mental depression, generalized weakness, and gastrointestinal signs (vomiting, diarrhea, and reduced appetite). Azotemia is frequently found along with electrolyte abnormalities.

19 If the ACTH stimulation test is normal, repeat the serum K^+ measurement, making sure that hemolysis does not occur in the sample. If the results are normal and the patient has no clinical signs, assume the original hyperkalemia to be a laboratory error. If the second sample shows hyperkalemia and all potential causes of hyperkalemia have been eliminated, suspect hyperkalemic periodic paralysis.

20 Hyperkalemic periodic paralysis is a rare condition precipitated by exercise, cold, or K^+ administration. It is diagnosed by eliminating other causes of hyperkalemia. Clinical signs often worsen with oral K^+ loading.

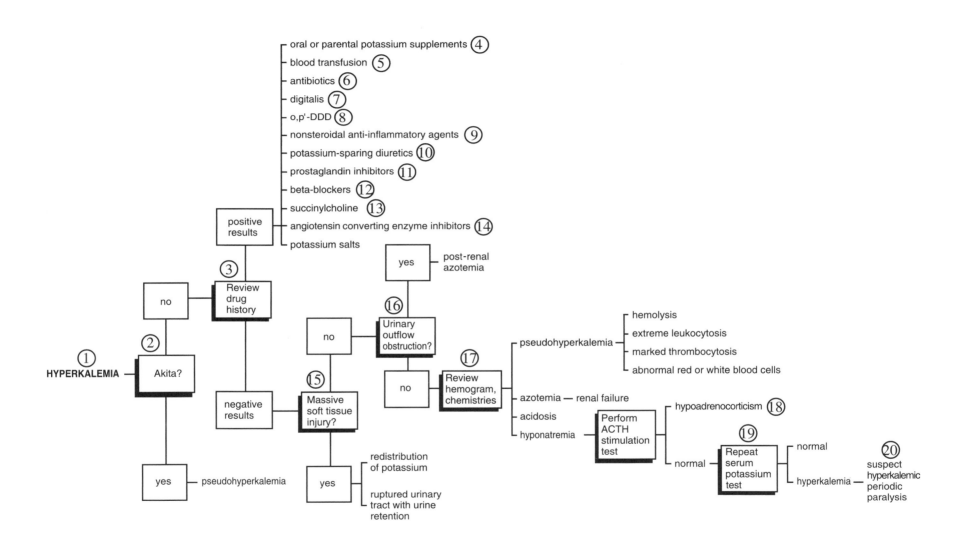

① **HYPERKALEMIA**

② Akita?

yes — pseudohyperkalemia

no

③ Review drug history

positive results

- oral or parental potassium supplements ④
- blood transfusion ⑤
- antibiotics ⑥
- digitalis ⑦
- o,p'-DDD ⑧
- nonsteroidal anti-inflammatory agents ⑨
- potassium-sparing diuretics ⑩
- prostaglandin inhibitors ⑪
- beta-blockers ⑫
- succinylcholine ⑬
- angiotensin converting enzyme inhibitors ⑭
- potassium salts

negative results

⑮ Massive soft tissue injury?

yes
- redistribution of potassium
- ruptured urinary tract with urine retention

no

⑯ Urinary outflow obstruction?

yes — post-renal azotemia

no

⑰ Review hemogram, chemistries

pseudohyperkalemia
- hemolysis
- extreme leukocytosis
- marked thrombocytosis
- abnormal red or white blood cells

azotemia — renal failure

acidosis

hyponatremia

Perform ACTH stimulation test
- hypoadrenocorticism ⑱
- normal

⑲ Repeat serum potassium test
- normal
- hyperkalemia — ⑳ suspect hyperkalemic periodic paralysis

1 For most laboratories, serum calcium (Ca^{2+}) concentrations below 8.5–9 mg/dl are considered lower than normal. In dogs, the serum Ca^{2+} concentration is closely linked to the serum albumin concentration. In hypoalbuminemic patients, serum Ca^{2+} needs to be corrected to determine whether patients actually are hypocalcemic. Clinical signs of hypocalcemia generally consist of acute-onset neuromuscular problems that worsen with exercise and excitement. Signs include restlessness, panting, nervousness, muscle twitching, and rubbing the face as if it is intensely pruritic. Patients also may appear to have diffuse pain. As serum Ca^{2+} falls, clinical signs progress to muscle tremors, ataxia, muscle rigidity, stiffening of the gait, facial rictus, seizure activity, or severe tetanic muscle spasms. Seizure activity due to hypocalcemia is unlikely to respond to anticonvulsants, although sedation may reduce muscle spasms temporarily. Severe clinical signs are most commonly seen in patients with puerperal tetany (eclampsia) and primary hypoparathyroidism and in patients that become hypocalcemic iatrogenically (after removal of productive parathyroid adenomas or accidental removal of the parathyroid glands in conjunction with thyroidectomy). Hypoalbuminemic patients who are hypocalcemic do not usually have clinical signs of hypocalcemia (because the ionized Ca^{2+} concentration is normal in the majority of these patients). Patients with true hypocalcemia resulting from renal failure (renal secondary hyperparathyroidism), pancreatitis, nutritional secondary hyperparathyroidism, and intestinal disease also rarely present with clinical signs of hypocalcemia, because generally hypocalcemia is mild (Ca^{2+} above 7 mg/dl).

2 Common causes of hypocalcemia include laboratory error, placing the sample in an EDTA-containing blood tube, and hypoalbuminemia. In any patient with low serum Ca^{2+} who is not exhibiting clinical signs, the Ca^{2+} concentration should be reevaluated in conjunction with measurement of serum albumin concentration to allow the correction to be made. Note that serum Ca^{2+} may still be low after correction; therefore, it should not be assumed that serum Ca^{2+} is low just because the patient is hypoalbuminemic. Measurement of ionized calcium is useful if it can be checked in house (on a blood gas machine) since it may be normal in patients that do not have appropriate clinical signs of hypocalcemia. Ionized Ca^{2+} concentrations represent Ca^{2+} actually available to the body.

3 Physical examination may indicate lactation (suggesting eclampsia), diarrhea (suggesting intestinal disorders), or oral ulceration, pale mucous membranes, and poor body condition (suggesting renal disease). Clients should be questioned about known preexisting conditions (e.g., renal failure); recent thyroid, parathyroid, or cervical surgery; diet (particularly unusual or homemade diets fed to young animals); recent whelping/kittening and heavy lactation; possible exposure to ethylene glycol; and concurrent drug administration.

4 Nutritional secondary hyperparathyroidism may develop in dogs and cats fed diets with a relative deficiency of Ca^{2+} and a high phosphorus concentration (e.g., liver, a meat-based diet with no bones/bone meal). Low Ca^{2+}-phosphorus ratios are particular problems in young animals on deficient diets and those fed such diets chronically. Problems generally do not arise as a result of hypocalcemia, which is either mild or transient, but are secondary to the body's efforts to maintain serum Ca^{2+} in the normal range in the face of dietary deficiency. As serum parathyroid hormone (PTH) concentrations rise, Ca^{2+} and phosphorus are removed from bone. Serum concentrations of Ca^{2+} are maintained and phosphorus is excreted. This leads to a chronic drain on bone stores of Ca^{2+} and phosphorus, progressive demineralization, bone pain, increased fragility, and eventually pathological fractures. Imaging bones (radiographically or via bone scans to demonstrate increased bone turnover) may be helpful in confirming the diagnosis, as may measurement of serum concentrations of PTH, ionized Ca^{2+}, and vitamin D.

5 Recent parathyroidectomy (for primary hyperparathyroidism) or thyroidectomy can result in hypocalcemia. In patients with primary hyperparathyroidism, removal of the abnormal (adenomatous) parathyroid gland temporarily removes the body's main source of PTH, which is responsible for maintaining serum calcium concentrations. The remaining normal glands are chronically suppressed by the abnormal tissue, and recovery of function in these glands may take 3 to 4 months. During the recovery period, patients need supplementation with vitamin D and sometimes also with calcium. Patients that have undergone thyroidectomy, particularly bilateral thyroidectomy for neoplasia or adenomatous hyperplasia of the thyroid gland, may lose all four parathyroid glands during the procedure, leading to permanent hypoparathyroidism and a need for lifelong supplementation with vitamin D and calcium. Clinical signs of hypocalcemia generally are severe in these patients and develop within 1 to 7 days of surgery.

6 Many therapeutic agents are known to cause hypocalcemia. In approximate order of likelihood of administration, these are glucocorticoids, anticonvulsants, phosphate-containing enemas, potassium phosphate (injectable), citrate-containing solutions (injectable), sodium bicarbonate (injectable), potassium EDTA (injectable), mithramycin, and salmon calcitonin. Phosphate-containing enemas may be a particular problem in cats, especially if used in dehydrated patients and those with megacolon.

7 Metabolites of ethylene glycol chelate Ca^{2+} and cause hypocalcemia. Often neurological signs such as muscle tremors and seizures develop quickly following patient exposure. They precede azotemia by 12 to 24 hours and may have resolved by the time that condition develops. If there is suspected exposure to ethylene glycol, either accidentally or maliciously, blood must be tested as soon as possible. This should be done even if exposure is unlikely because of the need for therapy to be initiated within 12 to 24 hours of exposure, and before patients become azotemic, to be successful. If there is no chance of exposure (i.e., the patient is indoors only, no ethylene glycol is available, the patient is closely observed, etc.), this step may be bypassed. Urine (if available) can be evaluated under ultraviolet light (e.g., a Wood's lamp) since many ethylene glycol–containing fluids also contain a dye that causes urine to fluoresce.

8 Eclampsia or puerperal tetany is an acute, life-threatening condition seen in lactating bitches and queens, especially those with large litters where the demand for milk is high. It is most common in small-breed dogs. Neuromuscular signs in lactating animals should be assumed to be due to eclampsia until proven otherwise.

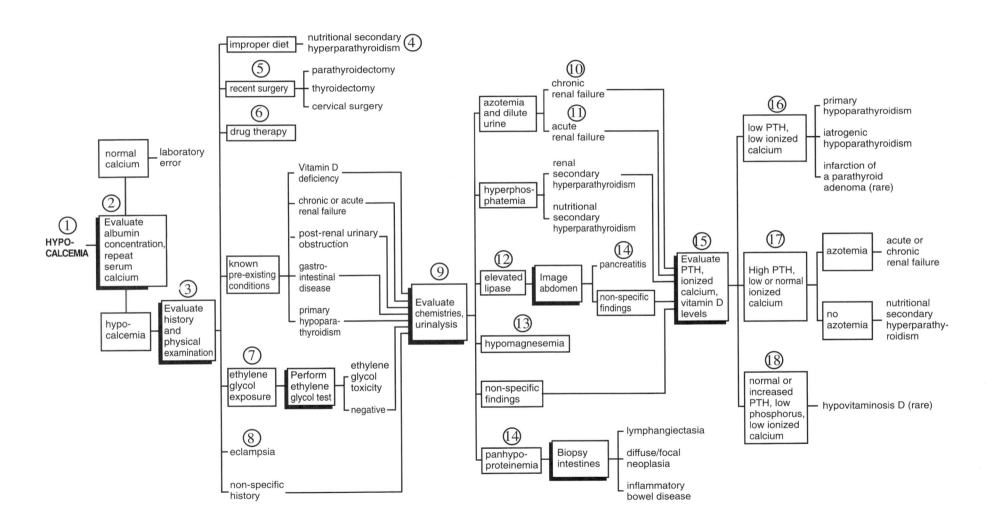

9 A minimum database of laboratory work is likely to have been obtained earlier in the diagnostic process and will be the source from which the original problem of hypocalcemia was generated. Laboratory findings should be combined with physical examination findings (e.g., diarrhea, abdominal pain) to guide diagnostic testing from this point.

10 Although hypocalcemia is not particularly common with CRF, the high frequency of CRF in the canine and particularly the feline population makes this a relatively common cause of hypocalcemia overall. Hypocalcemia is generally mild and rarely is associated with clinical signs unless chronic secondary renal hyperparathyroidism leads to severe bone loss and pathological fractures.

11 Hypocalcemia may be more significant in patients with acute renal failure (ARF) because of the dramatic, acute increase in serum phosphorus concentrations that develops with this condition and with blunting of compensatory mechanisms. Hypocalcemia is seen particularly with acute, life-threatening problems such as postrenal urinary obstruction, which leads to acute, dramatic hyperphosphatemia, hyperkalemia, azotemia, and hypocalcemia. Such patients also may develop seizures, although it is difficult to know whether these are related to hypocalcemia alone or are due to a combination of severe metabolic derangements.

12 In patients with elevated serum lipase on the chemistry profile, the history and physical examination findings should be reassessed for evidence of pancreatitis. This includes recent dietary indiscretion, exposure to drugs known to cause pancreatitis (L-asparaginase, azathioprine, and possibly glucocorticoids), vomiting, anorexia, fever, cranial abdominal pain, and tenderness. Laboratory results also should be evaluated for leukocytosis, elevated amylase (very nonspecific), and evidence of increases in bilirubin and alkaline phosphatase that might suggest biliary obstruction secondary to pancreatic swelling. Hypocalcemia resulting from pancreatitis is usually mild to moderate and is not associated with neurological or neuromuscular signs. The exact mechanism for the development of hypocalcemia is unknown, but theoretically it is related to precipitation of calcium secondary to saponification of fat around the inflamed pancreas.

13 Hypomagnesemia may result in hypocalcemia due to refractoriness to or reduced synthesis of PTH. Currently, this has not been proven to occur in veterinary patients, but it should be borne in mind if magnesium is particularly low on the serum chemistry profile.

14 Patients with low total serum protein (i.e., panhypoproteinemia) may have underlying gastrointestinal disease resulting in protein loss through the intestinal mucosa. Correction of serum Ca^{2+} for the low serum albumin may not raise Ca^{2+} to the normal range. Clinical signs of hypocalcemia are rare with gastrointestinal disease, but they have been reported with lymphangiectasia. In this condition obstructed intestinal lacteals leak chyle, resulting in protein and fat (chylomicron) loss into the bowel. It is postulated that in lymphangiectasia Ca^{2+} precipitates out in tissues around obstructed and inflamed lacteals in a process very similar to that of saponification of fat in pancreatitis. Further investigation of protein-losing enteropathy requires gastrointestinal biopsy via upper endoscopy or exploratory surgery.

15 When nonspecific results are obtained from the minimum database or conditions such as nutritional or renal secondary hyperparathyroidism are suspected but not confirmed, it is useful to measure serum concentrations of PTH, ionized Ca^{2+}, and vitamin D to facilitate the diagnosis of hypocalcemia.

16 Low PTH with low ionized Ca^{2+} confirms primary hypoparathyroidism (or iatrogenic hypoparathyroidism if there is an appropriate surgical history). Primary hypoparathyroidism is rare in both dogs and cats. Reported patient age range is wide (6 weeks to 13 years in dogs and 6 months to 7 years in cats). There are very rare case reports of patients with primary hyperparathyroidism that go on to develop acute hypocalcemia. It is postulated that this is due to infarction and acute necrosis of a parathyroid adenoma.

17 Patients with low or normal ionized Ca^{2+} concentrations and high circulating PTH concentrations are likely to have renal or nutritional secondary hyperparathyroidism.

18 Hypovitaminosis D occurs in patients that are young, receiving diets deficient in vitamin D, and that have no exposure to sunlight (rickets). Rickets and its adult equivalent (osteomalacia) are extremely rare in cats and dogs. Radiographs identify the characteristic skeletal abnormalities in young, growing patients, including axial and radial growth-plate thickening and cupping of adjacent metaphyses. Additional findings are osteopenia and bowed diaphyses. Affected animals may be lame or reluctant to walk. There may be enlargement of costochondral junctions and flaring of the metaphyses.

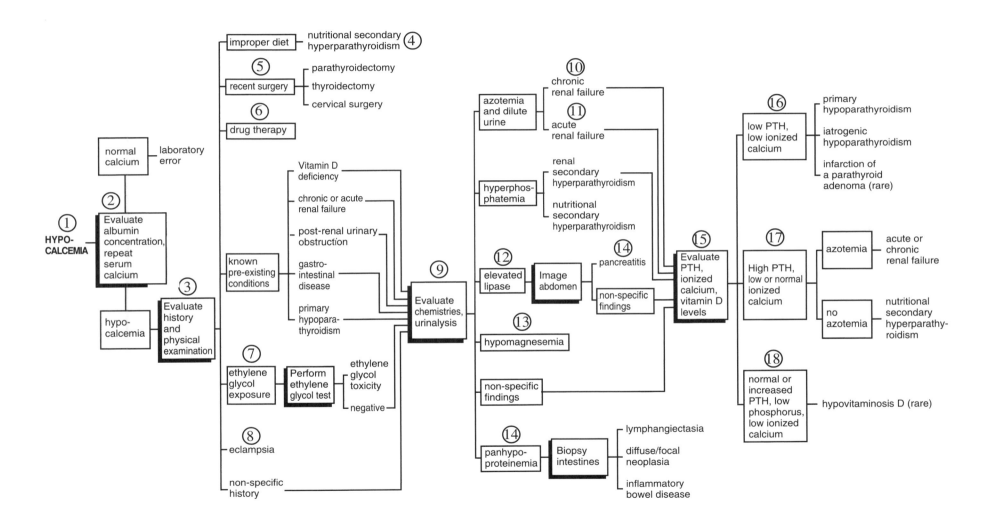

1 Ca^{2+} stores in the body are regulated by antagonistic activities of PTH and calcitonin. The former is produced from the parathyroid glands in response to low serum Ca^{2+}, thereby increasing Ca^{2+} removal from bone, intestinal absorption, and reabsorption from renal distal convoluted tubules. Usually increased serum Ca^{2+} exerts a negative feedback on parathyroid gland production of PTH. Most laboratories consider serum Ca^{2+} above 11–12 mg/dl to be elevated. In dogs, serum Ca^{2+} and albumin are linked, and a correction factor is applied in hypoalbuminemic dogs ([3.5 g/dl − actual serum albumin] + measured serum Ca^{2+} = actual serum Ca^{2+}). This formula has not been validated for cats or for cases in which albumin is in the normal range or high. Patients with elevated serum Ca^{2+} concentrations can have signs related to the underlying cause (e.g., peripheral lymphadenopathy with lymphoma, tenesmus due to an anal sac mass) or can present with nonspecific problems such as nausea, anorexia, and weight loss. Anorexia can be due to primary intestinal lymphoma, hypercalcemia, or renal failure secondary to hypercalcemia (especially if the Ca^{2+} × phosphorus product exceeds 70). Severe hypercalcemia causes muscle weakness, neurological problems, tachyarrhythmias, and premature heartbeats. Fluid diuresis is an effective method of reducing Ca^{2+} that does not interfere with diagnosis of the underlying condition.

2 Ca^{2+} should be rechecked with concurrent albumin to allow correction if needed. Serum should be evaluated for lipemia since this can artifactually increase Ca^{2+}. Normocalcemic patients with a history of hypercalcemia and appropriate clinical signs or underlying conditions should have Ca^{2+} evaluated several more times, as some tumors secrete PTH-related polypeptide (PTHrP) intermittently or produce other factors (interleukins, tumor necrosis factor) that cause hypercalcemia.

3 The history should include a review of preexisting conditions, toxin exposure, and drug use. Drugs causing hypercalcemia include testosterone, other anabolic steroids, progesterone, estrogen, vitamin D, and oral phosphate binders. Cholecalciferol-containing rodenticides cause vitamin D intoxication, anorexia, lethargy, weakness, hematemesis, and melena. Laboratory tests show hyperphosphatemia and hypercalcemia, and patients develop dystrophic tissue mineralization and ARF. Measure vitamin D, its metabolites, and ionized Ca^{2+} to confirm the condition. Preexisting conditions that can result in hypercalcemia include renal failure, neoplasia, hypoadrenocorticism, and various granulomatous diseases. Physical examination looks for masses because many underlying causes of hypercalcemia are neoplastic (lymphoma, plasma cell myeloma, anal sac apocrine gland adenocarcinoma). These induce hypercalcemia by release of PTHrP and other humoral effects. It is rare for primary bone tumors to cause hypercalcemia, but tumors with multiple bony metastases (e.g., mammary adenocarcinoma) can produce enough osteolysis to cause hypercalcemia. Plasma cell myeloma, bone marrow lymphoma, and cancer metastatic to bone are difficult to diagnose on physical examination alone. Patients may have nonspecific signs such as fever, hyperviscosity, and poorly localizable pain.

4 Dehydration and hemoconcentration can cause mild hypercalcemia. A history of water deprivation or heat shock is useful. Reassess Ca^{2+} after rehydration.

5 Screening for tumor metastasis involves three-view thoracic radiographs, abdominal ultrasound, and bone radiographs.

6 Excisional biopsy of single neoplastic masses should be performed when possible. After removal of neoplastic tissue, a fall in Ca^{2+} concentration into/below the normal range suggests that all neoplastic tissue has been removed. Ongoing elevation suggests residual tumor or another cause of hypercalcemia.

7 Peripheral lymphadenopathy (one or more nodes) or enlargement of hematopoietic organs (liver, spleen) is an indication for fine-needle aspiration and cytology. If cells suggest tumor other than lymphoma, go back to step 5. When tumor cells are found in a node, the regions drained by that node should be checked and the tumor should be considered to have metastasized regionally.

8 If lymphoma is diagnosed, assess the extent of tumor tissue within the body for the prognosis. Staging includes evaluation of other nodes, thoracic radiographs, abdominal ultrasound, and bone marrow aspiration. Test cats for FeLV/FIV since status can alter the prognosis. Hypercalcemia can be associated with shorter remissions.

9 When testing to this point is negative, reevaluate laboratory tests. Patients with normal or low phosphorus have hypercalcemia of malignancy or hyperparathyroidism. Elevated phosphorus suggests renal failure or osteolysis. The hemogram occasionally reveals neoplastic cells in the circulation (lymphoblasts in stage V lymphoma or lymphoblastic leukemia or occasionally other cell types in rarer leukemias). More commonly, the hemogram shows marrow suppression (because tumors decrease normal cell production without entering the circulation themselves) or nonregenerative anemia (because sequestration of iron within the marrow prevents RBC production). Elevated serum globulins result from inflammation, chronic antigenic stimulation, or neoplasia. Serum protein electrophoresis (SPE) can help the diagnosis (see the algorithm for hyperglobulinemia). Elevated Na^+ and low/normal K^+ and chloride suggest hypoadrenocorticism. Note that it is the glucocorticoid and not the mineralocorticoid deficiency that causes hypercalcemia; therefore, this can occur without the other electrolyte abnormalities. Patients with hypercalcemia, gastrointestinal signs, or episodic weakness and collapse should undergo ACTH stimulation testing. Azotemia with dilute urine is diagnostic of renal failure. This can be acute (secondary to hypercalcemia) or chronic (possibly causing hypercalcemia). Patients are hyperphosphatemic and hence hypercalcemic due to secondary renal hyperparathyroidism. Hypercalcemia is uncommon with CRF (10–20% of cases).

10 Urinalysis detects glomerular loss of albumin or sometimes other small proteins resulting from glomerular immune complex deposition in neoplastic or immune-mediated conditions. Urine dipstick evaluation is sensitive to albumin. If protein is detected via spectrophotometry (measuring urine protein/creatinine ratios), and especially if this is positive but the dipstick is negative, there may be Bence Jones proteinuria (rare in dogs and cats). This can be confirmed via urine protein electrophoresis looking for a monoclonal spike. In patients that fit the criteria for diagnosis of multiple myeloma (Bence Jones proteinuria, monoclonal spike on SPE, bone pain, lytic bone lesions), the clinician should progress straight to bone marrow aspiration.

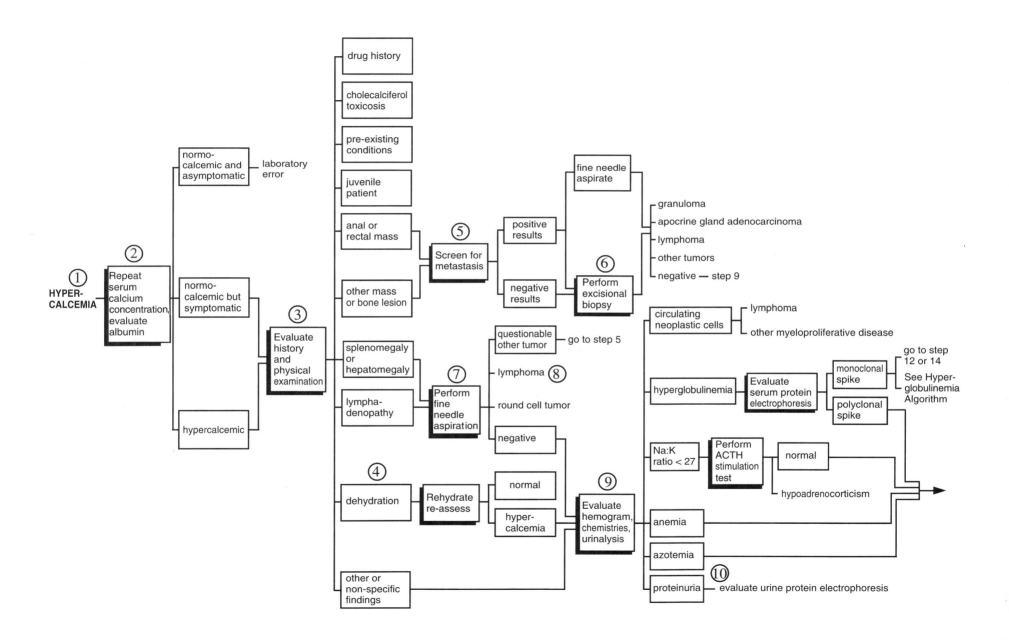

11 Low or normal ionized Ca^{2+} is present with high serum Ca^{2+} only in hypoadrenocorticism (rare) or renal disease.

12 In patients with hypercalcemia and nonspecific laboratory findings or renal disease, serum PTH and PTHrP should be evaluated (PTHrP is produced by some malignant cells) to try to determine the underlying cause of the hypercalcemia. Since this assay takes 5–10 days, is temperature sensitive, is not 100% accurate (like all assays), and is affected by azotemia, it may be appropriate to perform further tests while awaiting the results. The test is most useful to establish a diagnosis of primary hyperparathyroidism. Testing to be performed concurrently includes imaging the kidneys (especially with ultrasound) to evaluate for gross evidence of disease/structural changes. Note that increased cortical echodensity can develop secondary to hypercalcemia.

13 Low PTH with elevated PTHrP suggests malignancy as an underlying cause of hypercalcemia and patients should be reevaluated, starting with steps 3 and 4 and progressing to bone marrow evaluation.

14 If multiple myeloma or lymphoma confined to bone marrow is suspected based on the PTH/PTHrP assay and the results of prior diagnostic testing, radiographs of the skeleton (starting with the vertebrae and pelvis before going on to the long bones) may be indicated. However, finding lytic bone lesions will not confirm the diagnosis unless Bence Jones proteinuria and a monoclonal serum protein spike have been detected, in which case the majority of patients can be diagnosed as having multiple myeloma.

15 In patients without radiographic evidence of lytic bone lesions, it is necessary to progress to bone marrow evaluation. It may be appropriate to recheck the PTH/PTHrP assay for confirmation (usually unnecessary since the majority of hypercalcemic patients have underlying neoplasia). Bone scans (nuclear scintigraphy) may be contemplated to identify areas of increased bone turnover. In the majority of patients, bone radiographs or scans are used only to guide the area sampled for marrow evaluation since not all tumors extend to all areas of the marrow.

16 Bone marrow aspiration may be performed under general anesthesia or heavy sedation (good analgesia is required if sedation is elected, and this is not recommended for small dogs and cats).

17 "Cold" myeloma has lytic bone lesions or no obvious radiographic lesions and is negative on a bone scan (there is no evidence of bone turnover).

18 Chronic granulomatous conditions rarely result in hypercalcemia. These can be screened for by thoracic radiography, abdominal ultrasound, or other imaging modalities.

19 Vitamin D toxicosis/hypervitaminosis D causes hypercalcemia in the absence of elevations of PTH/PTHrP. This condition results from cholecalciferol-containing rodenticides, excessive vitamin D supplementation, and ingestion of plants such as *Cestrum diurnum*, *Solanum malacoxylon*, and *Trisetum flavescens*. The situation may be further clarified via the history and by measuring vitamin D and its metabolites as part of the PTH/ionized calcium assay.

20 Localized bone lesions can cause hypercalcemia with low PTH and normal PTHrP because of osteolysis. This is a very rare cause of hypercalcemia. Patients should be evaluated for single bone lesions (neoplasia, osteomyelitis) or hypertrophic osteodystrophy in young dogs. Occasionally, elevated serum calcium may be seen in giant-breed dogs 6 to 12 months of age. Rarely, hypercalcemia occurs with disuse osteoporosis.

21 Rarely, hypercalcemia has been seen with fungal infection (blastomycosis, coccidioidomycosis) without gross evidence of bone involvement.

22 Azotemic patients should be evaluated for renal disease as a cause of hypercalcemia. Evaluation can consist of renal ultrasound or tests that assess glomerular filtration (creatinine, inulin, or iohexol clearance testing) if appropriate.

23 If renal function appears normal or renal failure appears acute, and therefore secondary to hypercalcemia rather than the cause of the problem, the patient may have primary hyperparathyroidism. This generally is a disease of dogs older than 10 years, and poodles and keeshonds reportedly are overrepresented. In patients with appropriate signalment, the parathyroid glands should be evaluated by either cervical ultrasound or exploratory surgery. While ultrasound is ideal, being minimally invasive, a skilled and experienced operator is needed to obtain an accurate impression of the parathyroid glands. Exploratory surgery may worsen renal function in an azotemic patient because of the anesthesia, but it is a relatively straightforward procedure. Enlargement of all glands suggests that renal disease is the underlying cause of hypercalcemia. Enlargement of one gland suggests primary hyperparathyroidism, generally due to a benign adenoma. This tumor should be removed surgically and submitted for histopathology while serum calcium is closely monitored postoperatively.

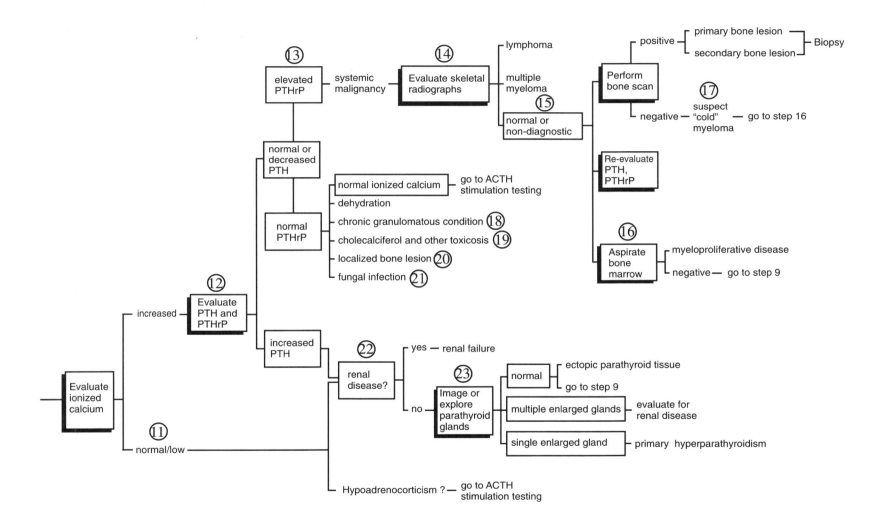

1 Hyperlipidemia is increased lipid in the blood. Lipid types include chylomicrons (triglyceride, cholesterol, and phospholipid combinations), very low density lipoproteins (VLDLs), low density lipoproteins (LDLs), and high density lipoproteins (HDLs). It is HDLs that predominate in dogs and cats, making them less predisposed to LDL-associated cholesterol elevations and atherosclerosis. Patients with grossly lipemic serum usually have elevated triglycerides. Hypertriglyceridemia can cause changes in serum ranging from mild haziness (triglycerides >300 mg/dl) to a very milky appearance (triglycerides >2500 mg/dl). Elevated serum cholesterol rarely affects serum opacity unless it is very severe. Hyperlipidemia most commonly is secondary to underlying metabolic problems. A variety of disease states (e.g., diabetes mellitus) may alter the lipoprotein profile. Patients may be asymptomatic, and abnormalities are picked up on routine laboratory tests. However, CNS depression, behavior changes, and seizures may occur with severe triglyceride and cholesterol elevations. These occur most commonly in patients with primary hyperlipidemias. There also may be peripheral neurological abnormalities as a result of xanthomas (lipid and cholesterol deposits) compressing individual nerves, especially around foraminae in the skull and spinal cord. Xanthomas also develop in the skin at sites of trauma. Other presentations of hyperlipidemia include nonspecific abdominal pain, pancreatic inflammation and diabetes mellitus (it is difficult to know whether hyperlipidemia is the cause or the result of the pancreatic inflammation), insulin resistance, glucose intolerance, and hypertension. There may be clinical signs of primary conditions underlying hyperlipidemia. These include PU, PD, and polyphagia in patients with diabetes mellitus and hyperadrenocorticism, muscle loss and weight gain with hyperadrenocorticism, weight gain and cold intolerance with hypothyroidism, weight loss and peripheral neuropathy with diabetes mellitus, and vomiting and fever with pancreatitis. Finally, patients may have ocular abnormalities including corneal opacities, lipid infiltration of the globe of the eye, and visible lipemia in aqueous humor and ocular blood vessels.

2 The first step in testing any patient with milky serum or high serum concentrations of triglycerides or cholesterol is to determine whether the patient has been fasted. If not, the patient should be fasted for 12 to 18 hours and laboratory tests rechecked. It is important to try to clear serum since gross lipemia may produce artificial elevations in bilirubin; lower cholesterol, chlorides, amylase, and lipase; and affect the ability of instruments to measure Hb and plasma proteins.

3 An extremely high-fat diet has to be fed to produce consistent hyperlipidemia; however, dogs fed diets with 67% of calories as fat (as opposed to the typical maintenance diet, which has 16% of calories as fat) show marked hyperlipidemia and a shift in lipoproteins to LDLs. Patients on very-high-fat diets (e.g., sled dogs) that have hyperlipidemia and associated clinical problems should be switched to lower-fat diets and reassessed in about 1 month. Patients suspected of having primary hyperlipidemia should be placed on a low-fat, high-fiber diet, and laboratory tests should be reassessed in a month.

4 Many secondary causes of hyperlipidemia (e.g., hyperadrenocorticism, hypothyroidism, diabetes mellitus, hepatic disease resulting in cholestasis) develop in middle-aged and older animals, while congenital or familial problems may be seen in younger animals. Hyperadrenocorticism and hypothyroidism are much rarer in cats than in dogs, while diabetes mellitus and cholestatic liver disease are fairly common in both species. Miniature schnauzers and beagles are predisposed to primary hyperlipidemias but also are commonly diagnosed with many secondary causes of hyperlipidemia. Further testing may be required to exclude these possibilities.

5 Glucocorticoid administration in both dogs and cats may lead to steroid hepatopathy and mild cholestasis. Glucocorticoids also stimulate lipolysis, causing mild to moderate increases in serum cholesterol. Progestogen-containing compounds such as megestrol acetate may result in hyperlipidemia, mainly because they are diabetogenic.

6 Evaluation of a serum chemistry profile and urinalysis helps the diagnosis of some causes of secondary hyperlipidemia, including diabetes mellitus, hepatobiliary dysfunction, and pancreatitis. The results also can increase the suspicion of hypothyroidism, hyperadrenocorticism, renal disease, and pancreatic inflammation, and allow determination of the magnitude of the hyperlipidemia and whether triglycerides, cholesterol, or both are contributing to it.

7 Diabetes mellitus is diagnosed by identifying persistent hyperglycemia (above the renal tubular threshold of 180–220 mg/dl in dogs and 290 mg/dl in cats) with concurrent glycosuria. It is a common cause of marked hypertriglyceridemia and moderate hypercholesterolemia. Insulin is needed for the normal production and activity of the enzyme lipoprotein lipase. Diabetic patients also may have changes in the normal distribution of lipoproteins. Persistent hyperlipidemia may result in pancreatic inflammation and transient diabetes mellitus. Therefore, it is important to do follow-up laboratory testing to determine which abnormalities are primary and which are secondary.

8 The serum chemistry profile may help to confirm the diagnosis of pancreatitis in a patient with an appropriate history, clinical signs (e.g., fever, lethargy, depression, vomiting, diarrhea, and cranial abdominal pain), and leukocytosis on a hemogram. The fasting serum chemistry profile may indicate elevation of serum lipase (and amylase), hypertriglyceridemia, and/or hypercholesterolemia. Note, however, that a conclusive diagnosis of pancreatitis can be difficult to make in dogs and particularly in cats. A percentage of animals with pancreatitis will exhibit only some of the clinical signs and laboratory findings noted above. Further evaluation, including abdominal radiographs, abdominal ultrasound, and even exploratory surgery for tissue biopsy, may be required to confirm the diagnosis (see the algorithm for elevated amylase and lipase). In addition, hyperlipidemia itself is thought to predispose patients to pancreatitis, possibly due to hyperchylomicronemia causing pancreatic ischemia and necrosis. It is important to follow up on patients after pancreatitis resolves to determine whether or not hyperlipidemia persists.

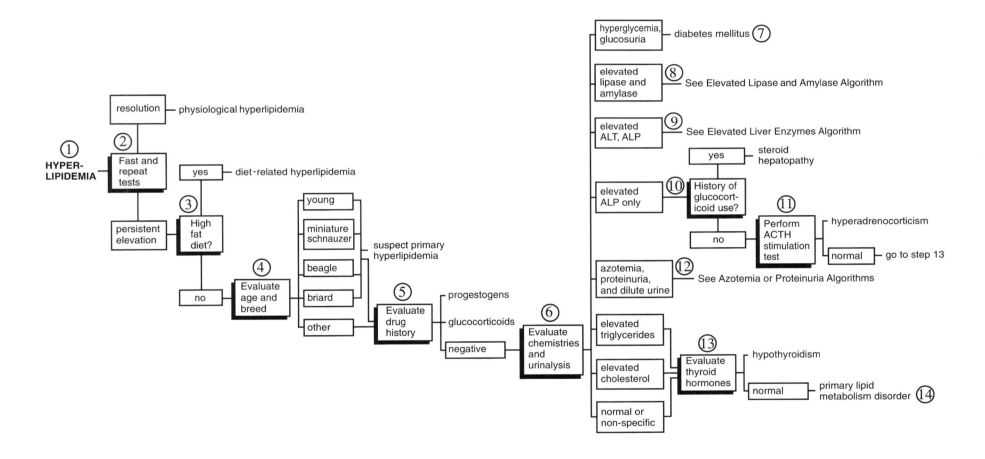

9 Liver disorders are common causes of hyperlipidemia. Cholestatic conditions mainly cause hypercholesterolemia. Cholestasis may be intrahepatic (as a result of hepatocyte inflammation and swelling obstructing biliary canaliculi) or extrahepatic (within the gallbladder and common bile duct). Elevations of serum concentrations of hepatic enzymes signal cholestatic and other hepatic disorders. Serum ALP frequently is increased, since this originates in cells lining the biliary system. However, there also may be ALT elevations because hepatocytes are secondarily affected by biliary system disease or because of primary hepatocellular damage and secondary intrahepatic biliary stasis. Serum bilirubin elevations also may develop in patients with significant hepatobiliary obstruction. Common hepatic diseases in dogs and cats that lead to hyperlipidemia include hepatic lipidosis in cats, acute hepatitis, and hepatic necrosis. Hepatobiliary problems include partial or complete obstruction of the extrahepatic biliary tree by neoplastic masses in the bowel, pancreas, or biliary system, pancreatic inflammation, immune-mediated or suppurative cholangiohepatitis, or, rarely, choleliths. Further diagnostic testing for hepatobiliary disease may include hepatic function testing, ultrasound or other diagnostic imaging, and hepatic biopsy (see the algorithm for liver enzyme elevations).

10 In patients with elevated ALP and cholesterol (and sometimes triglycerides) but no other indications of hepatobiliary disease (e.g., normal bilirubin, ALT), the drug history should be re-reviewed for exogenous glucocorticoid administration. Any exogenous glucocorticoid should be discontinued if possible and laboratory tests reassessed several weeks to months later (depending on the duration of action of the glucocorticoid preparation used) before pursuing further diagnostic testing.

11 If there is no history of exogenous glucocorticoid administration, the history and physical examination should be assessed for indications of endogenous overproduction of glucocorticoids. Suggestive findings include PU, PD, polyphagia, weight gain, muscle loss, changes in body shape (pot-bellied appearance) and reduced haircoat quality, alopecia, thinning of the skin, calcinosis cutis, comedones, hepatomegaly, excessive panting, and behavior changes. Patients should be evaluated for hyperadrenocorticism by means of appropriate screening tests (ACTH stimulation test, urine cortisol/creatinine ratio, low-dose dexamethasone suppression test and abdominal ultrasound to evaluate adrenal gland size and structure). Patients with hyperadrenocorticism generally develop mild hyperlipidemia, probably as a result of insulin resistance and alteration in the function of lipoprotein lipase. Hyperadrenocorticism is very rare in cats.

12 Patients with subclinical renal disease may only have persistently dilute urine. This requires further diagnostic testing (e.g., measurement of GFR or a renal biopsy). Patients with more overt renal disease have azotemia with dilute urine. Hypercholesterolemia (mild to moderate), proteinuria, hypoalbuminemia, and azotemia may develop with nephrotic syndrome (secondary to renal glomerulonephritis or amyloidosis). The serum albumin concentration is inversely correlated with the serum cholesterol concentration. Hypercholesterolemia in nephrotic syndrome is thought to be the result of a number of factors, including hypoalbuminemia stimulating VLDL production by the liver, reduced catabolism of lipoproteins, and a relative loss of low molecular weight proteins in the urine. It should be noted that restricted protein diets fed to patients with renal failure also have been implicated as a cause of hypercholesterolemia because of their higher fat content.

13 Canine patients with appropriate clinical signs (e.g., weight gain, poor haircoat, dermatological problems, lethargy, cold intolerance) and hypercholesterolemia or hypertriglyceridemia and those with no other specific findings on laboratory tests should be evaluated for hypothyroidism. Since concurrent disease states may suppress total thyroxine (T_4) and triiodothyronine (T_3) concentrations, a full thyroid panel (free T_4 measured by equilibrium dialysis, thyroid-stimulating hormone [TSH] concentration, and possibly T_3 and T_4 autoantibodies) should be evaluated. Hypothyroidism is very rare in feline patients. Even cats undergoing radioactive iodine therapy or surgery for hyperthyroidism rarely show clinical signs of hypothyroidism.

14 Very young animals with hyperlipidemia, breeds reported to have primary hyperlipidemia, and patients in which no other underlying cause of hyperlipidemia has been found should be evaluated for primary idiopathic hyperlipidemia and a number of other conditions resulting from abnormal lipid metabolism. Sometimes the breed suggests a likely disorder. Miniature schnauzers and beagles with primary idiopathic hyperlipidemia have moderate to severe elevations of serum triglycerides (and sometimes hypercholesterolemia) that may not respond to dietary management. Briard dogs with primary hypercholesterolemia have mild to moderate elevations of serum cholesterol and no hypertriglyceridemia. Other breeds and species may have abnormal lipid metabolism that results in elevations of triglycerides, cholesterol, or both. Cats are reported to have a primary inherited hyperchylomicronemia and other inherited disorders of lipid metabolism. Lipoprotein electrophoresis will help to map out the distribution of serum lipids and lipoproteins in such cases to see whether they fit previously described cases. Precipitation techniques allow more quantitation of the different lipid and lipoprotein classes found.

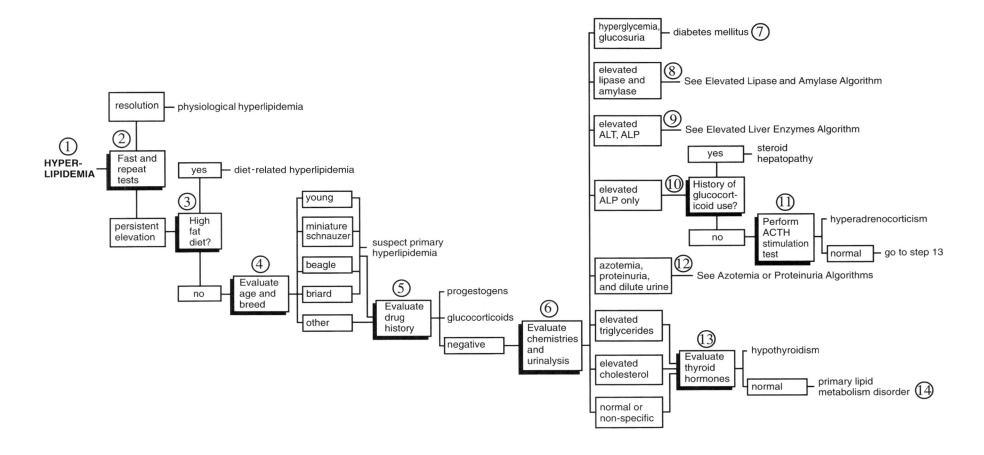

1 Amylase and lipase are enzymes produced by the exocrine pancreas to assist digestion of food in the small intestine (lipase digests fat; amylase, carbohydrate). Lipase is more specific for the pancreas but is also produced from the gastric mucosa in dogs. Amylase increases in pancreatic, intestinal, and hepatic disease. Serum concentrations of both enzymes increase when renal excretion is reduced. Thus, they are not highly sensitive for pancreatic disease, particularly in cats. The degree of enzyme elevation does not correlate with the severity of pancreatic inflammation; however, 5- to 10-fold increases are likely with true pancreatic disease, and very high elevations can be associated with pancreatic cancer.

2 Drugs causing lipase and amylase elevations include L-asparaginase, azathioprine, calcium, estrogens, furosemide, thiazides, glucocorticoids, tetracycline, metronidazole, azulfidine, and sulfonamides. Lipase increases with heparin administration. Only L-asparaginase and azathioprine have been shown to cause pancreatitis in dogs on reexposure. Although none of these drugs reliably causes pancreatitis in cats or dogs, they should be withdrawn in patients with pancreatitis. Dexamethasone may cause mild to severe (up to fivefold) elevations in amylase and lipase without histopathological evidence of pancreatic inflammation.

3 High-fat diets, table scraps, or trash ingestion may predispose the patient to pancreatitis. However, some patients with a tendency to develop pancreatitis do so even on low-fat, high-fiber diets.

4 Foreign body ingestion, especially with vomiting, suggests a gastrointestinal source of increased amylase or lipase.

5 Melena indicates bleeding into the upper portions of the bowel and suggests that these sites are sources of amylase or lipase (e.g., foreign body, bleeding ulcer, or tumor). However, gastric ulceration also can develop with severe pancreatitis.

6 Since the kidneys excrete amylase and lipase, reduced GFRs may cause mild to moderate enzyme elevations. Patients in renal failure who do not have fever, icterus, vomiting, and cranial abdominal pain are likely to have elevated amylase and lipase as a result of the renal failure. Also, in patients known to have gastric/duodenal ulcer disease or gastric neoplasia, these enzyme elevations may not need to be pursued. The index of suspicion for pancreatitis increases in patients that have had the problem before and in those with hyperadrenocorticism or other conditions causing hyperlipidemia. Hyperlipidemia may be a cause or an effect of pancreatic inflammation.

7 Pancreatitis is suspected if patients are febrile, nauseous, or have cranial abdominal pain on palpation. These findings also can occur with foreign body obstruction or peritonitis. In small dogs and cats, it may be possible to palpate a swollen pancreas. This cannot be distinguished from a pancreatic mass, pancreatic pseudo-cyst, or mass arising from other tissues. Physical examination is most useful when it identifies conditions other than pancreatic disease (e.g., an intestinal foreign body or mass).

8 If an intestinal foreign body can be palpated, abdominal radiographs are recommended to determine the location of radiodense material, obstructive intestinal gas patterns, bunching of intestines suggesting a linear foreign body, and free air in the abdomen due to intestinal rupture. A barium series may locate partial obstruction or outline a foreign body, but this should be avoided if perforation is suspected. Surgery is needed to remove intestinal foreign bodies and resect bowel.

9 If masses are detected outside of the pancreas, they may be pursued via abdominal imaging, needle aspiration, surgery, and so on. Mass lesions associated with elevations in amylase and lipase are found mainly in bowel and liver.

10 If abdominal fluid is detected, abdominocentesis should be performed if coagulopathy is not suspected. Fluid can be evaluated for cell counts and type, protein content, the presence of foreign material (suggests bowel perforation), lipase and amylase concentrations and bacteria. It also can be cultured.

11 A mixed bacterial population, degenerate neutrophils, and foreign material suggest bowel rupture. Patients should undergo surgery as soon as they are stable. Elevations of serum or fluid amylase and lipase are likely to result from damaged bowel or secondary pancreatic inflammation from the septic abdominal exudate.

12 A less florid exudate (e.g., degenerate neutrophils with bacteria outside of phagocytic cells in moderate numbers or inside phagocytic cells in small numbers) suggests sepsis, bowel perforation, or rupture of an infected pancreatic abscess. Abdominal imaging is indicated to determine the cause.

13 Sterile inflammatory effusions commonly are seen with moderate/severe pancreatitis. Fluid is generally an exudate, and appearances range from hemorrhagic through serosanguinous, opaque, and purulent to clear. Gross and microscopic appearances of fluid do not distinguish pancreatitis from other intra-abdominal problems. If neoplastic cells are found, abdominal imaging is recommended. A minimum database (step 15) might be important for decisions about suitability of the patient for surgery and to determine the tissue of origin of fluid.

14 Amylase and lipase concentrations can be measured on abdominal fluid. Clear effusions can be evaluated directly. Hemorrhagic/opaque effusions need to be spun down. High concentrations of amylase and lipase in fluid raise the suspicion of pancreatic disease or bowel perforation. Pancreatic disease may cause much greater lipase and amylase elevations in abdominal fluid than in peripheral blood.

15 The minimum database in patients with pancreatitis may show leukocytosis (with or without a left shift), as well as elevations in ALP and bilirubin secondary to obstruction of the common bile duct by the pancreas. Findings are not specific for pancreatitis and may be seen with bowel perforation, obstruction, ulcers, and neoplasia.

16 When the patient is azotemic but urine is appropriately concentrated, the patient is dehydrated secondary to the underlying condition. Azotemic patients with dilute urine are in renal failure, that is probably also causing mild to moderate elevations in amylase and lipase. This is especially the case in a patient with no clinical or laboratory signs consistent with pancreatitis/proximal gastrointestinal disease. Note that pancreatitis may cause secondary renal failure.

17 Although the pancreas is a difficult organ to image, abdominal radiographs and ultrasound may be able to differentiate other causes of elevated serum amylase and lipase.

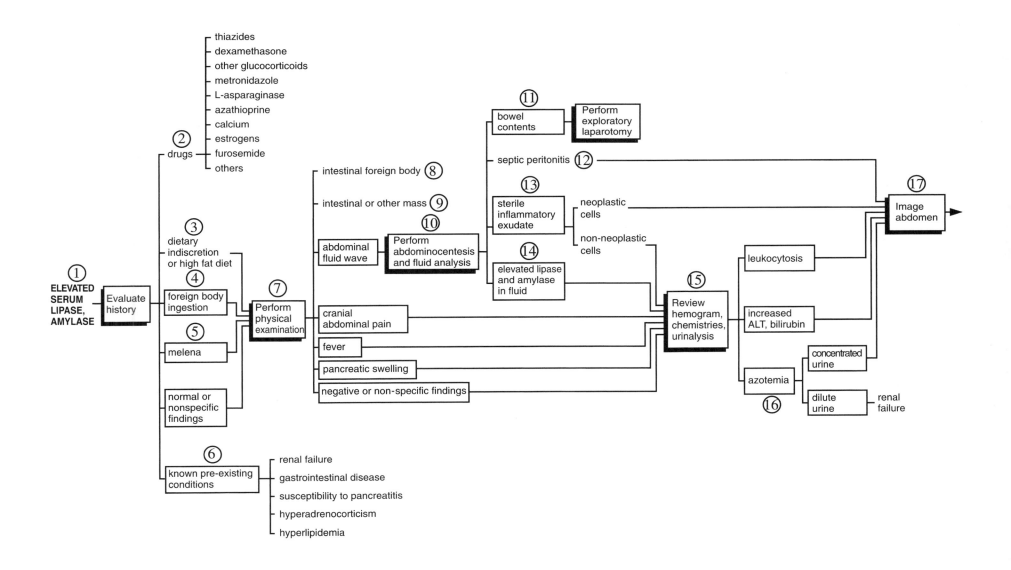

18 Free fluid on abdominal radiographs is an indication for abdominocentesis if this has not already been performed. Free air suggests gastrointestinal perforation, a penetrating abdominal wound, or, rarely, a ruptured abscess containing gas-forming organisms. Surgical exploration is indicated for free air. Radiographs also can show abdominal masses (although probably none associated with the pancreas), radiopaque intestinal foreign bodies, some radiolucent material (especially within the stomach), and obstructive intestinal patterns. Haziness or fluid limited to the right cranial quadrant of the abdomen and a static duodenal loop (a duodenal C in the right cranial quadrant on the ventrodorsal view of the abdomen) may suggest pancreatic inflammation.

19 Ultrasound may allow differentiation of pancreatic masses, abscesses, and pseudocysts, all of which have a different prognosis and some of which require different management techniques. Imaging an increased echodensity, especially in the right cranial quadrant of the abdomen and around the duodenum and common bile duct, is suggestive of pancreatitis. Other factors increasing the suspicion of pancreatic inflammation include generalized haziness of all tissues in this region, localized or generalized fluid accumulation, a thickened, echogenic pancreas, and common bile duct obstruction and tortuosity. The last condition may be due to primary obstruction of the duct and may not be secondary to pancreatic inflammation. Sometimes there are focal changes in echogenicity within the pancreas that suggest mass lesions or an abscess. Pancreatic pseudocysts are often very large and are filled with relatively echolucent fluid. Ultrasound also may be able to distinguish intestinal, gastric, and hepatic masses causing elevations in lipase and amylase. It is not always useful for imaging gastrointestinal wall thickness or masses because bowel is often filled with air, blocking the ultrasound beam.

20 Abdominal CT or MRI scans are probably the most precise and least invasive methods of identifying pancreatic swelling, inflammation, and masses and distinguishing these from other intra-abdominal causes of elevated amylase and lipase. Both require general anesthesia in veterinary patients, and not all such patients will be stable enough for anesthesia. Additionally, such scans are not always immediately available.

21 Measurement of serum trypsin-like immunoreactivity (TLI) is controversial in dogs and cats for detection of pancreatitis. Serum trypsin concentrations are thought to rise above the normal range with pancreatic inflammation, probably due to leakage into the blood from inflamed tissue. Like the other tests described so far, it can only contribute to the diagnosis. Normal or low concentrations of serum trypsin do not rule out pancreatitis or other pancreatic conditions. If the suspicion of pancreatic disease still remains, diagnostic alternatives include assessing the response to appropriate therapy for pancreatitis, CT or MRI imaging, or exploratory surgery. Other blood tests currently being evaluated in dogs include the measurement of serum phospholipase A_2 and trypsin-activating peptide. The only definitive method of confirming pancreatitis is pancreatic histopathology. This is not an appropriate initial step in the majority of clinical cases unless exploratory surgery is needed for other reasons. Surgical intervention and pancreatic biopsy should be considered for suspected abscesses, for pseudocysts not accessible for percutaneous drainage or recurring after drainage, for pancreatitis that has not responded to appropriate medical management, and to confirm suspected neoplasia.

22 If appropriate and accessible, pancreatic masses, pseudocysts, and possibly abscesses can be aspirated under ultrasound guidance to assist in making the diagnosis. Aspiration of potentially infected tissue carries the risk of rupture of the abscess and peritonitis, while aspiration of potentially neoplastic tissue carries the risk of disseminating the neoplasm throughout the abdomen.

23 Pancreatic tumors that cause elevations in pancreatic enzymes are generally carcinomas or, rarely, lymphoma. The prognosis is guarded to poor.

24 Pancreatic abscesses may be sterile or infected. Neither type is likely to resolve on its own, even with antimicrobial therapy. The majority require surgical drainage, with or without subsequent open abdominal drainage. The prognosis is fair to guarded, with an approximately 50% survival rate with surgery.

25 Identification of a cystic structure associated with the pancreas in patients with clinical signs of pancreatitis or a history of moderate to severe pancreatitis about 6 weeks prior to presentation suggests a pancreatic pseudocyst. Drainage of acellular fluid from the structure and sometimes the presence of high concentrations of amylase or lipase in that fluid are sufficient to make this rare diagnosis. Pancreatic pseudocysts are accumulations of pancreatic secretions within a cystic structure created by breakdown of pancreatic acini secondary to inflammation. The differential diagnosis includes cysts arising from other intra-abdominal tissues (e.g., the biliary system) and cystic neoplasms. Percutaneous drainage may cause the clinical signs to resolve and should be attempted before surgical intervention.

26 When the pancreas does not appear to be affected by any disease condition, and especially when a gastric or small intestinal problem is suspected, upper endoscopy or exploratory surgery is indicated to evaluate for primary gastrointestinal disease that may be associated with elevations in serum lipase and amylase. It also is the only definitive way of confirming pancreatic disease.

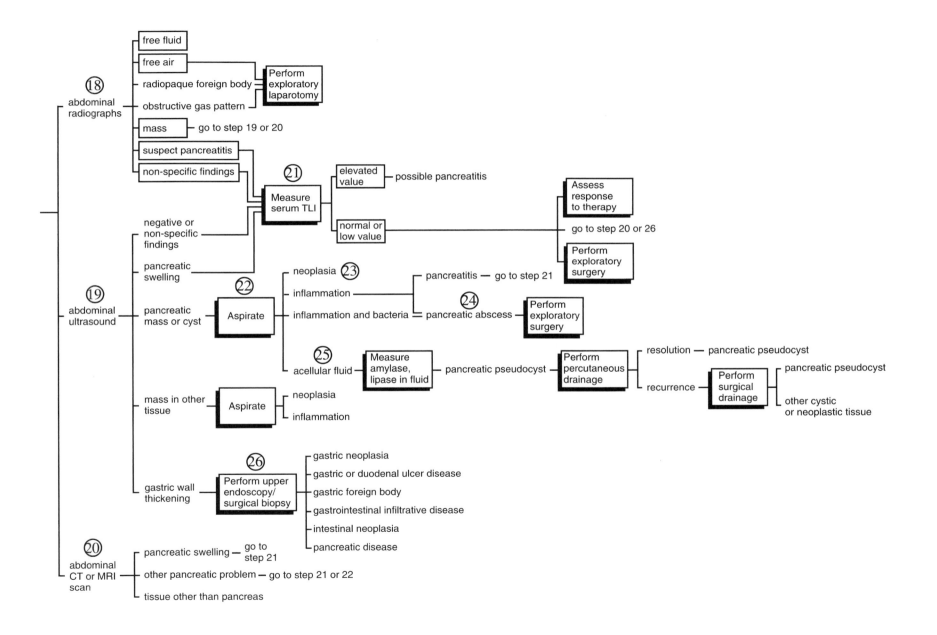

Hepatic Disorders

1 Hepatomegaly is enlargement of the liver. It is most commonly identified on physical examination or abdominal radiographs. Clinical signs may not be associated with hepatomegaly. If present, they often are related to liver disease (anorexia, weight loss, vomiting, diarrhea, icterus, PU, PD, encephalopathy, fever), right-sided heart failure, or systemic effects of nonhepatic disorders. Most cats with liver disease (cholangiohepatitis, hepatic lipidosis, amyloidosis, tumors, cirrhosis, or congestive disorders) develop pronounced liver enlargement.

2 The normal-sized liver lies within the costal arch and is generally not palpable. The liver is considered enlarged if anything other than the most distal margins can be palpated. Abdominal radiographs and ultrasound may be useful to distinguish among an enlarged liver, spleen, and cranial abdominal masses. Radiographically, generalized hepatomegaly is observed as extension of the liver beyond the costal arch, caudal rotation/displacement of the stomach, or rounding of the liver margins. The significance of mild hepatic enlargement in the absence of clinical signs is questionable.

3 Some drugs can cause hepatomegaly, most notably corticosteroids and anticonvulsants (e.g., phenobarbital). These rarely are associated with signs other than hepatomegaly unless long-term use of anticonvulsants results in liver failure. Phenobarbital causes hypertrophy of hepatocyte organelles and endoplasmic reticulum.

4 Other drugs occasionally cause acute hepatic damage and hepatomegaly. These include acetaminophen, halothane, methoxyflurane, ketoconazole, itraconazole mebendazole, griseofulvin, thiacetarsamide, phenylbutazone, potentiated sulfonamides, diazepam (cats), azathioprine, oxybendazole, carprofen, tetracycline, and L-asparaginase.

5 If the drug history is negative, evaluate the patient's history and physical examination for signs of cardiac disease, especially right-sided heart failure that might cause hepatic congestion and enlargement. Signs of right-sided heart failure include exercise intolerance, anorexia, weight loss, tachycardia, weakness, cardiac murmurs, and arrhythmias. If such signs are present, proceed with thoracic radiographs, testing for dirofilariasis, electrocardiography, and echocardiography to arrive at a diagnosis.

6 If there are no signs of cardiac disease, hepatomegaly should be further investigated via laboratory tests (hemogram, chemistry profile, and urinalysis). An FeLV/FIV test is recommended for cats since a positive result may cause the client not to pursue further diagnostic testing. Testing for *Dirofilaria immitis* (heartworm) disease also is a consideration in dogs even if signs of cardiac disease are absent.

7 Canine patients with hyperadrenocorticism have some or all of the following laboratory changes: mature neutrophilia, eosinopenia, lymphopenia, increased ALP and, to a lesser extent, ALT, hypercholesterolemia, mild to moderate elevations of glucose, proteinuria, bacteriuria, and hyposthenuria. Hepatomegaly in a middle-aged or older small-breed dog, accompanied by elevated ALP, is suggestive of hyperadrenocorticism. Other clinical signs include PU, PD, bilaterally symmetrical nonpruritic alopecia, pendulous abdomen, polyphagia, calcinosis cutis, and thin skin.

8 Although ultrasound scanning of the liver and adrenal glands contributes to the diagnosis of hyperadrenocorticism, definitive diagnosis requires a positive ACTH stimulation test. Low-dose dexamethasone suppression testing is not always definitive. If these tests are normal, abdominal ultrasound may be the next step in evaluating the enlarged liver.

9 Hepatomegaly resulting from diabetes mellitus is due to accumulation of lipid and glycogen in hepatocytes as a result of a variety of metabolic derangements. Diabetes mellitus is diagnosed by finding fasting hyperglycemia and accompanying glycosuria. Ketonuria may also be present but not in all cases. Because cats can develop hyperglycemia due to the stress of phlebotomy, persistent hyperglycemia should be documented by repeating the test after the cat has acclimated to the clinic's environment or by placing an intravenous catheter for blood sampling. The owner also can collect a urine sample at home to document the presence or absence of glycosuria.

10 Hepatomegaly can be the result of systemic illnesses such as fungal, protozoal, rickettsial, viral, or bacterial infections, but it is rarely the major clinical sign of such illnesses. Affected animals are usually obviously unwell, with fever, tachycardia, lethargy, and anorexia. If marked neutrophilia or neutropenia with a left shift is detected, then bacteremia or septicemia should be suspected and the source of the infection investigated via blood cultures, abdominal ultrasound, and thoracic radiographs.

11 If anemia or thrombocytopenia is found in patients with hepatomegaly, it is best to pursue those problems rather than hepatomegaly alone. Hepatomegaly can occur in patients with immune-mediated hemolytic anemia or thrombocytopenia due to destruction of RBCs and platelets by the liver. It may also occur with tick-borne diseases such as ehrlichiosis and Rocky Mountain spotted fever.

12 Hepatomegaly in an FeLV- or FIV-positive cat can either be a direct viral effect or the effect of a secondary problem such as neoplasia or infection. Depending on the client's concerns and the overall health of the cat, one can stop testing at this point or progress to ultrasound of the liver.

13 By this point in the algorithm, cardiac disease, effects of medication, hyperadrenocorticism, diabetes mellitus, systemic illness, tick-borne diseases, bone marrow failure, and immune-mediated hemolytic anemia/thrombocytopenia should have been eliminated as underlying causes of hepatomegaly. Ultrasound of the liver can identify masses, cysts, and choleliths. It can characterize the problem as focal or diffuse, as well as determining whether the hepatic parenchyma is normal or abnormal and the biliary system is patent or obstructed.

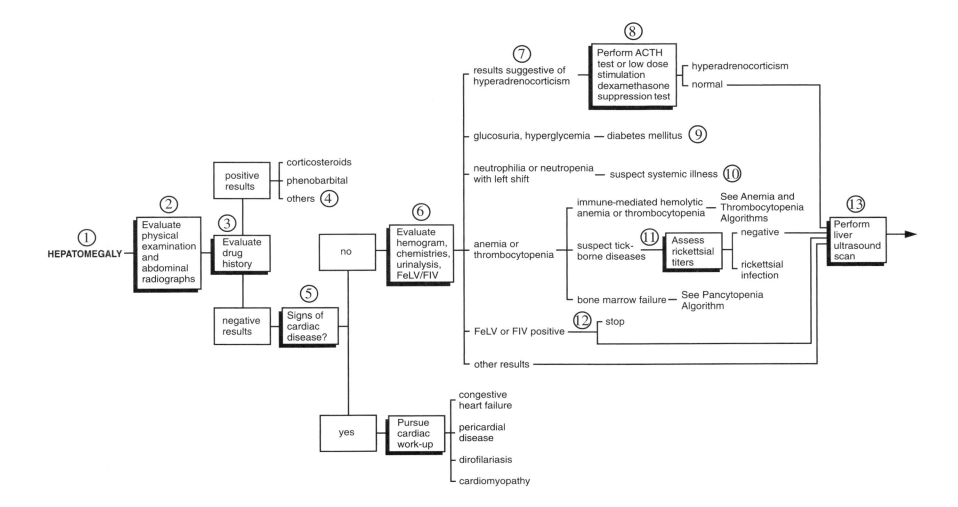

14 Ultrasonography is a noninvasive method of determining the presence of extrahepatic bile duct obstruction. This may be due to pancreatitis, choleliths, inspissated bile, or neoplasia of the biliary system or pancreas. Ultrasonographic findings with extrahepatic bile duct obstruction include gallbladder distention and enlarged/tortuous ducts (cystic duct, common bile duct, or intrahepatic bile ducts). Such cases may require exploratory surgery to determine the cause and to relieve the obstruction.

15 If the liver parenchyma appears normal on ultrasound and there are no other clinical signs, it may be prudent to wait and reevaluate the patient at a later date. The patient should be reassessed again in 3 months or sooner if clinical signs develop.

16 If the liver parenchyma appears normal on ultrasound but the patient has other clinical signs, consider pursuing these or reevaluate the patient for the possibility of infectious diseases common to the local area. Toxoplasmosis, blastomycosis, histoplasmosis, coccidioidomycosis, neosporosis, FIP, infectious canine hepatitis, CDV, salmon poisoning, ehrlichiosis, Rocky Mountain spotted fever, and leptospirosis are possible examples.

17 If the liver parenchyma appears abnormal on ultrasound, aspiration for cytology or biopsy for histopathology is the next appropriate step. However, a coagulogram should be evaluated before biopsy (surgical or ultrasound-guided) because the liver synthesizes many coagulation factors and severe liver disease often causes coagulopathy. Coagulation times also allow indirect measurement of the severity of liver dysfunction. If the PT or PTT is prolonged, aspiration and definitely biopsy should be avoided until the patient has been stabilized.

18 Aspiration of abnormal liver parenchyma is best done under ultrasound guidance to reach any focal abnormalities and to avoid blood-filled structures and the biliary system. Although aspiration cytology can be useful for the initial evaluation of hepatomegaly, it is not the same as a histopathological diagnosis. Nonetheless, some disorders (e.g., hepatic lipidosis in cats) can be diagnosed using this technique. If the results are nondiagnostic, liver biopsy is indicated.

19 Although liver biopsy permits a histopathological diagnosis of the underlying cause of hepatomegaly, the accuracy of the diagnosis depends upon sampling an adequate amount of tissue from the correct location with focal conditions and good histopathological interpretation by someone well versed in liver histopathology. Methods used to obtain hepatic biopsy specimens include ultrasound-guided percutaneous, blind percutaneous, keyhole approach and wedge biopsy, and exploratory laparotomy and wedge or excisional biopsy of focal lesions. Several samples should be collected in patients with diffuse liver disease to increase the chances of an accurate diagnosis. Samples are routinely fixed in 10% buffered formalin. In breeds predisposed to the toxic effects of copper accumulation (Bedlington terriers, West Highland white terriers, Dobermans, and some others), the clinician should request staining for copper-containing pigment. Some laboratories may measure hepatic tissue copper concentrations.

20 Hemochromatosis (iron overload and excessive storage in the liver) is a rare condition.

21 Glycogen storage diseases are inherited disorders resulting from deficiency of specific enzymes required for normal glycogen metabolism. Enzyme deficiency results in impaired glycogen mobilization and subsequent visceral glycogen accumulation. In dogs, three types of glycogen disease have been confirmed by enzymatic assays. Hepatomegaly caused by massive glycogen deposition is a consistent finding in types I and III.

22 In certain conditions (diabetes mellitus, hypothyroidism, hyperlipidemia), hepatic lipid accumulation occurs as an expected response but does not result in obvious hepatic dysfunction or hepatomegaly. Hepatic lipidosis occurs when lipid accumulation compromises the liver and causes clinical illness. Middle-aged cats, especially females, are commonly affected. Hepatomegaly is an inconsistent finding.

23 Amyloidosis is a progressive systemic disease associated with extracellular deposition of insoluble fibrillar proteins. The condition can result in dysfunction of the liver, spleen, kidneys, and adrenal glands. Clinical and biochemical evidence of hepatic dysfunction occurs more frequently in oriental and Siamese cats and less frequently in Abyssinian cats and Chinese shar-pei dogs. The liver is often pale, enlarged, and friable, with associated hemorrhage, hematomas, and capsular tears.

24 Microhepatica is a common radiographic finding in dogs with cirrhosis because parenchymal tissue is replaced by fibrous tissue. In contrast, cats with biliary cirrhosis often have hepatomegaly.

25 Extramedullary hematopoiesis can cause hepatomegaly. Causes of extramedullary hematopoiesis include bone marrow failure, severe chronic blood loss, and erythrocytic parasitemias.

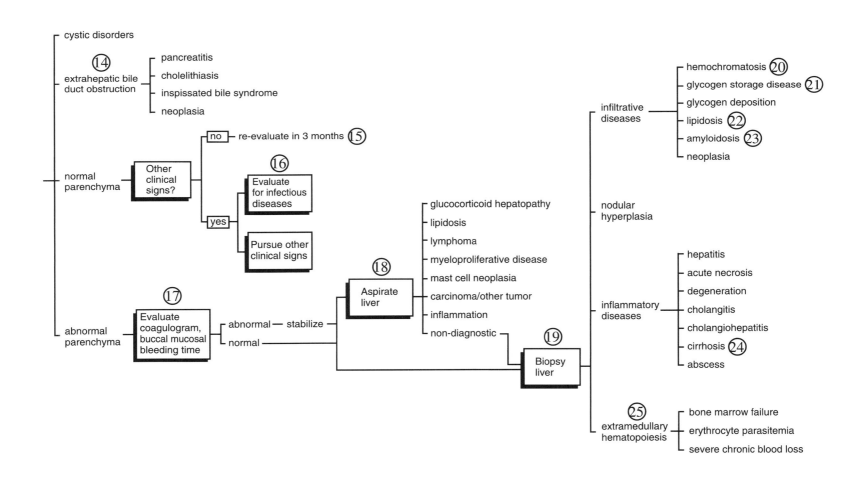

1 Icterus is yellow discoloration due to accumulation of bilirubin in plasma/tissue. Bilirubin is a breakdown product of Hb. Icterus results from excessive RBC destruction and from failure of the liver to remove bilirubin from blood or excrete it via the biliary system.

2 Check the PCV for anemia and total protein (TP) to see if anemia is due to bleeding (low TP) or hemolysis (normal TP). Mild decreases in PCV result from chronic disease or low-grade blood loss. Where PCV is low (<20% for cats, <25% for dogs) a hemogram, reticulocyte count, and other tests should be evaluated for RBC destruction.

3 A hemogram and a reticulocyte count assess for regeneration (corrected RC > 1–2% in dogs, >1% in cats). Regenerative anemia (RA) suggests RBC loss or destruction. In early cases of anemia, the bone marrow may not have mounted a regenerative response. Recheck the values in 24–48 hours.

4 If anemia is regenerative, blood loss should be excluded via urinalysis, checking stool for melena, and sequential monitoring of PCV/TP. If PCV decreases but TP does not, this suggests that anemia is due to RBC destruction. Blood loss results in anemia and low TP.

5 Clients should be questioned about drugs, foods, or toxins that cause RBC destruction. Agents causing hemolysis include zinc, onions, garlic, acetaminophen, methylene blue, propylene glycol, naphthalene (mothballs), benzocaine, and methionine. Some drugs (cephalosporins) are associated with immune-mediated RBC destruction, and any drug can cause hemolysis idiosyncratically. In the southern/southwestern United States, patients should be evaluated for RBC parasites. Flea control, indoor-outdoor status, recent vaccination, and the presence of *Dirofilaria immitis* infestation, neoplasia, or artificial heart valves should be determined to see whether there are any removable causes of anemia.

6 In patients with normal hematocrits or only mild anemia, a serum chemistry screen can define liver problems (primary hepatic disease or posthepatic obstruction) or other conditions causing icterus (e.g., pancreatitis, biliary system inflammation/obstruction causing posthepatic icterus). Low concentrations of substances produced by the liver (albumin, BUN, glucose, cholesterol) suggest primary liver disease. Proportional differences in hepatic enzyme evaluations help to determine the underlying causes of icterus. Marked elevations in ALT compared to ALP suggest a primary hepatic condition. If ALP is higher, biliary system problems (intra/posthepatic) are likely. Relative enzyme proportions are not as useful in cats as in dogs, as ALP has a short half-life in cats.

7 Review of the history and physical examination is unlikely to provide a definitive diagnosis of the underlying causes of icterus unless the patient is taking a hepatotoxic drug. The breed is important in dogs since cocker spaniels, Dobermans (especially females), and West Highland white and Bedlington terriers are at risk of breed-related hepatopathy. Golden retrievers and Labradors develop granulomatous hepatitis and may have an increased risk of developing carprofen-induced hepatotoxicosis. Older animals may be more likely to have neoplasia. In cats more than 8 years old or with a palpable thyroid nodule, thyroid concentrations should be measured, especially when icterus is mild and ALT is elevated. Recent changes in the environment, diet, or management are important in cats because these could cause anorexia and secondary hepatic lipidosis. Overweight cats are more at risk for lipidosis. The indoor/outdoor status of patients should be checked, as should recent introduction of new animals, for infectious disease (canine adenovirus infection and leptospirosis in dogs and FeLV, FIV, FIP, and toxoplasmosis in cats). Trauma should be considered. On physical examination almost all liver conditions, including cirrhosis, can cause hepatomegaly in cats. A palpable abdominal mass suggests primary or metastatic hepatic or posthepatic neoplasia.

8 If a known hepatotoxic agent is identified, therapy consists of drug withdrawal, supportive care, and monitoring. Acutely hepatotoxic agents include ketoconazole, itraconazole (to a lesser extent), trimethoprim sulfa (dogs), tetracycline, diazepam (cats), oral hypoglycemics such as glipizide (cats), griseofulvin (cats), excessive iron supplements, and NSAIDS (particularly carprofen in dogs). Many drugs have idiosyncratic hepatotoxicosis. When possible, medication should be withdrawn. More long-term hepatotoxicosis occurs with anticonvulsants (phenobarbital, phenytoin), oxibendazole-diethylcarbamazine (Filaribits Plus), and possibly carprofen (Rimadyl). Glucocorticoids induce the isoenzyme of ALP in dogs, so elevations do not necessarily indicate hepatobiliary disease.

9 Most findings from the signalment, history, and physical examination only suggest the underlying cause of icterus. The next step is hepatic imaging. Abdominal radiographs can identify focal masses, radiodense choleliths (rare), or, occasionally, other gallbladder problems. However, abdominal ultrasound provides more information about the structure and texture of the liver parenchyma, masses, the biliary system, pancreas, and proximal small bowel. Abdominal CT/MRI scans also can be used to evaluate the hepatobiliary system.

10 When increased RBC destruction is present, a peripheral blood smear allows diagnosis of spherocytes (small RBCs with no central pallor that have "rounded up" due to damage to membranes). Spherocytes are pathognomonic for immune-mediated RBC destruction, and further diagnostic testing is only confirmatory. A blood smear also identifies anisocytosis (variable RBC size), polychromasia, and intracellular parasites (such as *Babesia* spp. and *Haemobartonella* spp.). Special stains may be needed to identify RBC parasites (methylene blue for *Haemobartonella* spp.). Blood smears also allow identification of Heinz bodies (with onion or methylene blue intoxication). A small proportion of Heinz bodies may be normal in cats.

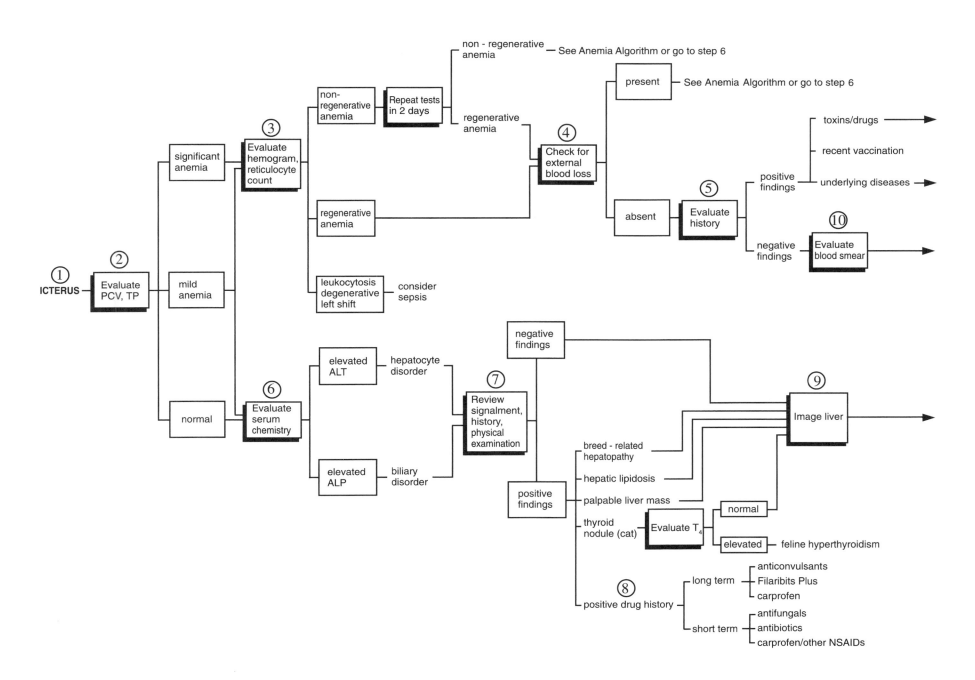

11 An abdominal radiograph quickly excludes the possibility of a metallic foreign body and the risk of zinc intoxication. Coins (U.S. pennies minted after 1983) and bolts cause zinc intoxication, as does ingestion of zinc oxide–containing ointment licked off wounds and hot spots.

12 If intracellular erythrocytic parasites are suspected, titers can be measured for *Babesia* spp. or polymerase chain reaction (PCR) can be done for *Haemobartonella felis*. Testing for *Dirofilaria immitis* is appropriate if vena cava syndrome is suspected (causes RBC destruction).

13 If immunological disease is suspected (e.g., IMHA), a Coombs' test can identify "anti-dog" antibodies on the surface of RBCs. This is not necessary when spherocytes are seen. An ANA titer can be considered if multiple organ system involvement is a concern.

14 Gallbladder abnormalities on ultrasound include thickening/increased echogenicity of the wall (suggests inflammation) and thickened/inspissated bile. Both findings may not be clinically significant, but if they are, ALP is likely to be greater than ALT. Choleliths are rare in dogs and cats and do not usually cause obstruction. However, there can be underlying hepatic disease and choleliths can act as foci of infection. If no other cause of icterus is found and there is no response to symptomatic therapy, liver biopsy and cholelith removal are recommended. Ultrasound also can identify masses involving the gallbladder. On occasion the gallbladder cannot be imaged. Causes include effacement by a mass or inspissated bile or gallbladder rupture. The last is likely to cause progressive abdominal fluid accumulation. Sometimes a collapsed gallbladder will be imaged, but often it is not visible. Gallbladder masses/ruptures are indications for a coagulogram and exploratory surgery to treat the primary condition and biopsy the liver.

15 Biliary system dilation greater than 4 mm suggests posthepatic obstruction. In cats the biliary system can remain dilated up to 4 mm after obstruction is relieved.

Obstruction may be due to focal lesions (masses in the biliary system, pancreas, or liver, or choleliths) or diffuse disease (pancreatitis, biliary inflammation, and bile sludging). If a focal mass is imaged, it may be aspirated for a cytological diagnosis. If there is no evidence of pancreatitis and obstruction is worsening, this is an indication for further imaging (CT/MRI if available) or exploratory surgery. At surgery, hepatic and pancreatic tissue should be biopsied, bile cultured, the biliary system catheterized to identify/treat obstruction. If necessary, the biliary system should be rerouted.

16 If masses are seen in the liver, pancreas, or elsewhere, or if hepatic parenchyma is diffusely hyper- or hypoechoic, a fine-needle aspirate of tissue can diagnose neoplasia, lipidosis, diffuse infection (histoplasmosis), or inflammatory infiltrates. Cytology will not diagnose neoplasms that do not exfoliate (many sarcomas), hepatic fibrosis, cirrhosis, or biliary hyperplasia. Inflammatory infiltrates also do not always correlate with underlying conditions (e.g., fibrosis may have an inflammatory component).

17 Hepatic lipidosis in cats often is diagnosed on the basis of the history, physical examination, laboratory tests, and hepatic parenchymal aspirates. Cytology reveals distended hepatocytes, vacuolization displacing hepatocyte nuclei, and no inflammation.

18 If cytology results are negative or questionable, or if the patient does not respond to therapy, liver biopsy is indicated. This should be preceded by a coagulogram, especially if done percutaneously with ultrasound. Surgical biopsy is necessary if the liver is small, if coagulation abnormalities are severe, or if there is a focal lesion that cannot be reached percutaneously. Percutaneous biopsy is useful for diffuse hepatic disease.

19 Severe inflammatory bowel disease and neoplasia can cause posthepatic biliary obstruction due to thickening of the duodenal wall around the common bile duct papilla.

20 Biliary flukes are a rare cause of biliary obstruction in cats. *Platynosomum fastosum* infects cats in the Caribbean, Florida, and Hawaii and is acquired by eating toads and lizards.

21 The liver can react only in a limited way to any insult; therefore, many causes of inflammation result in similar histopathological changes. Chronic hepatitis can be due to breed predisposition (step 7), copper storage disease (Bedlington and West Highland white terriers, Doberman pinschers), drugs, and infections (canine adenovirus, leptospirosis). Idiopathic chronic hepatitis and fibrosis are postulated to be autoimmune diseases. Lobular dissecting hepatitis is a chronic hepatitis in dogs less than 1 year of age and may be secondary to a variety of insults. In cats, chronic hepatitis often is secondary to cholangiohepatitis (either suppurative, due to ascending infection from the bowel, or lymphoplasmacytic, which is immune mediated).

22 FIP is definitively diagnosed by finding granulomatous hepatic inflammation.

23 Microvascular dysplasia is a congenital disorder in dogs. Many clinical signs and laboratory test results are similar to those of patients with congenital portal systemic shunts. Patients are initially asymptomatic but may progress to end-stage liver disease and icterus.

24 If percutaneous liver biopsy is negative in an icteric patient, exploratory surgery may be indicated for more extensive liver and biliary system examination. Patients should be reevaluated for sepsis since severe systemic infections can cause icterus. Septic patients often are febrile, collapsed, shocky, and icteric. They may have diarrhea, vomiting, heart murmurs, bleeding disorders, and anterior uveitis. Laboratory tests show leukocytosis (neutrophilia, often with a degenerative left shift), elevated ALP, and low serum albumin and glucose. With these findings, septic patients generally are detected early in the diagnostic process for icterus.

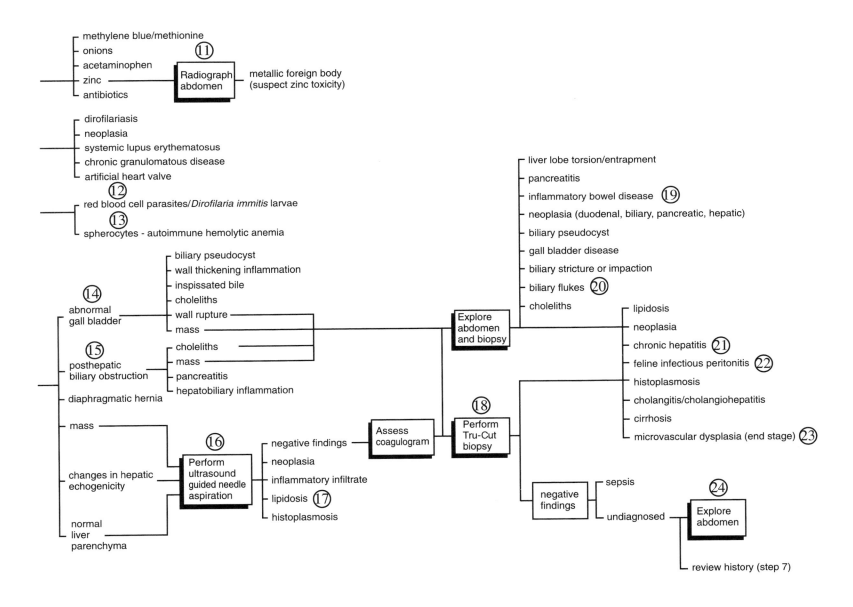

methylene blue/methionine
onions
acetaminophen
zinc — ⑪ Radiograph abdomen — metallic foreign body (suspect zinc toxicity)
antibiotics

dirofilariasis
neoplasia
systemic lupus erythematosus
chronic granulomatous disease
artificial heart valve
⑫
red blood cell parasites/*Dirofilaria immitis* larvae
⑬
spherocytes - autoimmune hemolytic anemia

⑭ abnormal gall bladder
biliary pseudocyst
wall thickening inflammation
inspissated bile
choleliths
wall rupture
mass

⑮ posthepatic biliary obstruction
choleliths
mass
pancreatitis
hepatobiliary inflammation

diaphragmatic hernia

mass

⑯ Perform ultrasound guided needle aspiration
negative findings
neoplasia
inflammatory infiltrate
lipidosis ⑰
histoplasmosis

changes in hepatic echogenicity

normal liver parenchyma

Assess coagulogram

⑱ Perform Tru-Cut biopsy

Explore abdomen and biopsy
liver lobe torsion/entrapment
pancreatitis
inflammatory bowel disease ⑲
neoplasia (duodenal, biliary, pancreatic, hepatic)
biliary pseudocyst
gall bladder disease
biliary stricture or impaction
biliary flukes ⑳
choleliths

lipidosis
neoplasia
chronic hepatitis ㉑
feline infectious peritonitis ㉒
histoplasmosis
cholangitis/cholangiohepatitis
cirrhosis
microvascular dysplasia (end stage) ㉓

negative findings
sepsis
undiagnosed

㉔ Explore abdomen

review history (step 7)

1 Increased liver enzyme activity is seen commonly but is not necessarily associated with clinically significant liver disease. Nor does it provide information on the liver's functional capabilities. In some cases (e.g., portosystemic shunt or cirrhosis), severe liver dysfunction can exist in the presence of normal or only mildly elevated enzyme concentrations. Nonetheless, liver enzyme elevations are associated with many liver, endocrine, and infectious disorders. There are numerous hepatic enzymes, but ALT and ALP are the most useful for evaluating hepatobiliary disease in dogs and cats. Increased ALT is generally associated with hepatocellular damage or regeneration, while increased ALP is associated with cholestasis, steroid use, bone growth or disease, and the use of many drugs. The half-life of ALP is short in cats, and the total liver content is 50% less than that in dogs. There is no corticosteroid-induced isoenzyme of ALP in cats. For these reasons, any ALP elevation in a cat should be considered significant and investigated. Clinically, the largest increases in ALP in cats are seen with intra- or extrahepatic cholestasis especially associated with hepatic lipidosis, cholangiohepatitis, or common bile duct obstruction.

2 Young, growing dogs up to 7 months of age often have slightly increased serum concentrations of ALP because of osteoclast activity.

3 Bone lysis, with osteomyelitis or osteosarcoma, can cause a two- to fivefold increase in ALP. However, the half-life of the bone-origin isoenzyme is short.

4 Hypoxia or hypotension often results in increased ALT and occasionally mild increases in ALP. Conditions associated with hypoxia include congestive heart failure; acute severe blood loss; status epilepticus; septic shock; circulatory shock; and hypoadrenocorticism.

5 Passive congestion of the liver from right heart failure can cause mild increases in ALP and ALT.

6 Many drugs can cause an elevation in ALP, ALT, or both. Glucocorticoids induce production of a unique liver isoenzyme of ALP in dogs. Elevations can persist long after discontinuation of the glucocorticoid. Gluco-corticoids also can induce hepatic production of ALT and produce pathological changes (steroid hepatopathy) that cause hepatocellular leakage of ALT. Anticonvulsants, notably phenobarbital, primidone, phenytoin, and carbamazepine, often cause increases in ALP and ALT. In cats, diazepam can induce hepatic necrosis and elevations of ALT and ALP. Other drugs that can elevate liver enzymes consistently include griseofulvin, phenylbutazone, thiacetarsamide, ketoconazole, mebendazole, and oxibendazole.

7 Hepatotoxins include aflatoxins, carbon tetrachloride, arsenic, chlordane, chlorinated hydrocarbons, mercury, mushrooms, tetrachloroethane, and many others.

8 Common infectious diseases that localize in the liver or infect the liver as part of a more systemic process include infectious canine hepatitis, canine herpes virus, FIP, histoplasmosis, toxoplasmosis, leptospirosis, and *Bacillus piliformis*.

9 Evaluating a cat's FeLV/FIV status is prudent since these viruses can affect the liver or influence how far the client is willing to pursue the problem of elevated liver enzymes.

10 The most common laboratory abnormalities in cats with hyperthyroidism are increased serum concentrations of ALT and sometimes ALP. Azotemia, hyperglycemia, hyperphosphatemia, and hyperbilirubinemia are seen at times. Any cat over 8 years of age with increased ALT and ALP should be evaluated for hyperthyroidism, although the mean age for the disease is approximately 13 years. The reason for hepatic degeneration and necrosis is unknown, but concurrent hepatic dysfunction is rare.

11 If elevated liver enzymes are found in a clinically ill dog or if the enzymes are more than 2.5 times normal in a healthy dog, evaluate a full serum chemistry profile and urinalysis. If the dog is healthy and enzymes are less than 1.5–2 times normal, then reevaluation in 2–3 weeks is in order. If the enzymes remain the same, either monitor them every 3–12 months as long as the dog is healthy or pursue further evaluation via a serum chemistry profile.

12 Diabetes mellitus is associated with increased ALT in dogs and cats and increased ALP in dogs. Increased ALP is less common in diabetic cats.

13 Pancreatitis causes increases in ALT and ALP by hepatic ischemia, exposure of the liver to toxic and inflammatory portal venous drainage of the inflamed pancreas, or posthepatic obstruction of the common bile duct. The entire abdomen should be imaged.

14 Hypercalcemia in conjunction with increased ALT and/or ALP should raise the suspicion of neoplasia, particularly lymphoma.

15 Hyperbilirubinemia in the face of normal RBC counts signifies inadequate uptake or conjugation of bilirubin (hepatocellular disease), inadequate excretion of bilirubin (biliary disease), or both. Neither the ratio of conjugated (direct) or unconjugated (indirect) bilirubin nor the measurement of urobilinogen has proved useful in differentiating intra- and extrahepatic causes of hyperbilirubinemia.

16 Increased cholesterol is associated with increased hepatic synthesis and/or decreased biliary excretion of cholesterol.

17 In the dog, both hypo- and hyperadrenocorticism can cause elevation of liver enzymes.

18 Hypoalbuminemia associated with liver disease suggests chronic, marked liver dysfunction. Inhibition of albumin release due to hyperammonemia and dilution in ascitic fluid can lower the serum concentration of albumin further. Hypoglycemia can result from diffusely impaired glycogen storage, gluconeogenesis, and insulin degradation or, rarely, as a paraneoplastic hepatic disorder. Low BUN occurs with liver failure, hepatic masses, or portosystemic shunting. Liver function testing should be pursued if any of these abnormalities are found.

19 Immunoglobulins are not synthesized in the liver but can increase in chronic inflammatory diseases. Hypergammaglobulinemia is found in about one-half of cats with cholangiohepatitis.

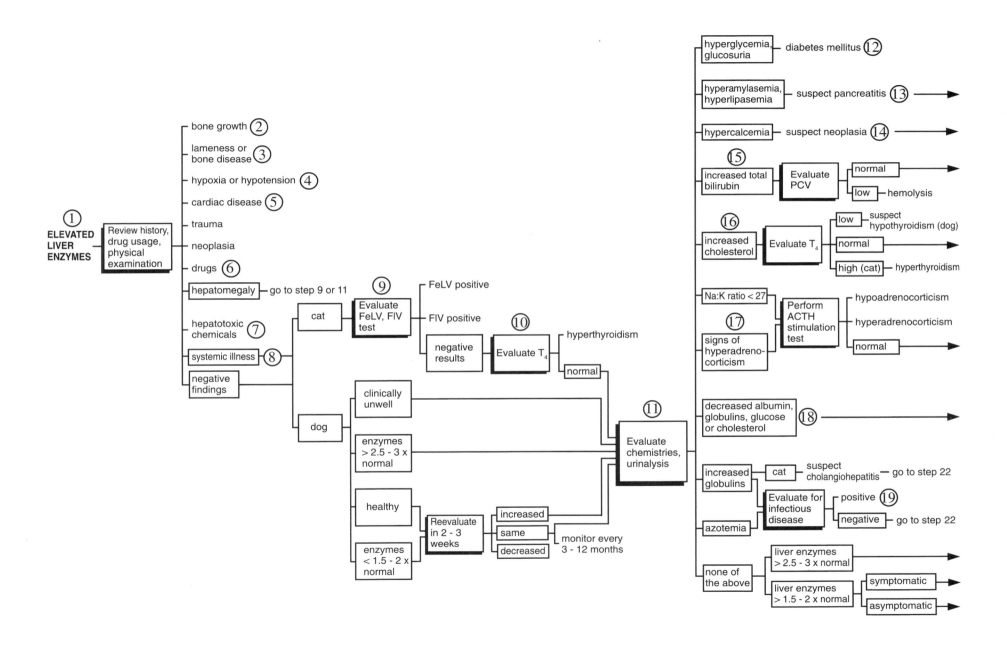

20 Liver function tests include measurement of serum bile acids (SBA) pre- and postprandial or fasting/postchallenge plasma ammonia concentrations. In the general practice setting, the SBA concentration is a practical and generally sensitive indicator of hepatocellular, biliary, and portal circulatory function. To evaluate SBA, fast the patient for 12 hours and take a serum sample (preprandial) for measurement of bile acid concentrations. Feed the patient to stimulate bile flow and gallbladder contraction and take another sample (postprandial) 2 hours after feeding. Evaluation of fasting pre- and postprandial SBA is particularly important in identifying abnormal hepatic blood flow. Bile acids do not always identify severe hepatic dysfunction, however. Fasting plasma ammonia concentration also is a fairly sensitive test of hepatic and portal circulatory function. However, false-positive results occur if stringent handling requirements are not followed. Plasma ammonia measurement is best reserved for rapid assessment of the critical patient with encephalopathic signs of unknown origin. Administration of oral or rectal ammonium chloride (the ammonia challenge test) also can assess liver function. However, this test should be performed with caution because of the risk of causing encephalopathy in seriously affected patients.

21 If liver function test results do not indicate liver dysfunction and the patient is asymptomatic, then monitoring for the development of clinical signs is a reasonable approach. Liver enzymes should be evaluated periodically to determine if they are decreasing or increasing. If enzymes increase over time, then progress to step 22.

22 Ultrasonography of the liver (as opposed to plain film radiography) provides more information about liver structure. Abnormalities commonly identified ultrasonographically include diffuse or focal parenchymal disease, changes in hepatic size and margination, cystic lesions, vascular disorders, distention or abnormal contents of the gallbladder, biliary obstruction or inflammation, perihepatic disease, masses, and abdominal effusion. Normal ultrasound examination results do not exclude hepatobiliary disease. Although in some instances a strong correlation can be made between changes in echogenicity and histological findings (notably hepatocellular carcinoma in the dog and hepatic lipidosis in the cat), a definitive diagnosis cannot be made by ultrasonography alone. The main uses of ultrasonography are to assist with biopsy planning, to identify surgically correctable vascular anomalies, and to differentiate intra- and extrahepatic causes of cholestasis.

23 The ability of ultrasonography to diagnose extrahepatic bile duct obstruction is hampered slightly by gallbladder distention and bile sludging that often is found in anorectic patients. Additionally, persistent dilation of bile ducts can be observed after resolution of chronic obstruction, especially in cats.

24 If the liver parenchyma appears abnormal, then liver aspiration for cytological examination is recommended. Because the liver produces many clotting factors, a coagulogram may be needed prior to aspiration.

25 Ultrasound-guided liver aspiration has the advantage of being a relatively noninvasive procedure and increases the probability of sampling discrete lesions, avoiding inadvertent puncture of major biliary or vascular structures, and obtaining representative specimens in diffuse hepatobiliary disease. While cytological findings of inflammation, cholestasis, necrosis, or hepatocyte hyperplasia or degeneration do not constitute a diagnosis, such findings can provide objective evidence of liver disease. The value of fine-needle aspiration cytology is that occasionally a definitive diagnosis of neoplasia (especially round cell tumors or carcinomas) or infection can be established. Because of the possibility of tumor seeding into the abdominal cavity or along the needle tracks, aspiration of a solitary hepatic mass is not advocated if surgical excision is planned.

26 If liver aspiration cytology does not yield a reasonable explanation for the increase in liver enzymes, then liver biopsy can be performed in patients whose clinical signs warrant further investigation. Indications for liver biopsy include persistently elevated liver enzymes, abnormal hepatic function, or ultrasonographically identified hepatic changes. Common methods of liver biopsy include needle biopsy (blind or ultrasonographically guided percutaneous, keyhole, laparoscopic) and surgical biopsy (requires exploratory surgery). In general, needle biopsies are useful for primary and diffuse parenchymal diseases. Anesthesia is often required even for percutaneous biopsies in small animals. Complications of needle biopsy include bleeding and bile peritonitis. Contraindications to needle biopsy include microhepatica, severe and uncorrectable coagulation abnormalities, large-volume ascites (which interferes with hemostasis and makes the liver lobes excessively mobile within the fluid), hepatic cysts or abscesses, vascular tumors, or a lesion adjacent to the major bile ducts. A surgical biopsy is warranted in such cases. Other indications for an exploratory procedure include a single resectable hepatic mass, mechanical extrahepatic bile duct obstruction, presumptive congenital vascular anomaly, septic cholangiohepatitis, and diagnostic failure of previous needle biopsy. Laparotomy offers advantages over percutaneous biopsy techniques, including the ability to evaluate the entire abdomen, prevent and control hemorrhage, collect bile for culture, perform manometry and portovenography, and correction of certain conditions (e.g., tumor excision or congenital portosystemic shunt ligation). However, many animals with chronic, severe hepatic dysfunction are in a relatively precarious state of compensation that could be overwhelmed by surgery.

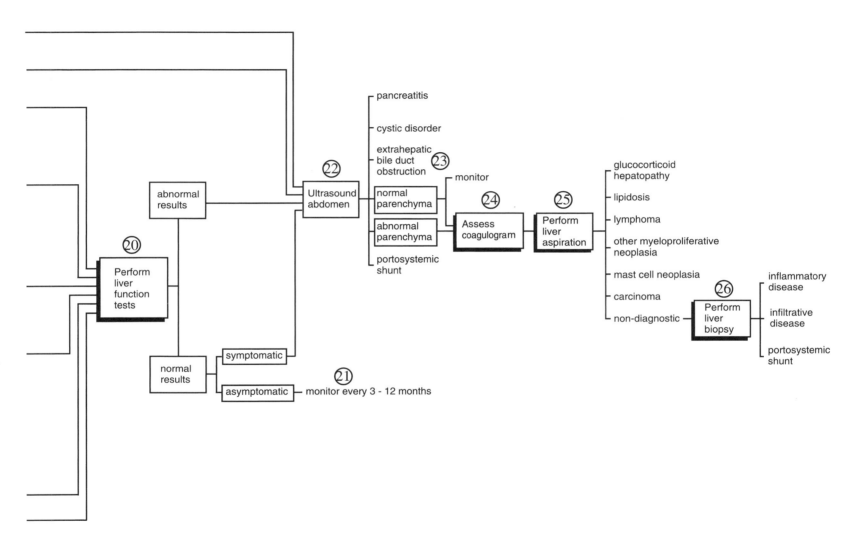

Gastrointestinal Disorders

1 Stomatitis is inflammation of oral mucosa, sometimes with extension to the tongue. It may be erosive, ulcerative, inflammatory, or proliferative, depending on the underlying disease. Causes are often species specific and occasionally breed specific. Stomatitis may be a local problem or may reflect more severe systemic disease. Stomatitis secondary to infection or debilitation is relatively common in cats. Stomatitis causes hyporexia, anorexia, ptyalism, dysphagia, and discomfort while chewing. Physical examination may reveal oral mucosal hyperemia, friability, proliferation, vesicles or bullae, mass lesions, raised plaques, or erosions and ulcers. The appearance is rarely disease specific. Vesicles or bullae, if seen, should increase the suspicion of immune-mediated disease in dogs and cats or of calicivirus infection in cats.

2 History of exposure to toxins or caustic substances (e.g., irritant chemicals, thallium, mercury, pesticides, herbicides, dieffenbachia, poinsettia, Christmas tree needles) is important. History also is important for recent drug therapy, vaccination, diet, and preexisting diseases that might cause oral ulcers (renal failure, neoplasia, immunosuppression). Dogs are more likely than cats to ingest toxins, caustic substances, and foreign bodies that directly irritate the oral mucosa. Cats are more likely to chew houseplants and may ingest chemicals on their fur while grooming. Things to look for on physical examination include signs of trauma (broken teeth), foreign material, and severe periodontal disease, and whether the problem is local, regional (enlargement of draining lymph nodes), or systemic (fever, petechiation, weight loss, generalized lymphadenopathy).

3 Drug therapy can cause reactions (idiosyncratically) that involve mucosal surfaces (erosion/sloughing) or skin (toxic epidermal necrolysis [TEN]). Drugs associated with TEN include cephalosporins, penicillins, sulfonamides, gold salts, and levamisole. Although biopsy may be required for diagnosis, development of lesions within 2 weeks of initiation of drug therapy and their resolution following drug withdrawal strongly suggest a drug reaction.

4 Young cavalier King Charles spaniels develop a necrotic and eosinophilic stomatitis. Ulcerative stomatitis is reported in Maltese terriers. Epidermolysis bullosa (in very young collies, Shetland sheepdogs, Siamese cats, and others) is a dermatosis causing oral vesicles/erosions. Collies and Shetland sheepdogs also develop dermatomyositis, which can cause oral ulcers. Biopsy is required for diagnosis.

5 Some home-prepared foods potentially cause vitamin A, D, or E deficiency, compromising mucosal integrity.

6 Cats and dogs develop oral lesions, burns, or necrosis of the hard palate, gums, and oral fornices from electrical cord bites. They may have noncardiogenic pulmonary edema.

7 A minimum database diagnoses neutropenia, which may cause stomatitis due to reduced mucosal immunity. Allergy-related oral lesions (e.g., eosinophilic granulomas) may be associated with peripheral eosinophilia. A chemistry profile and urinalysis diagnose renal failure, which causes mucosal ulceration due to bacterial metabolism of urea in saliva to ammonia. They also allow diagnosis of diabetes mellitus, which leads to immune system dysfunction and predisposes animals to infection of mucosal surfaces. Testing for FeLV and FIV is recommended since both may cause stomatitis directly, predispose to neoplasia, or cause immunosuppression and hence mucosal infections.

8 Full dental examination under general anesthesia allows assessment of all surfaces of the teeth for trauma, tartar, gingivitis, and diagnosis of subgingival "neck" lesions in cats that may be closely associated with stomatitis.

9 The majority of stomatitis cases require histopathology for confirmation of the underlying cause. Samples should be obtained for culture, cytology, histopathology, and IFA. The last is important when immune-mediated or viral disease is a concern.

10 Lymphocytic-plasmacytic stomatitis is a relatively common problem in cats and is suspected to be immune mediated, although upper respiratory tract viruses and secondary bacterial infections can play a role. Signs may be mild to severe, and lesions range from proliferative to ulcerative/erosive. It may accompany dental neck lesions.

11 Eosinophilic granuloma complex is a group of cutaneous/mucosal conditions in cats that may be manifestations of an allergic skin disease (e.g., flea allergy dermatitis, atopy). Skin lesions (e.g., linear granulomas) are most common. Oral lesions include eosinophilic ("rodent") ulcers on the upper lips and granulomas/plaques elsewhere.

12 Focal oral neoplasms generally consist of mass lesions that are easily identified. Diffuse neoplastic conditions include epitheliotropic lymphoma and oral mast cell tumors, which may mimic stomatitis. Therefore, all oral lesions should be biopsied if there is no obvious underlying cause.

13 Feline upper respiratory tract disease (herpesvirus, calicivirus, and *Chlamydia* spp.) commonly produces vesicles and oral ulcers. Lesions are most commonly seen with calicivirus and *Chlamydia* spp. Patients may have classical upper respiratory tract signs (oculonasal discharge, fever, lymphadenopathy) but may present only with stomatitis. Oral lesions should be biopsied. Viral inclusions may be seen. Laboratory confirmation of the infective organism can be made by IFA or virus isolation. Other viruses occasionally cause oral lesions in both dogs and cats (parvovirus and CDV in dogs and FIP, FeLV, FIV, feline syncytial virus, and FePLV in cats). Lesions generally are secondary to systemic immunosuppression or neutropenia.

14 Oral fungal infections (mainly *Candida* spp.) are rare in dogs and cats and are likely to be secondary to severe immunosuppression. Cytology and histopathology identify the organisms, but culture may be needed for confirmation.

15 Immune-mediated diseases such as SLE and some members of the pemphigus group are associated with oral lesions. These generally manifest as erosions and ulcers because the vesicles are extremely fragile and short-lived. Acantholytic cells within vesicles are the hallmark of immune-mediated diseases, allowing differentiation from other causes of oral vesicles and ulcers (especially drug reactions). IFA is required to establish patterns of antibody-antigen complexes in tissues and permit the diagnosis of a specific immune-mediated condition.

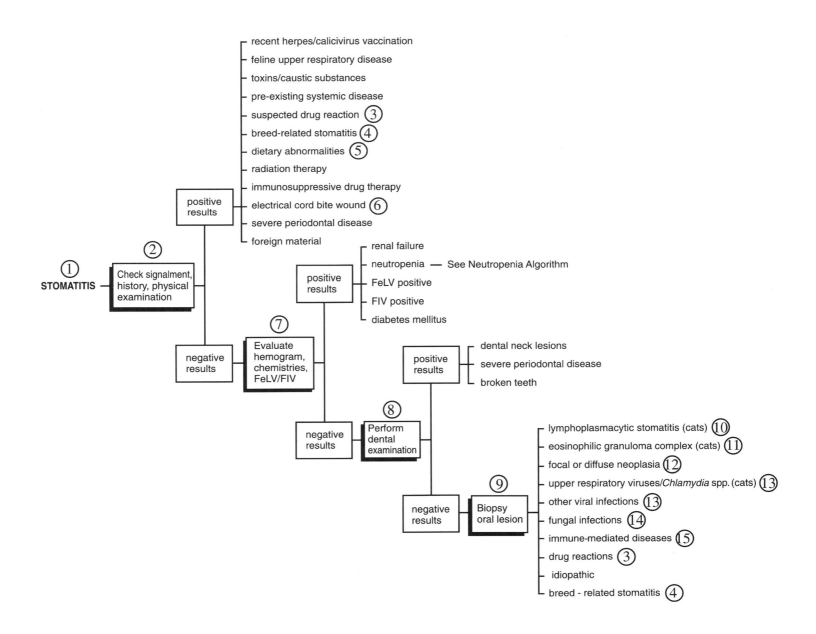

recent herpes/calicivirus vaccination

feline upper respiratory disease

toxins/caustic substances

pre-existing systemic disease

suspected drug reaction ③

breed-related stomatitis ④

dietary abnormalities ⑤

radiation therapy

immunosuppressive drug therapy

positive results — electrical cord bite wound ⑥

severe periodontal disease

foreign material

① STOMATITIS

② Check signalment, history, physical examination

positive results — renal failure

neutropenia — See Neutropenia Algorithm

FeLV positive

FIV positive

diabetes mellitus

negative results

⑦ Evaluate hemogram, chemistries, FeLV/FIV

positive results — dental neck lesions

severe periodontal disease

broken teeth

negative results

⑧ Perform dental examination

lymphoplasmacytic stomatitis (cats) ⑩

eosinophilic granuloma complex (cats) ⑪

focal or diffuse neoplasia ⑫

upper respiratory viruses/*Chlamydia* spp. (cats) ⑬

other viral infections ⑬

negative results — ⑨ Biopsy oral lesion — fungal infections ⑭

immune-mediated diseases ⑮

drug reactions ③

idiopathic

breed - related stomatitis ④

1 Regurgitation is passive backward movement of food or water from the esophagus into the pharynx, where a gag reflex is elicited, resulting in expulsion of the material. It must be differentiated from oropharyngeal dysphagia, vomiting, and, in some cases, expectoration by means of a careful history or observation of the event. With oropharyngeal dysphagia, repeated swallowing attempts occur before food or water falls from the mouth. Coughing precedes expectoration. Both regurgitation and vomiting can occur soon after swallowing or be delayed up to 24 hours after eating. The longer food is retained in the esophagus, the more "digested" it appears, giving the appearance of vomitus. Since vomiting is associated with nausea, frequent swallowing, lip licking, retching, and abdominal contractions should be observed. If the history and observation cannot distinguish regurgitation and vomiting, check the pH of the material produced via a urine dipstick. A low pH suggests acidic gastric contents and hence vomitus. Bile also suggests vomitus. Material that has not entered the stomach is alkali due to saliva.

2 If regurgitation begins before or soon after weaning, congenital megaesophagus and vascular ring anomaly are concerns. If the onset is acute in a previously normal patient, an esophageal foreign body is likely. Regurgitation developing 5 to 14 days after removal of an esophageal foreign body, after prolonged general anesthesia, or after a bout of severe vomiting leads to concern about esophageal stricture formation. In dogs with generalized/exercise-induced weakness, megaesophagus secondary to myasthenia gravis or polyneuropathy should be considered. A history of respiratory signs before the onset of regurgitation suggests possible extraluminal esophageal obstruction, while such a history after the onset of regurgitation suggests aspiration pneumonia secondary to megaesophagus.

3 Animals with regurgitation frequently have a history of weight loss or are very thin. Palpation of the cervical area may cause pain, suggesting esophagitis or a foreign body. A dilated esophagus also may be felt. Evaluation of the mouth for erosions can suggest ingestion of hot or caustic substance causing esophagitis. Auscultation of the thorax for crackles/wheezes may reveal aspiration pneumonia. In cats, a noncompressible cranial thorax or muffled lower respiratory sounds on auscultation can be associated with cranial mediastinal lymphoma and extraluminal esophageal obstruction.

4 An important initial diagnostic step in investigating esophageal problems is thoracic radiography. The esophagus is not usually seen unless air, food, or fluid is present in the lumen. Generalized esophageal dilation is seen with megaesophagus. Regional dilation occurs with stricture, a foreign body, extraluminal obstruction, or a vascular ring anomaly. If esophageal dilation is not seen directly, it should be suspected if there is mediastinal widening or displacement of the trachea (ventrally/to the right). Aspiration pneumonia, a common complication of regurgitation, appears as peribronchial or alveolar densities, especially ventrally in cranial/middle lung lobes. Cranial mediastinal masses and cardiomegaly can cause extraluminal obstruction of the esophagus.

5 If thoracic radiographs do not yield a diagnosis, evaluate the history for neurological disease and perform a neurological examination. Myasthenia gravis is the most common specific neurological disease causing regurgitation/megaesophagus. Others are polyneuritis and possibly hypothyroid neuropathy. If the neurological examination is normal, pursue esophageal disease.

6 A barium contrast esophagram with liquid barium then barium mixed with food is a sensitive method of assessing esophageal size, mucosal damage, and motility. Contrast fluoroscopy is the best technique for subtle motility problems, but radiographs are a good start. If esophageal perforation is suspected, barium should be avoided since it can cause severe mediastinitis. Aqueous iodine-based contrast should be used instead.

7 If a diagnosis cannot be obtained/confirmed via contrast esophagography, esophagoscopy is the next step. Esophageal foreign bodies can be diagnosed and removed in most cases. Strictures can be diagnosed and dilated with balloon catheters of appropriate sizes. More subtle conditions affecting the mucosa of the esophageal lumen such as esophagitis and intraluminal masses can also be visualized and confirmed.

8 Positive findings on the neurological examination include lower motor neuron (LMN) or upper motor neuron (UMN) diseases. LMN signs include muscular wasting, exercise-induced weakness, and normal to depressed spinal reflexes. Mentation usually is normal. If weakness is induced with exercise, myasthenia gravis and polymyositis become the primary differentials. If the patient began regurgitating within weeks of birth, congenital myasthenia gravis is more likely than the acquired form. UMN signs include increased spinal reflexes and weakness with little or no muscle loss (unless signs are chronic or the patient is unable to ingest sufficient food).

9 Occasionally, megaesophagus can be caused by primary brainstem disease. If test results up to this point are negative, a CT/MRI brain scan and spinal fluid analysis should be considered, especially if other cranial nerve signs are present. Since UMN causes of megaesophagus are due mostly to brainstem lesions, asymmetrical signs of weakness and other cranial nerve deficits are apparent.

10 In most cases of generalized megaesophagus and if endoscopy proves negative, the "myasthenia gravis titer" should be assessed. Serum is evaluated for anticholinesterase (ACH) receptor antibodies, which can confirm the diagnosis of acquired myasthenia gravis. However, about 15% of myasthenic dogs do not have elevation of this antibody and require immunological testing of muscle samples to make the diagnosis. Congenital cases of myasthenia gravis do not show an increase in antibody on peripheral blood samples because there is a congenital (probably inherited) lack of acetylcholine receptors rather than immune-mediated destruction of receptors in this form of the disease.

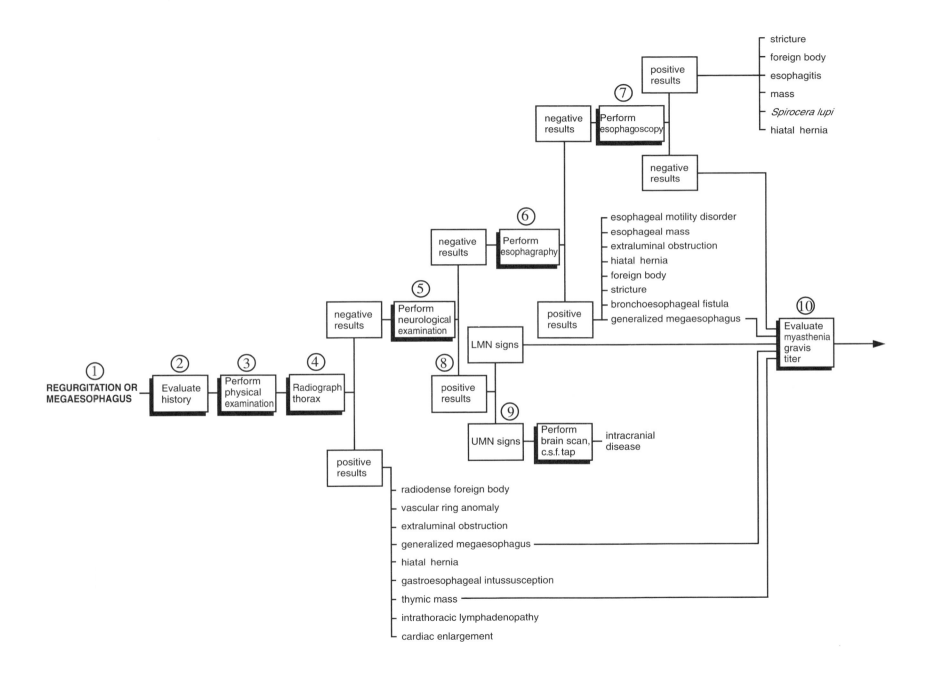

11 Evaluation of a serum chemistry profile, including CK, screens for hypoadrenocorticism and polymyositis. Hyponatremia in conjunction with hyperkalemia raises the index of suspicion for hypoadrenocorticism as an underlying cause of megaesophagus. If CK is elevated, polymyositis should be considered. There are a variety of infectious and immune-mediated causes, but idiopathic immune-mediated disease is probably the most common. Some degenerative myopathies also present with elevated CK, but megaesophagus is an uncommon sign associated with degenerative myopathy.

12 Hypoadrenocorticism is an extremely rare cause of megaesophagus. However, if the Na^+:K^+ ratio is less than 27 on the serum chemistry screen, it should be evaluated further by means of an ACTH stimulation test.

13 If serum CK is elevated, degenerative polymyopathy or polymyositis should be considered. Muscle (and/or nerve) biopsy of striated muscles that are more accessible than the esophageal muscle is the next consideration for diagnostic testing.

14 If the chemistry screen and serum CK concentrations are normal, then further testing can include serum ANA titer to increase the suspicion of immune-mediated disease, a resting serum thyroid concentration or full thyroid profile, including free T_4 by equilibrium dialysis and thyroid-stimulating hormone concentration, and measurement of serum lead concentration. Two of these tests evaluate for very uncommon causes of megaesophagus: lead intoxication and hypothyroidism. Although the connection between hypothyroidism and megaesophagus has not been proven or is very rare, it is worth testing for since the condition should be treated (although it may not result in resolution of megaesophagus). Immune-mediated disease is suspected to be a relatively common cause of esophageal and other neurological dysfunctions. A positive ANA titer supports a diagnosis of immune-mediated disease, but the trigger for this problem may not be apparent.

15 In teaching hospitals and specialty referral practices, needle electromyography (EMG) can be performed to look for denervation potentials or evidence of muscle inflammation. Any EMG testing should be performed prior to a nerve/muscle biopsy. Although muscle and/or nerve histopathology can confirm or exclude involvement of these tissues in the condition, a cause for the abnormalities is often not found. If inflammation is detected, considerations include infectious, neoplastic, and immune-mediated disorders. *Toxoplasma* spp. and *Neospora* spp. titers can be evaluated in serum. In older patients, underlying neoplasia is a consideration and should be evaluated for via thoracic radiographs and abdominal ultrasound.

16 If the only clinical sign found is megaesophagus, and if common and even uncommon differentials have been eliminated, the diagnosis is idiopathic megaesophagus. This is by far the most common underlying cause of generalized megaesophagus. Probably 80–90% of cases are supposedly idiopathic.

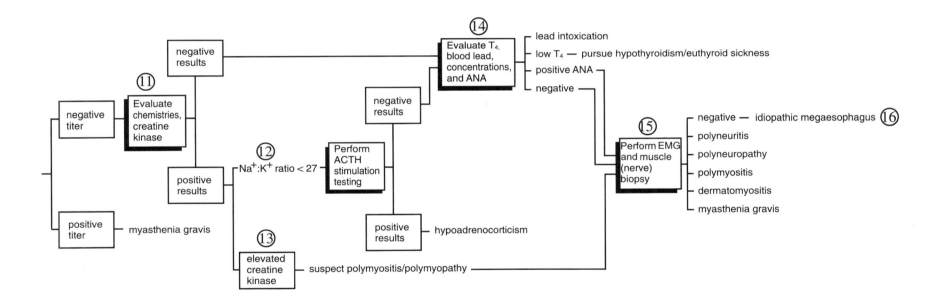

1 Vomiting is forceful expulsion of gastric contents from the body. It is usually associated with active abdominal contractions, retching sounds, a digested appearance of the vomitus, and the presence of yellow bile mixed with food or fluid. Such characteristics allow vomiting to be distinguished from regurgitation. However, both processes may occur immediately after feeding or hours later, and both may be accompanied by retching and discomfort. It is very important to determine initially whether the patient is vomiting or regurgitating, as these problems have markedly different underlying causes and there is little overlap in the initial diagnostic testing. If there is doubt about which process is occurring, the patient should be hospitalized and observed. Finally, a urine dipstick or litmus paper can be placed in any material produced to determine whether the pH is neutral (regurgitated material) or acidic (vomitus). Once it is established that the patient is vomiting, the chronicity and severity of the problem should be determined. The distinction between acute and chronic vomiting is often important to determine the underlying cause of the problem and decide about initial diagnostic testing, while the distinction between life-threatening and non-life-threatening vomiting is used to determine the need to pursue testing. Acute, non-life-threatening vomiting often is due to gastritis or dietary indiscretion and therefore requires only supportive care. However, acute, severe vomiting may be related to toxin ingestion, bowel obstruction, or anuric renal failure and requires immediate initiation of diagnostic testing and therapy. Acute vomiting is defined as vomiting developing within or lasting for less than 2 weeks. When the problem is not severe, limited or no diagnostic testing is required. Patients should have the initiating problems removed and be fasted for 24 to 48 hours. Intravenous or subcutaneous fluids may be necessary during that period. A bland diet should be used when feeding is reinstituted. If patients have more severe clinical signs initially or develop them in the course of therapy, then more aggressive diagnostic testing is required.

2 In young patients and those with incomplete vaccination against canine and feline gastrointestinal viruses, it should be determined whether they have been exposed to other animals whose clinical signs of disease (fever, vomiting, diarrhea, lethargy) suggest infectious causes.

Neutering status may be important in determining the likelihood of prostatic abscessation, prostatitis, or pyometra as a cause of acute vomiting in older patients.

3 It is easier to diagnose definitively viral diseases that cause vomiting in canine patients. Feces may be tested via an ELISA test for parvovirus. A positive test suggests either active infection or recent vaccination with a modified live virus.

4 An ELISA test does not exist for CDV. Acute infection mainly causes upper respiratory and neurological signs. However, it can also affect bone marrow and the gastrointestinal tract, and in patients with an oculonasal discharge, vomiting, and diarrhea, IFA should be performed on conjunctival swabs to evaluate for CDV inclusions. It should also be remembered that young canine patients with vomiting and diarrhea also may have a variety of other gastrointestinal viruses (rotavirus, adenovirus, and coronavirus), not all of which are included in standard vaccination protocols and which are not easy to diagnose without tissue biopsy.

5 Definitive diagnosis of viral causes of acute vomiting in young or poorly vaccinated feline patients is harder to achieve. FePLV infection can manifest with vomiting and diarrhea. Patients also are systemically ill, febrile or hypothermic, and leukopenic. No blood test exists for this virus. Both FeLV and FIV can be tested for, and the ELISA combination test should be part of the minimum database in vomiting feline patients that have not been previously tested. Often, however, neither infection is the actual cause of the clinical signs, and a positive test merely indicates that other tests should be performed or limits the client's desire to pursue the problem.

6 Older cats and dogs are less likely to present with infectious causes of acute vomiting unless they are very old or immunosuppressed due to concurrent disease or drug therapy. However, exposure to animals with vomiting or diarrhea still should be assessed as part of the initial history. Older patients are more likely to vomit as a result of organ failure, neoplasia, or drug exposure.

7 The history should be evaluated for drugs, gastrointestinal irritants, and toxins. Drugs may cause vomiting

due to direct irritant effects on the gastrointestinal mucosa or by affecting the brain's chemoreceptor trigger zone. Drugs that commonly cause vomiting are nonsteroidal anti-inflammatory drugs (NSAIDs), glucocorticoids, antimicrobials (e.g., erythromycin, cephalosporins, tetracyclines), cardiac glycosides, and chemotherapeutics. In most instances, there is a relatively close association between administration of the drug and induction of vomiting. However, chronic administration of both NSAIDs and glucocorticoids may cumulatively cause gastrointestinal irritation and vomiting. Toxins that cause acute gastrointestinal signs as well as other clinical problems include plant alkaloids, solanines, mushrooms, insecticides (amitraz, methaldehyde, naphthalene, nicotine, pyrethrins), and heavy metals (lead, zinc, iron). Potential toxins in garbage (garbage can intoxication) include preformed bacterial enterotoxins, mycotoxins, and fermentation products.

8 If no drugs or toxins are identified in the patient's history, evaluate for recent dietary changes or dietary indiscretion. Some patients develop gastrointestinal signs when switched to another diet. This may represent sensitivity to dietary constituents, changes in fat and protein content, or true food allergy. Other patients develop gastrointestinal signs after ingesting inappropriate foods (e.g., table scraps), getting into the garbage, or ingesting other inappropriate substances. If this is the case, patients should be fasted for 24 to 48 hours and switched back to their original diet, if possible, prior to further testing. The history also should be assessed for ingestion of nondigestible foreign material that may cause bowel obstruction or irritation.

9 Patients with no history of drug administration, toxins, foreign body ingestion, recent dietary changes, or inappropriate diets should undergo a detailed physical examination for lethargy, depression, fever, icterus, abdominal distention or fluid, abdominal masses, foreign bodies, and abdominal pain in an attempt to guide further diagnostic testing. Positive findings may be specific (i.e., they guide further diagnostic testing and therapy) or nonspecific (i.e., they identify problems but do not necessarily suggest a specific next step).

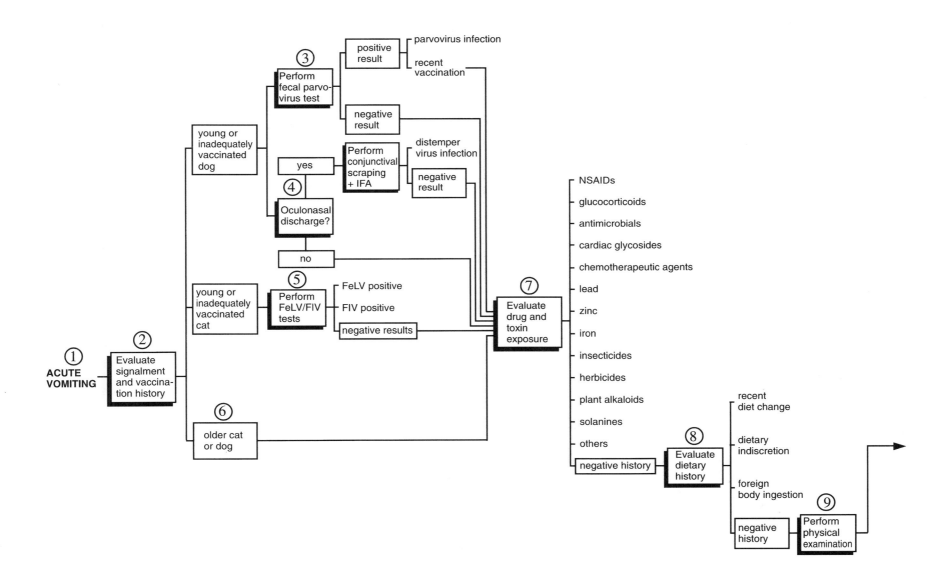

10 Positive specific findings include abdominal distention due to masses, fluid, or gas-filled viscera, a palpable abdominal mass, intussusception, intestinal foreign body, an enlarged, painful prostate that suggests prostatitis or a prostatic abscess, or a vaginal discharge suggesting an open pyometra. All these findings guide the clinician toward some type of abdominal imaging as the next diagnostic step.

11 Abdominal radiographs are likely to prove most useful in identifying gas-filled viscera (e.g., gastric dilation, gastric dilation and torsion, bowel obstruction, bowel torsion, and possibly intussuscepted bowel). Contrast studies may be required to identify partial gastric or bowel obstruction. However, contrast may prove difficult to administer to a vomiting patient. Water-soluble (iodine-based) contrast should be used if bowel perforation is suspected, despite the fact that the images obtained are not as good as those obtained when insoluble contrast such as barium sulfate is given. Abdominal ultrasound is more useful for patients with mass lesions (to identify the structure involved, tissue of origin, and consistency), intussuscepted bowel, pyometra, or prostatic enlargement (either due to focal abscesses or general prostatic hypertrophy and inflammation or infection). Ultrasound also may indicate the formation of abscess-like structures in other tissues (e.g., liver and pancreas), generalized pancreatic inflammation, or renal pelvis dilation that might suggest pyelonephritis or obstruction. Note that many of the above conditions may be suspected from abdominal imaging, but they require cytology, culture, or histopathology of affected tissues to confirm the problem.

12 Other positive findings on physical examination include acute onset of neurological signs that might suggest toxin exposure or vestibular lesions. Vestibular disease causes vomiting due to a syndrome akin to motion sickness. Underlying causes of acute vestibular signs include brainstem lesions (especially neoplasia and inner ear disease) and middle ear disease (infection, damage resulting from ear cleaning, tympanic membrane rupture, and administration of ototoxic drugs such as aminoglycosides).

13 Positive but less specific findings on physical examination include fever, icterus, oral ulcers, weakness, weight loss, and abdominal pain. In patients with non-specific or negative findings, a minimum database (hemogram, chemistry profile, and urinalysis) should be performed to try to identify systemic (i.e., nongastrointestinal) causes of vomiting. These include renal failure, pancreatitis, hypoadrenocorticism, diabetic ketoacidosis, and hepatitis. Note that finding some of these conditions may require further follow-up by abdominal imaging (e.g., ultrasound) if this has not already been done. Other conditions may require cytology or histopathology to confirm the problem.

14 Hypoadrenocorticism may manifest as acute vomiting, diarrhea, cardiovascular collapse, and shock accompanied by bradycardia, hypothermia, and electrolyte imbalances. It should be noted that while mineralocorticoid deficiency produces the classical electrolyte imbalances characteristic of hypoadrenocorticism, it is the glucocorticoid deficiency that causes gastrointestinal signs. Therefore, it is possible for patients to present with nonspecific signs, including vomiting and diarrhea, and have only the glucocorticoid deficiency (see the algorithm for chronic vomiting). Hypoadrenocorticism is extremely rare in feline patients unless it is iatrogenic.

15 Canine patients with severe clinical signs that include vomiting and bloody diarrhea, and with evidence of severe hemoconcentration (PCVs of 55–70% and very high total serum protein), may have hemorrhagic gastroenteritis (HGE). The actual cause of HGE has not been defined. *Clostridium* spp. enterotoxins and enterotoxigenic *Escherichia coli* have been suggested as etiological agents. The condition is classically described in middle-aged, small-breed dogs, and the clinical course of the disease is short (72 hours), provided that appropriate, aggressive fluid and antimicrobial therapy is instituted.

16 Sepsis (endotoxemia, septicemia) may lead to vomiting as a symptom of generalized, severe illness, gastric

mucosal compromise, or failure of other organs (e.g., liver and kidneys). Patients usually have evidence of other severe systemic problems that help to guide this diagnosis. Blood cultures (three samples taken within a 24-hour period, preferably at the time that the patient is febrile) and urine cultures may prove useful in determining the organism(s) involved.

17 In patients with acute vomiting and diarrhea that prove negative on diagnostic testing to this point, three zinc sulfate fecal flotation tests should be performed at least 24 hours apart, as well as a direct fecal smear to evaluate for gastrointestinal parasites. Some of these parasites may cause vomiting, particularly in young animals. Parasitic causes of vomiting include a very heavy burden of intestinal ascarids in dogs and cats, *Physaloptera* spp. infestation of the stomach in dogs, and *Ollulanus tricuspis* in cats. *Dirofilaria immitis* antibody and antigen testing may be appropriate in feline patients in endemic areas, since about one-third of cats with dirofilariasis present with acute or, more commonly, chronic vomiting.

18 Patients with acute vomiting rarely need upper endoscopy, exploratory surgery, or gastric and small bowel biopsies. Probably the one indication for upper endoscopy in an acutely vomiting patient is a known or suspected gastric foreign body. Indications for surgery include intestinal obstruction (which has a multitude of causes including foreign bodies, masses, and intussusceptions) and gastric and intestinal torsions. The last requires very rapid intervention (within 30 to 60 minutes of presentation) to have any chance of saving the patient. Endoscopy also may be important in patients presenting with acute hematemesis to determine the extent of any gastric or duodenal lesion. *Helicobacter* spp. gastric inflammation may be a cause of acute vomiting; however, it is more likely to be a chronic problem. Many causes of acute vomiting that require upper endoscopy or surgery and gastrointestinal biopsies are likely to have become chronic problems by the time the diagnostic algorithm has been worked through to reach this stage (see the algorithm for chronic vomiting).

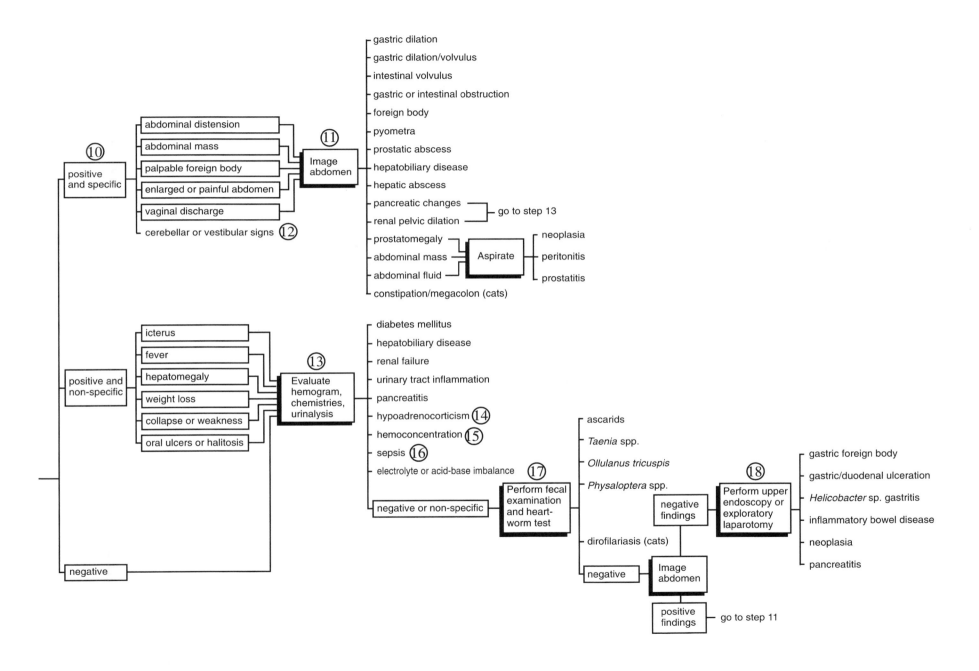

1 Chronic vomiting is defined as vomiting that has occurred intermittently or continuously for a period of 4 or more weeks. This leaves something of a gray area in terms of time between acute and chronic vomiting. Vomiting that is acute in onset (e.g., due to inflammatory bowel disease, *Helicobacter* spp. gastritis, or partial foreign body obstruction) may, over time, become chronic. Patients with chronic vomiting may be healthy, show no weight loss, and have no signs of systemic disease. Under these circumstances, the problem is most likely to be gastrointestinal and particularly gastric in origin (e.g., partial gastric outflow obstruction by benign masses or pyloric hypertrophy, motility disorders, bilious vomiting, *Helicobacter* spp. gastritis). Patients with more severe gastrointestinal signs accompanying vomiting (e.g., diarrhea, anorexia, weight loss) either have a more severe, generalized gastrointestinal condition or a systemic disease (e.g., CRF, liver disease). Although a good dietary history should be taken during the initial evaluation of any patient with chronic vomiting, it is not as useful in making up an initial differential diagnosis list as it is in patients with acute vomiting. However, the dietary history is useful for deciding on a hypoallergenic exclusion diet after a diagnosis of inflammatory bowel disease or suspected food allergy has been made.

2 Initial evaluation of patients with chronic vomiting should include determination of exposure to drugs and toxins. Although administration of many drugs is generally associated with acute vomiting, some drugs (e.g., NSAIDs, prednisone, and azathioprine) can cause chronic gastritis, erosions, ulceration, and more long-term signs. Although these patients may eventually need upper endoscopy or exploratory surgery to confirm the diagnosis or treat the problem, it is valid to withdraw drug therapy whenever possible and see whether clinical signs resolve. Few toxins are likely to result in chronic vomiting without more severe clinical consequences. However, chronic exposure to small amounts of both lead and arsenic may result in chronic gastrointestinal signs.

3 Signalment is important in diagnosing the chronically vomiting patient. For example, pyloric hypertrophy is more likely to be a congenital condition in a young Siamese cat or an acquired problem in an older small or toy-breed dog. Certain breeds also appear to have a predisposition to lymphoma and small intestinal bacterial overgrowth. The history is useful to determine chronicity of the problem and the presence of other signs such as diarrhea and weight loss. Physical examination is important in determining the presence of oral ulcerations, lymphadenopathy, uveitis, poor body condition, or mass lesions within the abdomen or in the skin that may suggest more severe systemic conditions causing vomiting, and in detecting colonic dilation/obstipation (particularly in cats, in which the colon is easy to palpate).

4 Small-breed dogs (miniature poodles, bichons frises, and Shetland sheepdogs) are prone to bilious vomiting syndrome. They vomit on an empty stomach, particularly just before the next meal (e.g., overnight or in the early morning). The problem is caused by excessive reflux of alkaline bile into the empty stomach from the small bowel when the pylorus relaxes because digestive processes in the stomach have ceased. Alkaline bile irritates the gastric mucosa, which is equipped to cope with acidity but not excessive alkalinity. Therapy includes multiple small meals during the day and late evening so that the stomach is rarely empty and gastric acid is present to neutralize any alkaline bile that refluxes.

5 Cutaneous or subcutaneous lesions, however small, should be aspirated and evaluated cytologically for mast cells. Systemic spread of mast cell tumors increases circulating histamine, which boosts gastric acid production by binding to H_2 receptors in the gastric mucosa and hence predisposes to gastric irritation and ulceration.

6 Discovery of neoplastic mast cells in a cutaneous or subcutaneous mass should be followed by a buffy coat examination (on a concentrated preparation of WBCs from peripheral blood) for evidence of circulating mast cells, abdominal ultrasound, cytological evaluation of the spleen and other organs for mast cell infiltration, and/or bone marrow examination, all to look for evidence of systemic spread of the tumor. Note that occasionally patients with severe gastrointestinal inflammation that is not related to mast cell tumors may have increased numbers of mast cells in the circulation, complicating the diagnosis of disseminated mastocytosis.

7 Feline patients more than 8 years of age that present with chronic vomiting should be evaluated for hyperthyroidism. Hyperthyroid cats usually, but not always, have a normal to increased appetite, weight loss, and changes in the nature of the stool (ranging from diarrhea to more bulky and poorly digested stool). Laboratory tests often also reveal increased liver enzymes, especially ALT.

8 In chronically vomiting patients with no specific history or physical examination findings or weight loss alone, at least three zinc sulfate fecal flotations should be performed. Parasite overload (roundworms in very young animals) or specific parasites of the stomach (*Physaloptera* spp., *O. tricuspis*) may cause chronic vomiting. This is usually a problem in younger animals that tend to have high worm burdens or eat unusual intermediate hosts.

9 In patients that are negative to this point on all diagnostic tests, a minimum database (hemogram, chemistry profile, and urinalysis) should be assessed to occlude metabolic causes of vomiting. This will identify various forms of hepatobiliary disease, hormonal problems, renal disease, and renal infection, all of which may lead to chronic vomiting. Once metabolic problems are identified, further imaging (e.g., abdominal ultrasound) and testing may be required (e.g., to differentiate vomiting due to pancreatic inflammation from that due to pancreatic neoplasia).

10 In feline patients with no underlying cause of chronic vomiting detected at this point, serum antibodies and antigen titers should be evaluated to establish exposure to *Dirofilaria immitis*. Although cats are not the primary host of this parasite, outdoor cats in endemic areas, and occasionally those from other regions, may develop infestation. Up to one-third of feline patients with heartworm disease present with clinical signs of vomiting alone.

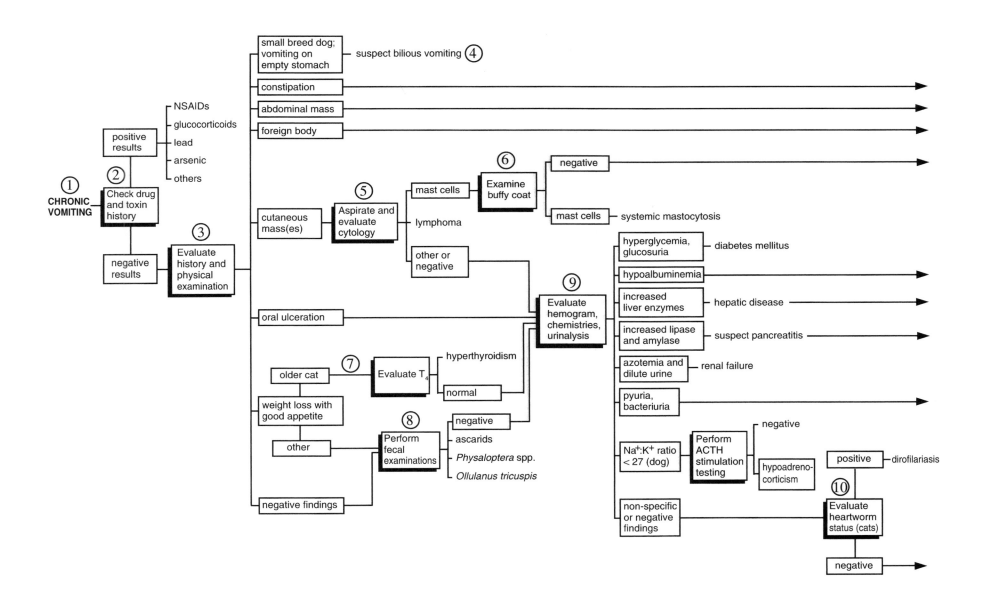

① **CHRONIC VOMITING**

② Check drug and toxin history
- positive results
  - NSAIDs
  - glucocorticoids
  - lead
  - arsenic
  - others
- negative results

③ Evaluate history and physical examination
- small breed dog; vomiting on empty stomach — suspect bilious vomiting ④
- constipation →
- abdominal mass →
- foreign body →
- cutaneous mass(es) → ⑤ Aspirate and evaluate cytology
  - mast cells → ⑥ Examine buffy coat
    - negative →
    - mast cells — systemic mastocytosis
  - lymphoma
  - other or negative
- oral ulceration
- older cat → ⑦ Evaluate T₄
  - hyperthyroidism
  - normal
- weight loss with good appetite
- other → ⑧ Perform fecal examinations
  - negative
  - ascarids
  - *Physaloptera* spp.
  - *Ollulanus tricuspis*
- negative findings

⑨ Evaluate hemogram, chemistries, urinalysis
- hyperglycemia, glucosuria — diabetes mellitus
- hypoalbuminemia →
- increased liver enzymes — hepatic disease →
- increased lipase and amylase — suspect pancreatitis →
- azotemia and dilute urine — renal failure
- pyuria, bacteriuria →
- Na⁺:K⁺ ratio < 27 (dog) → Perform ACTH stimulation testing
  - negative
  - hypoadreno-corticism
- non-specific or negative findings

⑩ Evaluate heartworm status (cats)
- positive — dirofilariasis
- negative →

11 Patients with an intra-abdominal mass, foreign body, intussusception, or colonic dilation/impaction should undergo abdominal imaging. Survey radiographs are useful to identify complete bowel obstruction, radiodense foreign bodies, obstipation, or megacolon. Contrast may be needed for partial obstruction, radiolucent foreign bodies, and motility disorders. Abdominal ultrasound diagnoses intestinal masses or intussusceptions and lesions in other organs and may identify pyelonephritis, gallbladder inflammation/partial obstruction, and small adrenal glands.

12 Chronically vomiting patients with negative or nonspecific findings on the minimum database probably have primary gastrointestinal disease, which can be further pursued by upper endoscopy or exploratory celiotomy. Upper endoscopy has the advantage of being relatively quick and noninvasive, and it allows direct visual evaluation of gastric and proximal enteric mucosa. Biopsy specimens are small but likely to be representative. Disadvantages include the inability to evaluate anything but the proximal portions of the small bowel, remove linear or intestinal foreign bodies, and evaluate the outer surfaces of the bowel for disease extension or extraintestinal conditions. Gross endoscopic diagnoses include pyloric hypertrophy, gastric antral polyps, other gastric/duodenal mass lesions, alterations in the normal anatomy of the stomach and pylorus due to prior surgery, gastric nematodes, gastroduodenal ulceration/erosion, and evidence of gastroduodenal reflux. Histopathology is required to determine whether a mass lesion is benign or malignant, the presence of lymphoplasmacytic or eosinophilic inflammatory bowel disease (IBD), or granulomatous gastritis. Histopathology and *Campylobacter*-like organism (CLO) testing may be required to make a diagnosis of *Helicobacter* spp. gastritis. Depending on the pathologist, histopathology may help confirm pyloric hypertrophy.

13 Large, focal gastroduodenal ulcerations are most commonly the result of drugs (NSAIDs or prednisone) or neoplasia. Rarer causes are disseminated mastocytosis, gastrinoma/other neuroendocrine tumors, and stress. Small ulcerations and erosions may be due to drug therapy, infiltrative neoplasia, disseminated mastocytosis, ingestion of caustic substances, *Helicobacter* spp., or IBD. Rare cases of gastritis do not have an obvious cause. Atrophic gastritis is associated with thinning of gastric mucosa and hyposecretion of acid and may be immune mediated. Generalized hypertrophic gastritis, excessive thickening of gastric mucosa, and multiple types of inflammatory cell infiltrates in the absence of mastocytosis or an amine precursor uptake and decarboxylation tumor (APUDoma) is seen in basenjis and small-breed dogs such as Lhasa apsos, miniature poodles, and Maltese terriers. The condition is probably hereditary and immune mediated.

14 Finding *Helicobacter* spp. in the stomach does not always mean this is causing vomiting. *Helicobacter* spp. and related spiral organisms may be normal gastric flora in dogs and cats. Reports exist of vomiting patients that are positive for *Helicobacter* spp., but do not have gastric inflammation yet respond to specific therapy for that infection.

15 IBD generally manifests as lymphocytic and/or plasmacytic infiltrates in mucosa of bowel or stomach. The condition is thought to be the result of inappropriate or excessive immune system responses to food proteins and bacterial antigens within the bowel lumen. The etiology of eosinophilic infiltrates is probably similar, although parasitic infestation may play more of a role. Eosinophilic infiltrates are more likely to cause obstruction and may prove less responsive to immunosuppression and hypoallergenic diets. Eosinophilic bowel infiltrates in cats may be a manifestation of hypereosinophilic syndrome, which affects multiple organs, causes peripheral eosinophilia, and is difficult to treat.

16 Granulomatous gastritis is a rare condition characterized by localized masses or diffuse microscopic granulomas. It is reported in association with eosinophilic infiltrates, fungal infections (histoplasmosis, phycomycosis), FIP, parasites, and neoplasia.

17 Pyloric hypertrophy causes outflow obstruction from the stomach and vomiting, which is often projectile. Obstruction may be the result of hypertrophy of the muscularis layer of the pylorus, the overlying mucosa, or both. It may be acquired (in older, male, small-breed dogs and rarely in cats) or congenital (particularly involving the muscle layer) in Boston terriers, Boxers, and Siamese cats.

18 Patients with gastric or duodenal ulceration, especially if severe and poorly responsive to appropriate therapy, should be evaluated for APUDomas. Most commonly these arise in the pancreas, but they also may be found in other neuroendocrine tissue. They secrete substances such as gastrin, stimulating gastric hyperacidity and ulceration. Fasting serum gastrin concentrations usually are elevated, but occasionally provocative testing (using injections of calcium or secretin) may be needed to stimulate excessive gastrin production and confirm the diagnosis. Abdominal ultrasound, CT scans, or MRI scans may be useful to identify lesions and determine their extent prior to surgical resection.

19 Canine and feline patients with no underlying cause of vomiting identified, with inflammatory infiltrates in bowel that do not appear significant or that do not respond to appropriate therapy, should be evaluated for true dietary allergies. Previous dietary constituents should be evaluated, and patients should be placed on a true hypoallergenic diet, containing proteins to which they have not been previously exposed. Diet trials should be continued for at least 10 weeks before determining success or failure. If a good response is seen, individual proteins may be reintroduced to the diet to expand the range of what the patient can eat and to identify the proteins that cause recurrence of vomiting.

20 In patients with no findings to this point, consider small intestinal bacterial overgrowth (SIBO) as a potential cause of vomiting. The condition predominantly causes diarrhea and weight loss, but it also may lead to vomiting. It is a particular problem in German shepherd dogs. Associated inflammatory infiltrates in the small bowel may be minimal. Diagnosis is based on the history, signalment, presenting signs, quantitative cultures of duodenal fluid, and response to appropriate therapy.

21 Finally, vomiting patients with no identified underlying cause should be evaluated for motility disorders, especially if gaseous bloating is present, if radiographs indicate an abnormal gas pattern in bowel, or if there is unusual positioning of a gas-filled viscus. Contrast studies using liquid barium and/or barium-impregnated spheres and either sequential radiographs or fluoroscopy may be useful in identifying motility problems. However, it should be noted that the stress of administering contrast and repeatedly radiographing the abdomen may slow gastric emptying in nervous patients.

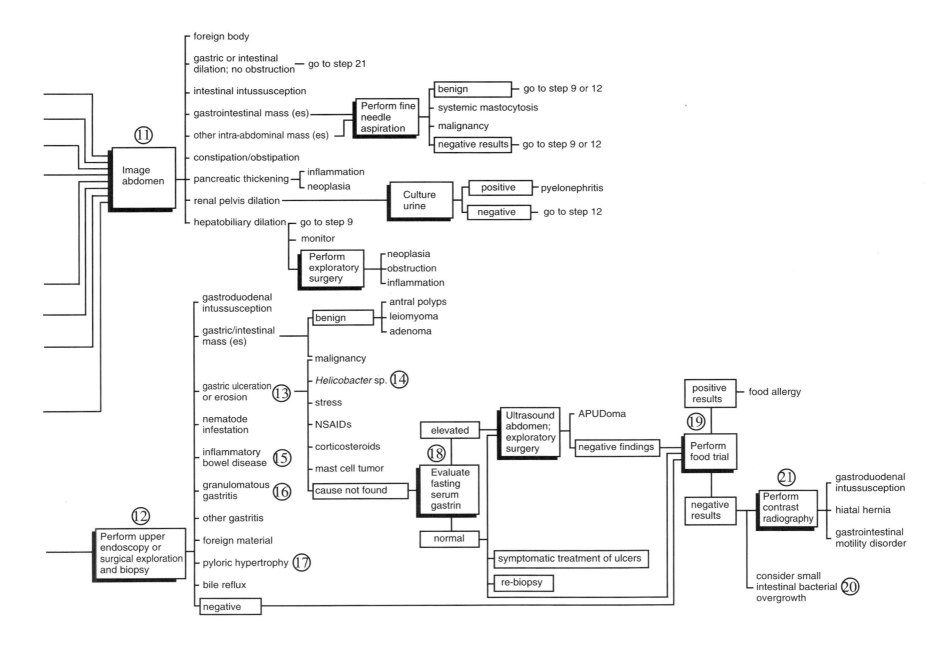

1 Hematemesis is vomitus that contains blood. Blood may be fresh (frank red clots) or digested (with a black or "coffee ground" appearance). Melena is the dark/black coloration and tarry appearance of stool containing digested blood. Both hematemesis and melena are manifestations of moderate to severe bleeding into upper portions of the gastrointestinal tract (esophagus, stomach, and small intestine). Loss of small amounts of blood tends to manifest more as chronic iron deficiency anemia. Bleeding may be focal or diffuse from disrupted areas of gastrointestinal mucosa (e.g., due to NSAIDs, mast cell tumors, severe liver disease, renal failure, or pancreatic gastrinoma). Bleeding also may occur from apparently normal mucosal surfaces in patients with underlying coagulopathies. Gastric ulcers are relatively common in dogs but less so in cats.

2 The history is important for ulcerogenic medications (NSAIDs, glucocorticoids, azathioprine), and prior diagnosis of hepatic and renal failure, and systemic mastocytosis, which predispose to gastrointestinal bleeding, ingestion of foreign material, or "stress ulceration." Stress ulcers in dogs and cats may develop in association with changes in blood flow to the gastric mucosa (e.g., consequent upon head or spinal trauma, sepsis, hypovolemia, or hypotension).

3 Physical examination also may help diagnose the causes of melena or hematemesis. Superficial petechial or ecchymotic hemorrhages on skin and mucous membranes often indicate platelet problems (deficiency/ functional failure) leading to gastrointestinal mucosal bleeding. Chorioretinitis suggests systemic conditions such as disseminated or gastrointestinal fungal infection (e.g., *Histoplasma capsulatum*).

4 Bleeding oral, nasal, or pharyngeal lesions may result in patients swallowing blood and presenting with melena or hematemesis. Such lesions may be neoplastic, traumatic, or fungal, or the result of foreign bodies or coagulopathies.

5 Cytological evaluation of cutaneous masses allows the diagnosis of mast cell tumors. If one is found, the patient should be evaluated for systemic spread. Regional lymph nodes should be palpated and aspirated; buffy coat examination of blood may detect mast cells in the

circulation; ultrasound-guided aspiration of liver and spleen, as well as bone marrow examination, may be appropriate to look for mast cell infiltration. Note that gastrointestinal inflammation may increase mast cells in peripheral blood without systemic mastocytosis being present. Disseminated mastocytosis may lead to infiltration of abdominal organs or bone marrow by neoplastic cells. Degranulation of mast cells releases histamine, causing gastric hyperacidity and ulceration by its action on H_2 receptors in the stomach. Mast cell granules also contain heparin, which may affect blood clotting.

6 Patients presenting with coughing and hematemesis or melena may have a source of blood loss besides the gastrointestinal tract. They may be bleeding into airways (e.g., due to coagulopathy, primary/metastatic neoplasia, or have a foreign body, abscess, or granuloma eroding blood vessels). Patients cough up blood (hemoptysis), which is then swallowed and either vomited or digested.

7 Esophageal problems may present as retching or gagging. Any blood appears fresh because it is not exposed to gastric acid. Patients also may vomit fresh or digested blood due to irritation of the stomach by blood from esophageal lesions and may have melena. Radiographs may identify radiodense foreign bodies and focal esophageal masses or nodules (e.g., due to *Spirocerca lupi*). They also may identify esophageal dilation due to masses, foreign body impaction, esophagitis, or motility disorders. Contrast esophagography or esophagoscopy can identify some masses, radiolucent foreign bodies, and esophagitis.

8 Young canine patients with melena should be tested for parvovirus enteritis. Hematemesis is unlikely unless there is severe esophagitis secondary to vomiting. Parvovirus testing also may be appropriate for older patients with immunosuppressive conditions or outdated vaccinations, those receiving immunosuppressive drugs, and those that have been exposed to dogs suspected of having parvovirus.

9 If the underlying causes of gastrointestinal bleeding are not immediately obvious, a minimum database may identify thrombocytopenia and metabolic problems compromising mucosal integrity. When this suggests problems likely to cause gastrointestinal ulceration, further

testing may be required to determine the severity of the problem and confirm it as the cause of clinical signs. Hematemesis or melena in a patient with renal failure requires little further evaluation. However, hematemesis or melena in a patient with only liver enzyme elevations may require abdominal ultrasound to determine the presence of masses, as well as liver structure and size. Liver function testing may be needed to establish the severity of the problem, as well as hepatic cytology or histopathology. Neutropenia implies sepsis, bone marrow problems, viral infection (CDV, parvovirus, FePLV), or salmonellosis. Electrolyte imbalances may suggest hypoadrenocorticism, although gastrointestinal signs associated with this condition are related to the glucocorticoid and not the mineralocorticoid deficiency and may, therefore, be seen in patients without electrolyte changes. Severe vomiting and diarrhea also may cause electrolyte abnormalities mimicking hypoadrenocorticism.

10 Intestinal parasites do not usually cause gross bleeding into the upper intestinal tract unless the parasite burden is large or causes direct mucosal damage, or unless there is larval migration within the bowel wall. Hookworms cause significant blood loss anemia in dogs by ingesting blood, but melena is unlikely unless there is a lot of bleeding from sites when the parasites detach. Ideally, three zinc sulfate fecal flotations, a direct fecal smear, and prophylactic deworming should be performed to exclude gastrointestinal parasites. Bacterial infections are unlikely to cause melena alone; therefore, fecal cultures are rarely indicated at this point.

11 If the minimum database is normal or shows nonspecific abnormalities (e.g., panhypoproteinemia), the majority of remaining patients with hematemesis/ melena have primary gastrointestinal lesions and testing should progress to abdominal imaging, upper endoscopy, or exploratory celiotomy. Both of the last two procedures are somewhat invasive and require general anesthesia. A much smaller number of patients have coagulation abnormalities (DIC, anticoagulant rodenticide exposure, or abnormalities secondary to hepatic failure). When patients are so seriously affected that they are not stable for anesthesia or need blood transfusion, or when there is a strong historical suspicion of coagulopathy, a coagulation panel is appropriate. Otherwise, this step may be bypassed.

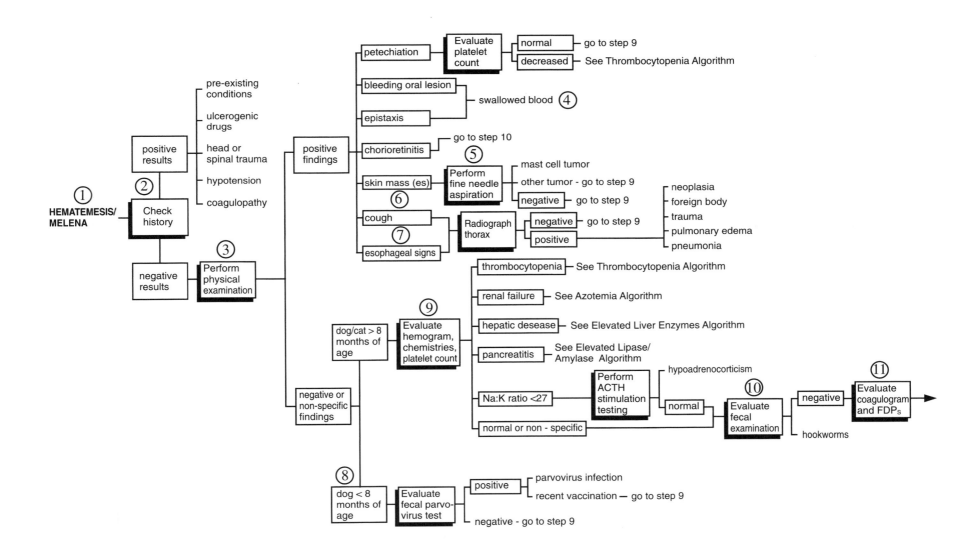

12 Imaging the gastrointestinal tract may be appropriate to pursue the causes of hematemesis or melena prior to upper endoscopy or exploratory celiotomy. Imaging may range from plain abdominal radiographs, contrast radiographs, and abdominal ultrasound to specialized biliary imaging, CT, MRI, and nuclear scintigraphy scanning in difficult or obscure cases. Imaging is, however, unlikely to provide a specific diagnosis of the cause of gastrointestinal bleeding. For example, a barium upper gastrointestinal tract study may reveal a thickened area in the gastric antrum with contrast adhesion, probably representing an ulcer and hence the source of blood loss. However, it will not determine whether the ulcer is due to administration of NSAIDs, stress factors, *Helicobacter* spp., or neoplastic tissue compromising the gastric mucosa. The value of imaging lies in determining whether the lesion is better addressed endoscopically or surgically. Surgery is needed when the lesion is located too far down the intestinal tract to be reached with an endoscope, if there is involvement of structures outside the gastrointestinal tract, or if the underlying condition may be corrected surgically. Plain abdominal radiographs identify some intestinal masses, intussusceptions, abdominal fluid, radiodense foreign bodies, and intestinal dilation. Contrast studies of the abdomen aid in diagnosis of ulcers, obstruction, nonradiodense foreign bodies, masses, and motility disorders. However, they may be difficult to perform in vomiting patients. Ultrasound of the abdomen is not always useful for primary gastrointestinal problems, mainly because the bowel lumen often contains gas, which blocks the ultrasound beam. Intestinal contents also may confuse the diagnosis. However, ultrasound is useful for involvement of tissues outside the bowel, especially pancreatic and gallbladder lesions and lymphadenopathy, and to evaluate liver size and structure. It also may be useful for measuring bowel wall thickness, finding focal bowel masses, and determining how far down in the bowel a lesion is located. More involved imaging techniques are indicated to look at difficult areas such as the pancreas or biliary system and to assess the extent of involvement of tissues prior to endoscopy or surgery.

13 Upper endoscopy, specifically esophagoscopy, is indicated in any patient suspected of having an esophageal abnormality unless there is involvement of the medi-

astinum or pleural space. In the latter case, surgical intervention is required and the prognosis is very guarded. Esophagoscopy allows diagnosis of esophagitis, strictures, and mass lesions, and permits removal of foreign material with minimal risk to the patient compared to surgery.

14 Immediate diagnosis of some conditions causing hematemesis or melena may result from surgical or endoscopic evaluation. Direct results are likely to consist of identification of the source of blood loss into the gastrointestinal tract, finding *S. lupi* nodules in the esophagus, primary or secondary esophagitis, foreign bodies anywhere in the upper portions of the gastrointestinal tract, any obstructive or partially obstructive conditions, or ulceration compromising mucosal integrity.

15 Histopathology is required to distinguish among diffuse or focal neoplasia, infectious conditions, and IBD. Adenocarcinoma is the main primary neoplasm of the stomach and small bowel. Lymphoma and mast cell tumors may affect the gastrointestinal tract as primary conditions or may compromise bowel integrity secondary to their systemic effects. Leukemia may result in bowel infiltration and compromise, along with that of many other organs. Metastatic tumors to bowel are very uncommon. Histopathology and impression smears of biopsy specimens also may identify *Helicobacter* spp. or *H. capsulatum*.

16 If *Helicobacter* spp. are seen on gastric biopsy specimen (usually identified with a silver stain) and are accompanied by lymphoid infiltrates or frank erosion/ulceration of the mucosa, the bacteria may be the cause of hematemesis or melena. Note that they also may be normal gastric flora in asymptomatic patients. Histopathology should be combined with testing of biopsy samples for urease production (CLO test) to increase detection of *Helicobacter* spp. in patients with gastric and proximal duodenal ulcers.

17 If endoscopic or surgical biopsies are negative or inconclusive in a patient with hematemesis or melena and the patient has diarrhea, fecal culture may be appropriate. Cultures evaluate mainly for overgrowth of a particular bacterium (e.g., *Salmonella*, *Campylobacter*, *Shigella*, and certain strains of *E. coli*. Growth of mixed cultures

probably represents normal enteric flora. Enteropathogenic bacteria are unlikely to cause melena alone, since they affect the distal small intestine and colon and are therefore likely to cause mixed bowel diarrhea with both digested and fresh blood present.

18 Like fecal cultures, an ACTH stimulation test is likely to be a relatively low-yield procedure, especially in a patient without a sodium/potassium ratio suggestive of hypoadrenocorticism. However, isolated glucocorticoid deficiency is a rare cause of hematemesis or melena, with or without diarrhea.

19 Elevated fasting serum gastrin concentrations may be found in conjunction with certain neuroendocrine tumors (APUDomas). APUDomas (usually gastrinomas) often arise from the pancreas but can potentially develop in neuroendocrine tissue elsewhere. These tumors often secrete gastrin continuously, leading to excessive gastric acid production, esophagitis, ulceration, hematemesis, diarrhea, melena, and mucosal fold hypertrophy. Abdominal imaging, endoscopy, and exploratory celiotomy may be employed to further diagnose and treat these tumors. Note that excessive use of H_2 blockers and conditions causing gastric outflow obstruction also may increase fasting serum gastrin concentrations. Occasionally, gastrin hypersecretion by an APUDoma is intermittent and a stimulation test with secretin or calcium is required.

20 If serum gastrin concentrations are normal, exploratory celiotomy should be considered if upper endoscopy was the diagnostic technique used previously. Lesions causing melena may be further down the small intestine or within the bowel wall and thus inaccessible with an endoscope. Alternatively, either a lesion was missed (unlikely if there is a lot of bleeding and a surgical procedure was performed), or the patient has idiopathic gastrointestinal ulceration (reported, but careful reevaluation of drug history and other factors is required before making this diagnosis), or there is an APUDoma secreting something besides gastrin (e.g., pancreatic polypeptide or other potentially ulcerogenic hormones).

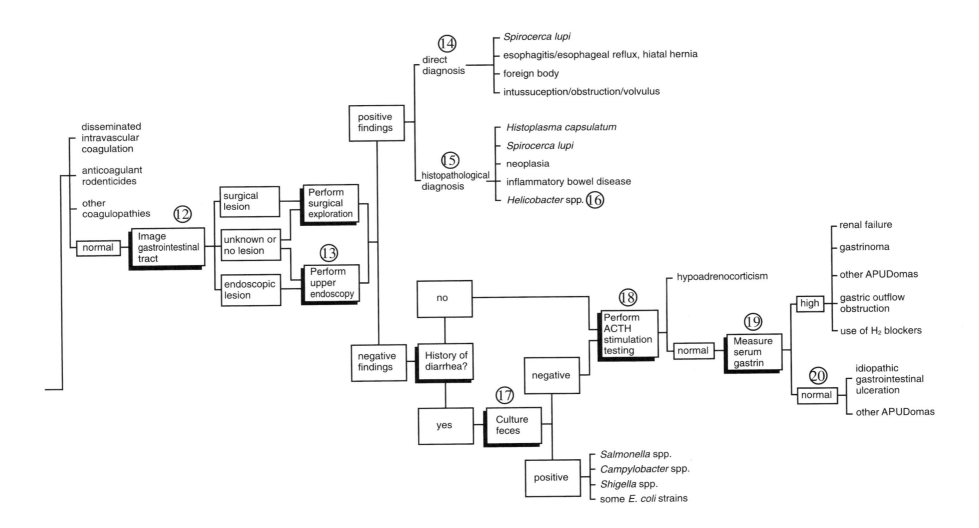

1 Diarrhea is a change in the consistency of stool from normal and formed through mild softening of stool with some retention of form, loss of form but retention of some consistency ("cowpie" stool), to very watery stools. Diarrhea is the result of primary gastrointestinal disease or systemic conditions that secondarily affect the gastrointestinal tract (e.g., renal failure, feline coronavirus infection, or sepsis). It can be an acute or chronic condition and may be self-limiting or life-threatening. It is important that the clinician consider these variants when first approaching a patient with diarrhea. For example, a patient with acute diarrhea that is not systemically affected and is likely to have a good response to supportive care alone (e.g., temporarily holding off food, subcutaneous or intravenous fluids) has an acute, self-limiting problem. Such a patient probably does not need to be tested or treated further unless the problem recurs. A patient that has continuous or recurrent diarrhea, whether or not this is associated with systemic illness, is likely to need more in-depth evaluation.

2 Diarrheic stool originates from either the small or large intestine. Features that allow distinction of small and large intestinal diarrhea are determined from the initial history of the problem and observation of the patient. A component of both forms can be present (mixed intestinal diarrhea). This algorithm divides patients primarily into those with small intestinal and large intestinal diarrhea and, subsequently, acute and chronic diarrhea. Conditions such as IBD or lymphoma that either can or will affect both the small and large intestines appear in both branches of each algorithm and cause mixed diarrhea.

3 Features of small intestinal (SI) diarrhea include weight loss (the result of failure to digest and absorb food or decreased SI transit time), increased stool volume, markedly watery stool, and normal to slightly increased frequency of defecation (one to three times daily). In some instances, stool will bear a close resemblance to undigested food. On occasion there will be clinical illness, including vomiting, anorexia or polyphagia (depending on the underlying cause), and the presence of melena (representing digested blood). Less common presenting complaints include abdominal discomfort, borborygmus, halitosis, and development of ascites (as a result of intestinal protein losses). The normal functions of the SI include continuation of the digestive process started in the stomach and absorption of nutrients. SI diarrhea results from conditions that alter SI function. Examples include changes in SI motility (dysmotility diarrhea), problems with absorption of nutrients, water, and electrolytes (osmotic diarrhea), and excessive secretion into the SI as a result of mucosal and submucosal inflammation (secretory diarrhea). Other forms of SI diarrhea result from loss of intestinal surface area for absorption, local (brush border or pancreatic) enzyme failure, overgrowth of SI flora leading to inappropriate fermentation of intestinal contents, and problems with intestinal permeability (exudative diarrhea).

4 Features of large intestinal (LI) diarrhea include increased frequency of defecation (six or more times daily), an urgent need to defecate, tenesmus (resulting from irritation of the colon and rectum), presence of fresh blood in or around the stool, mucus, and increased flatulence. Patients do not lose weight and usually are clinically well unless the problem is a manifestation of a more severe and generalized condition. Some feline patients vomit in association with colonic problems, including diarrhea. Since the main functions of the LI include storage of fecal material and absorption of water from the stool, derangement of these functions results in failure to store stool (increased urgency of defecation) and production of soft to watery fecal material. A more secretory or osmotic form of LI diarrhea may result from conditions that allow SI contents, including bile salts, to pass into the LI. This leads to irritation of the mucosal surfaces, which are not designed to cope with the presence of these substances. It also provides an unusual substrate for fermentation by colonic bacteria.

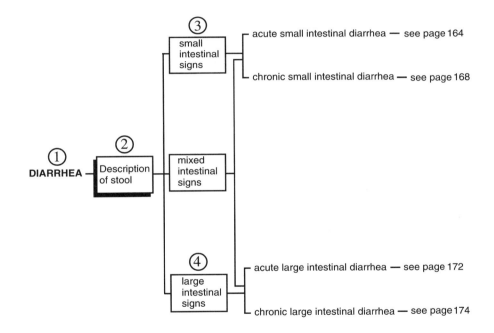

① **DIARRHEA**

② Description of stool

③ small intestinal signs

acute small intestinal diarrhea — see page 164

chronic small intestinal diarrhea — see page 168

mixed intestinal signs

④ large intestinal signs

acute large intestinal diarrhea — see page 172

chronic large intestinal diarrhea — see page 174

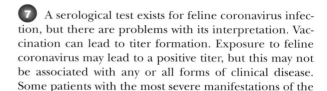

1 Small intestinal (SI) diarrhea may be acute or chronic. Generally, acute problems are continuously present for less than 2 weeks or intermittently present for less than 4 weeks. While it is tempting to include all causes of SI diarrhea in the acute category (because they all have to start at some point), this section has tried to include only conditions that present acutely and have a short clinical course. They should resolve rapidly with supportive care or appropriate, specific therapy or progress rapidly to a crisis point (as in FePLV infection, CDV infection, ARF, or peritonitis). There is considerable overlap between the causes of acute and chronic SI diarrhea, and conditions such as canine parvovirus infection that present acutely can so debilitate patients and structurally damage the intestinal tract that more chronic signs develop later.

2 The initial step in evaluating patients presenting with acute SI diarrhea is a thorough review of their history. This helps the clinician to establish that the diarrhea is indeed acute and SI in origin. Additionally, it determines whether there has been a recent diet change or ingestion of foreign substances (trash, rotten foodstuffs, chocolate, material with potential for causing intestinal obstruction). The history also establishes whether the patient roams without supervision, allowing ingestion of foreign material, spoiled foodstuffs, and so on without the client's realization.

3 An important part of the history is drug administration, especially recent initiation of therapy in patients developing acute SI diarrhea. Causes of acute SI diarrhea include drugs that target the gastrointestinal tract such as laxatives (castor oil, bisacodyl, dioctyl sodium sulfosuccinate) and motility modifiers (anticholinergics cause ileus, and motility promoters such as cisapride cause excessively fast transit times). Other causes of acute SI diarrhea include many antibiotics that alter intestinal bacterial flora and, in some instances, increase gastrointestinal motility (erythromycin). Other drugs that cause acute SI diarrhea include antifungals, cardiac glycosides, antiarrhythmic agents, ACE inhibitors, and NSAIDs.

4 The history should show whether the patient has had contact with animals of the same species with similar signs. This is especially important if the patient is young and debilitated, has an immunosuppressive disease or takes immunosuppressive drugs, is housed in a large group or in poor conditions, or has a poor vaccination history. Testing of patients suspected to have contracted an infectious cause of SI diarrhea varies with the suspected infection. Hopefully, if the problem has occurred previously in a group of contact animals, there will be a known disease agent and testing will be done to confirm the diagnosis. Clinical signs also may prove helpful. For example, dogs that contract parvovirus infection often start by vomiting and then develop more severe signs, including depression, dehydration, and bloody diarrhea. Dogs with acute CDV infection in addition to diarrhea often have mucopurulent ocular and nasal discharges and may develop neurological signs. In some cases of infectious diarrhea there is no specific, noninvasive test for the suspected cause (e.g., canine adenovirus infection), and clinical suspicions are based on the history, presenting signs, and possibly finding viral inclusions in biopsy or autopsy specimens. Scanning electron microscopy can identify virus particles in feces or intestinal biopsy specimens if samples are taken into appropriate transport media.

5 Pathogenic bacteria such as *Salmonella* spp. and *E. coli* are relatively uncommon causes of acute SI diarrhea in dogs and cats. If such infections are identified in animals that have contacted the patient, or if a patient with SI or mixed intestinal diarrhea is febrile, has melena or hematochezia, or has signs of severe systemic infection, fecal cultures might be indicated sooner than usual. Fecal culture generally grows a variety of organisms that are considered normal fecal flora. The microbiology laboratory will report overgrowth of a specific bacterium. If *Salmonella* spp. or a pure growth of *Campylobacter* spp. is found, this is likely to be a pathogen. Finding *E. coli* is less definitive since this is part of normal fecal flora, and culture alone is insufficient to determine whether this is an enterotoxigenic or enteropathogenic strain.

6 In the case of FIV and FeLV infections, a positive test means either that the virus is the cause of SI diarrhea or that it is predisposing the patient to infections or other problems that cause SI diarrhea.

7 A serological test exists for feline coronavirus infection, but there are problems with its interpretation. Vaccination can lead to titer formation. Exposure to feline coronavirus may lead to a positive titer, but this may not be associated with any or all forms of clinical disease. Some patients with the most severe manifestations of the infection with this virus never develop titers at all.

8 Patients with no history of exposure to specific infections should undergo a detailed examination to assess their physical status (bright and healthy versus clinically unwell, dehydrated, and endotoxemic). Examination should include abdominal palpation for masses, foreign bodies, intussusceptions, and areas of discomfort. It also should include oral and rectal examinations for foreign material.

9 The underside of the tongue should be examined, particularly in cats, for material such as string, thread, and cassette tape that can catch under the tongue and extend into the intestines. This can lead to intestinal plication, partial obstruction, and eventually perforation.

10 In patients that have diarrhea and are also clinically unwell, a minimum database of laboratory tests should be assessed (hemogram, serum chemistry profile, urinalysis, and FeLV/FIV tests for cats). This database detects metabolic abnormalities that can indicate the underlying causes of diarrhea (e.g., renal failure, liver disease) and highlights problems such as severe dehydration and life-threatening electrolyte imbalances that require immediate therapy.

11 In patients with abnormalities on abdominal palpation or that are clinically ill but have no specific metabolic abnormalities, testing should progress to abdominal imaging. Imaging will vary with what is available to the clinician. In most instances, abdominal radiographs will be obtained first and may be the best studies for conditions involving the bowel. They are useful for radiodense and some radiolucent foreign bodies, obstructive bowel patterns, and bowel plication, torsion, or intussusception. Mass lesions arising from many organs also may be visible. Abdominal ultrasound is excellent for evaluating the internal structure of solid organs, but it is not

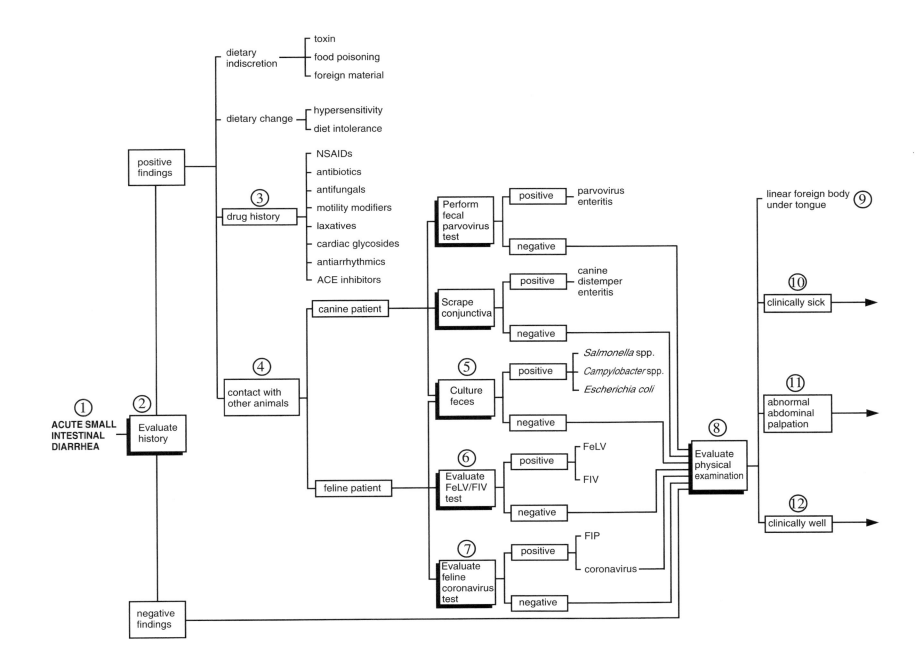

always best for bowel wall or obstructive conditions since gas in the bowel interferes with the ultrasound beam. Abdominal ultrasound is useful for determining the extent of masses and structures associated with them. It detects fluid-filled viscera (prostatic abscesses, fluid in the uterus), organ enlargement (prostatomegaly), renal pelvis dilation (which might suggest pyelonephritis), pancreatic thickening, and increased echodensity of tissue suggesting inflammation. It locates small amounts of fluid in the abdomen that would not be visible radiographically and evaluates structures within the fluid that would be obscured on radiographs.

12 In patients that are clinically well apart from acute SI diarrhea, three fecal samples should be evaluated by zinc sulfate flotation. The samples should be obtained at least 24 hours apart. This allows diagnosis of SI parasitic infections, including those with parasites that only shed eggs intermittently. A wet-mounted fecal smear also should be evaluated for *Giardia* spp.

13 Leukopenia is characteristic of several canine and feline viral infections that attack bone marrow stem cells (canine parvovirus, CDV, and FePLV). It also occurs with severe systemic infections, peritonitis, acute overwhelming bacterial sepsis, and some cases of salmonellosis.

14 Hemoconcentration (elevated hematocrit and protein) occurs with dehydration. Severe hemoconcentration accompanying acute hemorrhagic diarrhea is characteristic of hemorrhagic gastroenteropathy (HGE). This condition particularly affects small-breed dogs; the underlying cause is unknown. Acute hypersensitivity reactions to food or to the enterotoxin produced by *Clostridium perfringens* are possible underlying causes. Patients can be severely affected, with acute abdominal pain, vomiting, depression, and shock. There can be marked shifts of fluid into the gastrointestinal tract and acute bleeding. The diagnosis is based on the clinical presentation and the presence of PVCs of 55–65%. The response to aggressive supportive care is generally very good.

15 Patients with acute, severe SI diarrhea and melena whose laboratory tests show low Na^+ and elevated K^+ ($Na^+ : K^+$ ratio < 27:1) should be tested for hypoadrenocorticism (Addison's disease). Patients also may be azotemic due to dehydration, may be hypercalcemic as a result of glucocorticoid deficiency, and may have circulating lymphocytes and eosinophils despite being severely stressed. Note that it is glucocorticoids that maintain bowel integrity and normal appetite, and prevent vomiting and diarrhea. Therefore, it is possible for a patient to have clinical signs due to isolated glucocorticoid deficiency (atypical Addison's disease) without electrolyte abnormalities.

16 There are a few severe infectious conditions that require a very specific exposure history to increase clinical suspicion of the problem. Because these conditions may be rapidly fatal, they should be considered early on in the algorithm, despite their relative rarity.
A) Salmon poisoning is caused by two neorickettsial organisms acquired from a fluke (*Nanophyetus salmincola*) found in salmon in the Pacific Northwest. Dogs acquire the infection from eating raw salmon, and the *Neorickettsia* spp. cause hemorrhagic diarrhea, vomiting, fever, lymphadenopathy, oculonasal discharge, and severe lethargy. The condition can be mistaken for parvovirus infection, but mortality is very high if it is not treated appropriately. Diagnosis requires a history of eating raw fish, lymph node aspirates, and finding fluke eggs on fecal examination.
B) Most patients infected with any of the serovars of *Leptospira* spp. have hepatic or renal problems or both. Acute, severe diarrhea also can result from septicemia or renal/hepatic failure. The exposure history includes a rural location, drinking from slow-moving water (ponds, lakes, slow streams), and contact with or exposure to the same environment as rodents. It is important to test a full panel of serovars since it is unusual for canine patients to have disease due to the two serovars they are vaccinated against (*L. icterohamorrhagia* and *L. canicola*).
C) Blue-green algae bloom on ponds and lakes and cause acute, fatal gastroenteritis, liver and kidney failure, and neurological signs in dogs that drink the water. Diagnosis requires an exposure history and identification of the algae.
D) *Bacillus piliformis* is a rare infection carried by rodents. It causes acute, fatal (within 48 hours) SI diarrhea in puppies and kittens (Tyzzer's disease). It also causes hepatic necrosis. The diagnosis is usually made postmortem.

17 Finding a resectable mass lesion, a fluid-filled uterus in an intact female with signs of clinical illness, a radiodense foreign body, or an obstructive gas pattern in bowel is an indication to progress to exploratory surgery. Moderately to massively distended SI suggests obstruction or SI torsion. SI torsion presents very acutely, with patients exhibiting severe abdominal pain, shock, and bloody diarrhea. The condition usually progresses rapidly and is acutely fatal.

18 Finding pancreatic thickening or masses on ultrasound may lead to further evaluation for pancreatic inflammation (amylase, lipase, and serum TLI). Fine-needle aspiration of specific abnormal areas can be attempted for cytology. Patients also may be treated for suspected pancreatitis and their progress reassessed or exploratory laparotomy can be performed as appropriate.

19 Cytology on a fine-needle aspirate is appropriate in patients with more equivocal lesions, with evidence of tumor metastasis, or when the underlying tissue type may determine the prognosis.

20 Renal pelvis dilation suggests the need for urine culture, culture of fluid from the renal pelvis or a renal biopsy, or a therapeutic trial of antimicrobials for suspected pyelonephritis.

21 In patients with negative fecal evaluations, testing could progress to evaluate laboratory tests, looking for systemic conditions that cause SI diarrhea with no other clinical signs (e.g., some cases of renal failure, atypical Addison's disease). If there is a history of a recent diet change, the original diet should be reintroduced. If dietary hypersensitivity is suspected, an exclusion diet may be attempted. Alternatively, patients may be treated symptomatically and supportively (giving nothing by mouth, administering intravenous or subcutaneous fluids, and gradually reintroducing a bland diet and antibiotics or motility modifiers if appropriate). Patients that do not respond may be candidates for upper endoscopic evaluation or other tests. The algorithm for chronic SI diarrhea should be followed from this point.

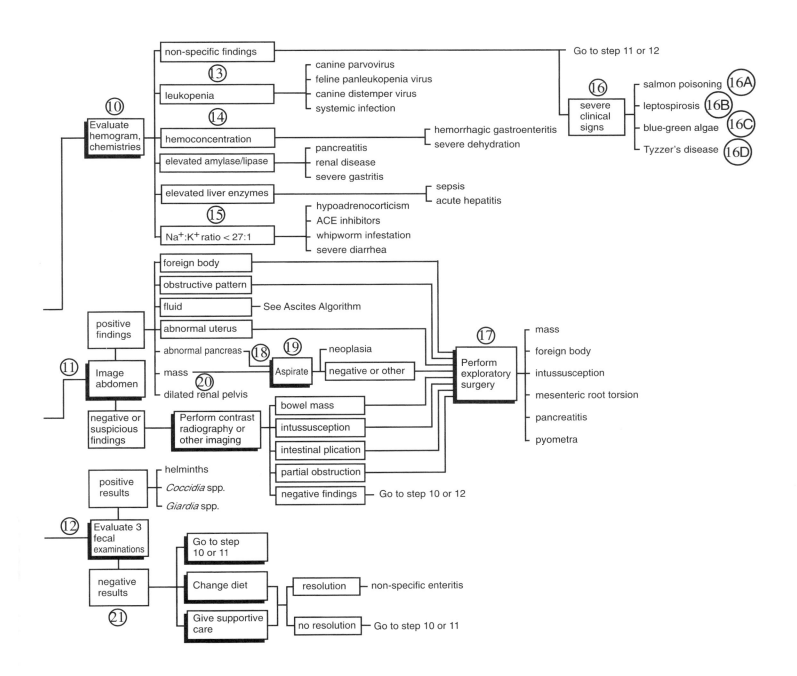

1 Chronic SI diarrhea is diarrhea that has been present continuously or intermittently for 2–4 weeks and has not responded to symptomatic therapy/supportive care. Some conditions that cause acute SI diarrhea become chronic (food allergies/intolerance if the diet is continued, parasitic infections).

2 The history should include diet changes made before the onset of diarrhea, the patient's usual diet (hypersensitivity develops with chronic exposure to food proteins), a history of poor supervision, contact with affected animals, chronic drug administration, and other medical conditions. The environmental history is particularly important and includes access to toxins, water sources, pesticides, carrion, or spoiled foods. Toxin exposure must be ongoing to cause chronic SI diarrhea (e.g., a bag of contaminated feed which is still in use). Determine whether the patient lives in dirty surroundings, which increases the chances of bacterial or parasitic infection.

3 Chronic drug administration can cause SI diarrhea. Anticholinergics in some antidiarrhea medications cause motility problems, ileus, and hence diarrhea. Antimicrobials cause SI diarrhea by altering normal bacterial flora and allowing pathogen overgrowth. Excessive levothyroxine supplementation in dogs causes diarrhea. Measuring serum T_4 concentration 4–6 hours after administration detects this condition.

4 Right-sided heart failure causes congestion/edema of the bowel wall and diarrhea. Often patients also are on cardiac medications (ACE inhibitors, digoxin) that cause diarrhea.

5 Hepatic cirrhosis/failure causes SI diarrhea by affecting intestinal function and repair, reducing endotoxin removal from blood, and causing intestinal edema due to portal hypertension.

6 Neurological problems (spinal trauma, surgery, diffuse neurological disease) affect intestinal innervation. This is likely to be the problem if other autonomic nervous system functions are affected (generalized dysautonomia or urinary bladder involvement). Patients develop SI ileus and diarrhea.

7 Patients who have undergone extensive abdominal surgery or have had extensive intra-abdominal inflammation (e.g., peritonitis) are likely to develop regional or generalized SI ileus and diarrhea. This is less of a problem in cats and dogs than in horses or human beings. Resection of more than two-thirds of the SI may cause *short bowel syndrome* and chronic diarrhea as a result of insufficient SI length to absorb fluid and complete digestion. The problem may be transient, as the remaining SI can make large adaptive changes.

8 Certain dog breeds are predisposed to conditions causing SI diarrhea. While the diagnosis is not likely to be based on the breed alone, this factor can guide testing. Breeds with specific gastrointestinal conditions include basenjis (immunoproliferative lymphoplasmacytic enteritis), German shepherds (idiopathic antibiotic-responsive diarrhea/SI bacterial overgrowth [SIBO], exocrine pancreatic insufficiency [EPI], and a predisposition to fungal infection), Lundehunds, Yorkshire terriers, and rottweilers (lymphangiectasia), and Irish setters (gluten sensitivity).

9 Physical examination determines how aggressively initial testing needs to be pursued. Patients that are unwell (fever, other body system involvement, shock, collapse, melena, hematochezia) need laboratory tests, possibly fecal cultures, ACTH stimulation testing, abdominal imaging, exploratory surgery, or upper endoscopy while supportive care is initiated. Clinically well patients need only a few tests initially (e.g., fecal flotations).

10 Sick patients need a hemogram, serum chemistry profile, and urinalysis, plus FeLV/FIV testing in cats. This can provide a specific diagnosis (renal failure, hepatic disease) or guide the clinician toward certain conditions (e.g., lymphopenia with low cholesterol and low albumin, and pleural or peritoneal transudates suggest lymph-angiectasia). Neutropenia can suggest viral infection or sepsis. Microcytic anemia suggests chronic blood loss. Low cholesterol, albumin, BUN, and glucose and high bilirubin suggest liver failure. In rare cases, increased K^+ and low Na^+ are due to severe gastrointestinal disease or whipworm infestation. It is more likely to indicate hypoadrenocorticism. ACTH stimulation testing differentiates these conditions. Chronic, poorly regulated diabetes mellitus can affect gastrointestinal motility and cause SI diarrhea (commonly it causes gastroparesis and vomiting).

11 In sick patients with negative or nonspecific findings on the minimum database, it is necessary to progress to abdominal imaging, endoscopy, or exploratory surgery as appropriate.

12 Young animals, those with hematochezia, melena, or fever, or those known to have contacted other affected animals may need fecal cultures. Only a few bacteria cause chronic diarrhea and wasting (e.g., *Yersinia pseudotuberculosis* in cats and *Actinomyces* spp.). These are unlikely to grow on routine fecal culture due to slow multiplication rates and overgrowth by normal flora.

13 Clinically healthy patients with chronic SI diarrhea should have three fecal examinations on samples obtained 24 hours apart, and a fresh fecal smear should be reviewed for parasite ova. This is sufficient to diagnose roundworms (*Toxocara canis/cati*, *Toxascaris leonina*), hookworms (*Ancylostoma* spp., *Unicinaria* spp.), tapeworms (mainly *Dipylidium caninum*, various *Taenia* spp.), coccidia (*Isospora* spp., *Cryptosporidium* spp., *Balantidium* spp.), and *Giardia* spp. A fecal antigen test exists for *Giardia* spp., but three fecal examinations are equally sensitive in making this diagnosis.

14 Rectal cytology is more useful for large intestinal (LI) diarrhea. It detects *Giardia* spp., *Campylobacter* spp., fungi (*H. capsulatum*), algae (*Prototheca* spp.), and abnormal bacterial populations (a preponderance of one type of bacterium suggests the need for fecal culture).

15 If abdominal palpation is abnormal (painful, palpable mass or foreign body) or a patient is unwell, abdominal imaging (radiographs, ultrasound) is needed. Radiographic contrast studies are required if the results of initial imaging are equivocal. These studies identify partial obstruction, masses, some ulcers, and increased intestinal transit times due to functional ileus. Liquid contrast and/or barium-impregnated polyethylene spheres (BIPS) are used. Liquid contrast adheres to ulcers or inflamed areas, although contrast studies are not really sensitive for such problems. Stress can slow rates at which contrast passes through the gastrointestinal tract. Therefore, finding normal transit times is helpful but delayed transit times suggest either patient stress or true problems with gastrointestinal motility that could be an underlying cause of diarrhea.

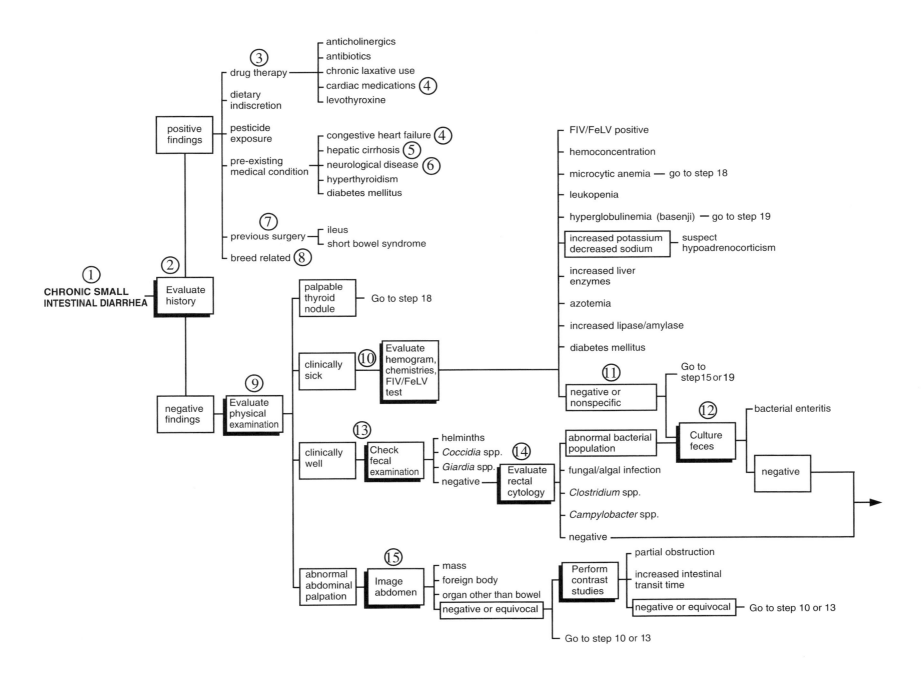

16 In cats more than 8–10 years old with weight loss and SI diarrhea, thyroid function should be tested, especially if they have polyphagia, poor haircoat, vomiting, irritability, a palpable thyroid nodule, and increased liver enzymes.

17 In dogs with marked weight loss, steatorrhea, ravenous appetite, and SI diarrhea, serum TLI should be measured. Low TLI indicates EPI, and SI maldigestion and malabsorption. The condition can arise in dogs of any age but particularly in young, adult German shepherds. It is very rare in cats.

18 If testing to this point is negative, the next step usually is SI biopsy. Other tests depend on the patient's signalment and history. Ancillary tests identify functional problems and the location of some SI abnormalities. These tests are noninvasive but can be difficult to perform, requiring substrates and equipment not always available in practice. Few of them definitively diagnose an underlying condition. Biopsy, medication, or exclusion diet trials will still be required. Fecal occult blood can be measured for microscopic intestinal blood loss. The test is affected by meat protein, so dogs need to be fed a vegetarian diet for 4–5 days before obtaining samples for valid results. The test is not appropriate for cats.

19 Upper endoscopy allows evaluation of SI mucosa for ulcers, bleeding, altered granularity/friability, mucosal or submucosal masses, and lacteal dilation. The disadvantage is that only the duodenum and the first 20–30 cm of the jejunum can be examined. Distal or submucosal lesions can be missed, as can tumors with an extensive fibrous tissue reaction.

20 If idiopathic, antibiotic-responsive diarrhea (also called SIBO) is a concern, duodenal aspirates should be obtained at surgery or during endoscopy for culture. Criteria for diagnosis of SIBO are controversial in veterinary patients. The bacterial counts initially published are probably too low. Numbers as high as 10^7 (dogs) and 10^7 to 10^9 (cats) may be normal. Increased bacterial counts also occur with abnormal SI motility, stagnant intestinal loops, and if maldigestion provides increased substrate for bacterial growth.

21 IBD is a histopathological condition with a complex pathogenesis. It is a collective term for a group of diseases characterized by inflammatory infiltrates, SI diarrhea, vomiting, anorexia, colitis, weight loss, and protein-losing enteropathy. Idiopathic IBD is an inappropriate immune response to normal dietary proteins, microbial antigens, or self-antigens. Lymphoplasmacytic enteritis (LPE) is the most common form in both dogs and cats. Eosinophilic enteritis is a severe, proliferative, segmentally distributed form of IBD that may be seen more frequently in young boxer dogs and responds poorly to treatment. Eosinophils in the circulation can be associated with hypereosinophilic syndrome in cats. Rare forms of IBD in dogs include regional (granulomatous) enteritis (similar to Crohn's disease) and basenji ileal proliferative enteropathy (hyperglobulinemia and progressive SI diarrhea). Both conditions respond poorly to therapy.

22 SI ulcers (mainly duodenal) are rare in dogs and cats compared to human beings, and mainly cause vomiting and anorexia. Cats with SI ulcers may be FIV positive.

23 Lymphangiectasia is associated with marked intestinal protein loss and low-protein ascites. Obstruction of lymphatics that absorb fat from the bowel causes mucosal lacteals to dilate with fat and protein-rich fluid and eventually rupture. Lymphatic obstruction can be mucosal (lymphoma, IBD, histoplasmosis, idiopathic) or distant (due to granulomas on serosal surfaces/in mesentery, lymph node inflammation/neoplasia, or congestive heart failure).

24 Diffuse SI neoplasia is a relatively common cause of chronic diarrhea.

25 Infectious chronic SI diarrhea is rare in dogs and cats. *H. capsulatum* causes diarrhea, weight loss, and hepatic problems in dogs. Pyogranulomatous thickening and bowel obstruction occur with pythiosis. The prognosis for patients with fungal/algal infection is poor. *Y. pseudotuberculosis* from birds and rodents causes chronic SI diarrhea in cats. Various forms of *Mycobacterium* spp. and higher bacteria (*Nocardia* spp., *Actinomyces* spp.) affect both dogs and cats.

26 Exploratory surgery and full-thickness SI biopsies may be needed if endoscopy does not provide a diagnosis. Gastrointestinal or systemic conditions can also cause diarrhea with normal or mild histopathological changes. The signalment, history, and results of prior tests determine further testing.

27 Tumors of neuroendocrine tissues in the gastrointestinal tract (APUDomas) overproduce hormones and cause chronic, intermittent SI diarrhea. These tumors are rare and hard to diagnose. Gastrinoma, a pancreatic islet cell tumor, produces gastrin and causes gastric acid hypersecretion as well as esophageal, gastric, and peptic ulcers. Abdominal ultrasound, fasting serum gastrin concentration, response to secretin/calcium administration, scintigraphy, exploratory surgery, and biopsy diagnose this tumor.

28 Dietary hypersensitivity, especially type I (immediate) hypersensitivity, is rare and difficult to diagnose in dogs and cats. Skin tests, and serum radioallergosorbent (RAST) or ELISA tests are disappointing. Diagnosis relies on observation, the dietary history, clinical suspicion, and use of exclusion diets for at least 10 weeks. Resolution of SI diarrhea on an exclusion diet is followed by challenge testing with individual proteins. Gluten sensitivity is a severe form of dietary hypersensitivity in Irish setters and is possibly associated with protein-losing enteropathy in soft-coated wheaten terriers.

29 Gastrointestinal motility disorders are hard to diagnose due to normal variation in transit times in stressed patients. Ileus can develop postoperatively and with metabolic problems (hypokalemia, diabetes mellitus), inflammation, severe parvovirus infection, or systemic neurological problems (dysautonomia). Ileus may be severe enough to cause signs of intestinal obstruction (pseudo-obstructive disease). Patients also can have excessive SI motility and cramping similar to irritable bowel syndrome (IBS) in human beings. Despite being SI in origin, IBS is associated mainly with LI signs. However, patients can have SI diarrhea and vomiting. Diagnosis of IBS is by exclusion. It can be associated with nervous or high-strung patients or stress. Therapy with a sedative/anticholinergic preparation can be helpful, but the results are inconsistent.

30 Gastric diseases that reduce preliminary digestion of food (decreased gastric acidity, premature gastric emptying) can cause SI diarrhea, either because digestion and absorption cannot be completed in the normal SI transit time or because presentation of unusual dietary components to the SI leads to bacterial overgrowth. These conditions are poorly documented in dogs and cats, as are brush border enzyme deficiencies and true autoimmune bowel diseases.

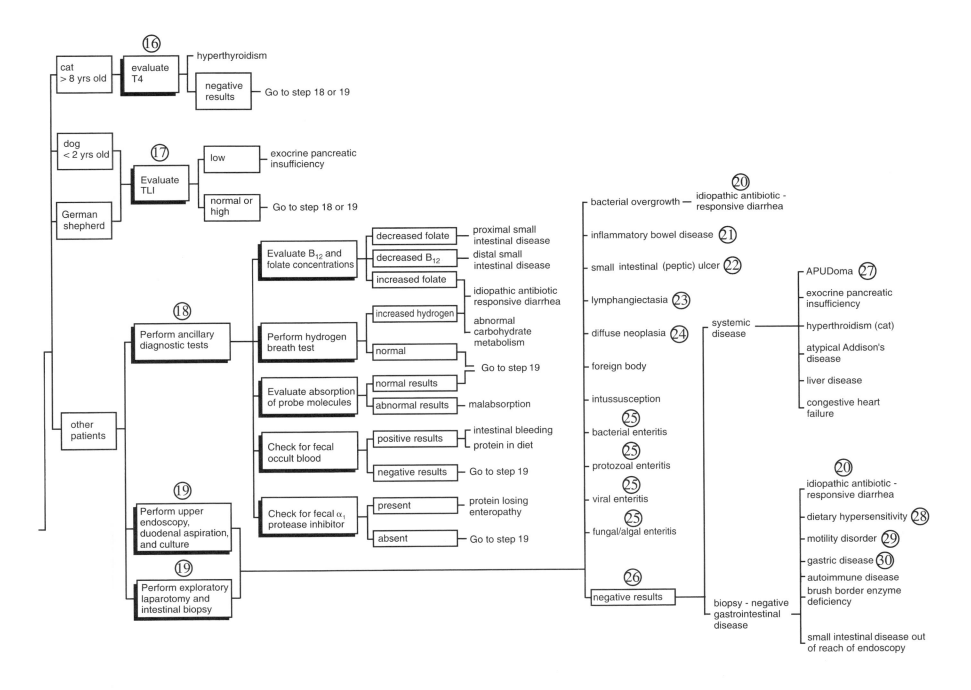

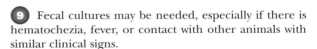

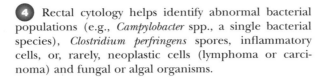

1 LI diarrhea can be acute or chronic. The time frame is very similar to that of SI diarrhea. Relatively few causes of acute LI diarrhea exist, and many can be excluded with a good history. Dietary and parasitic causes probably constitute over 50% of acute colitis cases.

2 An important historical issue is drug therapy, looking for antibiotics that change bacterial flora, motility modifiers such as narcotics and prokinetics, and dexamethasone administered for neurological problems. The clinician should also ask about dietary indiscretion (bacterial toxins in spoiled foodstuffs, ingestion of foreign material), lack of patient supervision (potential for ingestion of toxins and spoiled foodstuffs), and recent diet changes (dietary hypersensitivity, true allergy). The environment should be evaluated for contamination (fecal material and the potential for parasitic infestation and reinfestation). It is important to assess animals in contact with the patient to assess for potential infectious conditions. Finally, the client should be questioned about stressful situations that could contribute to *Clostridium* spp. overgrowth and enterotoxin production, a potential cause of colitis and hematochezia.

3 Patients that are clinically well should have three or more zinc sulfate fecal flotations and a fecal smear evaluated for parasites. Whipworms (*Trichuris vulpis*), in particular, only shed ova periodically in feces and are a common cause of LI diarrhea. Other potential parasitic causes of LI diarrhea in dogs include hookworms (mainly *Ancylostoma* spp.) and whipworms (*T. vulpis*). In dogs and cats *Giardia* spp., other protozoa, and various species of *Coccidia* cause LI diarrhea. Parasitic infestation is a particular problem in very young, old, debilitated, and immunosuppressed patients and those living in contaminated environments.

4 Rectal cytology helps identify abnormal bacterial populations (e.g., *Campylobacter* spp., a single bacterial species), *Clostridium perfringens* spores, inflammatory cells, or, rarely, neoplastic cells (lymphoma or carcinoma) and fungal or algal organisms.

5 *C. perfringens* is part of the normal flora of the large bowel. Under certain conditions it sporulates and, if it is a toxigenic strain, produces enterotoxin A. This causes signs of colitis, often with frank blood. It should be noted that the presence of spore-forming bacteria and even the finding of *C. perfringens* enterotoxin in stool is not specific for clostridial colitis, and spores or enterotoxin may be present in patients that do not have diarrhea or have diarrhea for other reasons.

6 When rectal cytology is negative, the patient's clinical condition should be evaluated. Patients that are clinically unwell (febrile and depressed), or that have hematochezia or a palpable abdominal mass, should be evaluated further.

7 Patients that are clinically well and are normal on abdominal palpation should receive supportive care and be monitored for resolution of clinical signs. Therapy includes fasting the patient for 12 to 24 hours, followed by reintroduction of a bland, easily digestible diet, with or without antibiotics such as metronidazole or amoxicillin for clostridial colitis.

8 In sick, febrile patients with no palpable abdominal lesion, a minimum database of laboratory tests should be evaluated to exclude sepsis, uremia, pancreatitis, hepatic disease, and other severe systemic conditions as a cause of acute LI diarrhea.

9 Fecal cultures may be needed, especially if there is hematochezia, fever, or contact with other animals with similar clinical signs.

10 Patients with abdominal tenderness or a palpable lesion and acute colitis signs should undergo abdominal imaging, bypassing much of the previous evaluation (e.g., fecal flotations and smears). Radiographs of the abdomen identify radiodense foreign material in the colon that may be causing mucosal irritation and may even suggest radiolucent foreign bodies.

11 Rarely, patients with acute mechanical obstructions such as SI mesenteric root torsion or ileocolic or cecocolic intussusception can present with signs of acute colitis. Abdominal radiographs can indicate severe, generalized SI distention (mesenteric root torsion) or a soft tissue mass lesion. The latter, if associated with a cylindrical midabdominal mass, suggests an ileocolic or cecocolic intussusception. Ileocolic intussusceptions are the most common. They are most frequently seen in young dogs and are commonly associated with underlying conditions that affect intestinal motility (e.g., parvovirus enteritis, whipworms). In older dogs they may be associated with mass lesions arising from the intestinal wall. Occasionally, long intussusceptions protrude from the anus, mimicking a rectal prolapse. All conditions causing intestinal obstruction require surgical correction. Foreign material in the LI is unlikely to require removal unless the patient is severely obstipated.

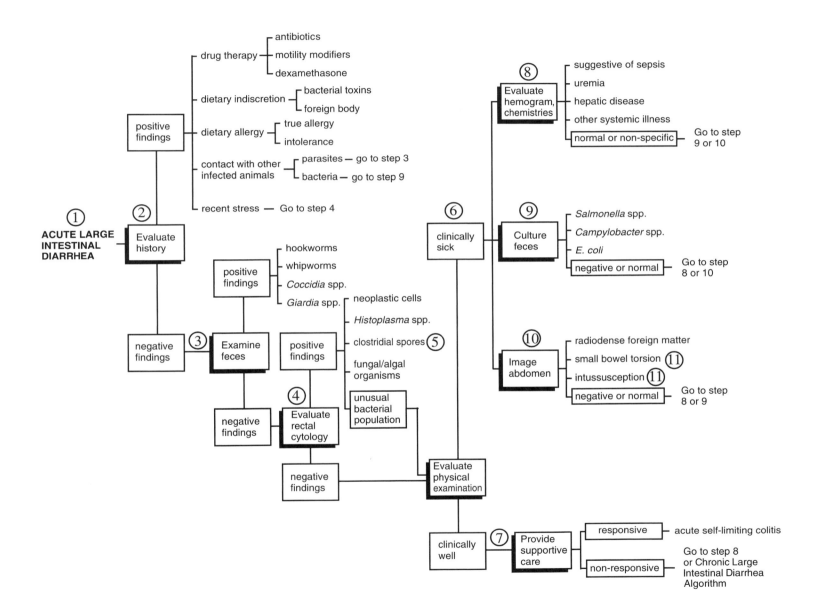

1 Chronic LI diarrhea is diarrhea that has been present for more than 2 to 4 weeks and has not responded to symptomatic therapy. These cases require more aggressive evaluation. Patients generally are clinically well apart from diarrhea, are eating normally, and do not exhibit weight loss. Rarely, patients with neoplasia or infectious conditions affecting the bowel (*Yersinia* spp., *Mycobacterium* spp., *Actinomyces* spp., *Nocardia* spp., fungal infections, protothecosis, and pythiosis) are clinically unwell. Such patients may be emaciated, have signs of other organ system involvement, and SI signs as well as colitis.

2 The history is important in patients with chronic LI diarrhea, but usually it only contributes to the diagnosis of the underlying cause. It is important to determine what the usual diet is in case of acquired intolerance after prolonged exposure to certain dietary proteins. It also is important to determine whether there is ongoing dietary indiscretion that might lead to chronic, intermittent LI diarrhea. Information should be obtained about the environment, patient supervision, or whether the patient is from an area where certain infections (fungal and algal) are prevalent. It also is important to determine whether patients have contact with environments that predispose them to infectious conditions. For example, a highly contaminated environment increases the risk of parasitism and certain bacterial infections, contact with pigs can predispose to infection with *Balantidium coli* and *Yersinia enterocolitica*, and contact with other animals of the same species with similar clinical signs also suggests a transmissible condition. Another historical finding is chronic antibiotic administration. Generally, signs of colitis associated with antibiotic use are mild. Penicillins and cephalosporins often are incriminated in dogs and cats. Signs of severe colitis occur rarely and can be associated with overgrowth of pathogenic bacteria such as *Clostridium difficile* and *Pseudomonas aeruginosa*. *C. difficile–*associated colitis in human beings can be very severe and even fatal. Although the organism and the enterotoxin have been reported in the feces of dogs and cats with diarrhea, they also have been found in asymptomatic animals; therefore, their significance is uncertain.

3 Physical examination is important to determine how severely the patient is affected. Most patients with chronic colitis are clinically well apart from having diarrhea. These patients can undergo methodical evaluation, including evaluation of fecal flotations, direct fecal smears, and rectal cytology, before abdominal imaging or colonoscopy is considered. Patients that are clinically unwell, especially with hematochezia, fever, and other systemic signs, or those with palpable rectal or abdominal lesions, need to be evaluated more aggressively.

4 A minimum database of laboratory tests is important for any patient that is clinically unwell. While unlikely to provide a specific diagnosis, the information obtained can help to increase the suspicion of a systemic problem (e.g., sepsis, pancreatitis, peritonitis, multiple organ failure) as an underlying cause of LI diarrhea. Additionally, it allows the clinician to determine how sick the patient is and how rapidly intervention and diagnostic testing should progress.

5 In selected clinically affected patients suspected of having an infectious cause of colitis, fecal cultures should be evaluated on selective culture media for *Salmonella* spp., *Campylobacter* spp., and *C. difficile*. This is particularly important for febrile patients or those in which an unusual bacterial population is seen on rectal cytology.

6 *Y. enterocolitica* is rarely found in dogs. It may be seen most frequently in animals living in close association with pigs. The organism produces enterotoxins, resulting in acute or chronic LI diarrhea. The prognosis is unknown because such cases are rare.

7 Patients suspected of having an abdominal mass lesion on physical examination should undergo abdominal imaging using either ultrasound or radiographs as appropriate and available. Radiographic studies may include administration of contrast (barium enema), which is administered after clearing the colon with multiple enemas to reduce the chance of creating artifacts. Contrast is most useful for mass lesions, partially

obstructive foreign bodies, and intussusceptions. Ultrasound is useful for differentiating true mass lesions from intussusceptions. When imaging identifies a suspected impacted foreign body (unusual in the colon but possible when clinical signs are chronic), a mass lesion, or an intussusception, abdominal exploratory and corrective surgery is appropriate. However, if imaging studies are negative or equivocal, the next step is colonoscopy.

8 In patients with signs of chronic colitis, mass lesions can be identified on rectal examination. If accessible, such lesions may be aspirated for cytology or biopsied for histopathology under sedation. Otherwise, or if the condition is suspected to extend from the rectum into the colon, the patient should undergo colonic preparation and colonoscopy for tissue biopsy.

9 Mass lesions within the colon and rectum can be benign adenomatous polyps. Unlike such lesions in human beings, these are usually isolated (although some cats have multiple polyps). Other possibilities include benign tumors such as leiomyomas and malignant tumors that have not yet spread through the bowel wall (carcinoma in situ).

10 Malignant tumors may be isolated (adenocarcinoma, leiomyosarcoma, lymphoma, plasmacytoma, mast cell tumor) or diffuse (lymphoma, mast cell tumor, and occasionally adenocarcinoma). The prognosis depends on the tumor type and the extent of spread.

11 In clinically well patients with LI diarrhea and no abnormalities on physical examination, three fecal samples, obtained 24 hours apart, should be evaluated for parasite larvae and *Giardia* spp. In addition, a direct fecal smear should be examined for protozoa.

12 Rectal cytology is useful for identification of spores of *C. perfringens*. Enterotoxigenic strains of *C. perfringens* are suspected of being associated with chronic LI diarrhea. Rarely, neoplastic cells and fungal or algal organisms also may be seen on rectal cytology.

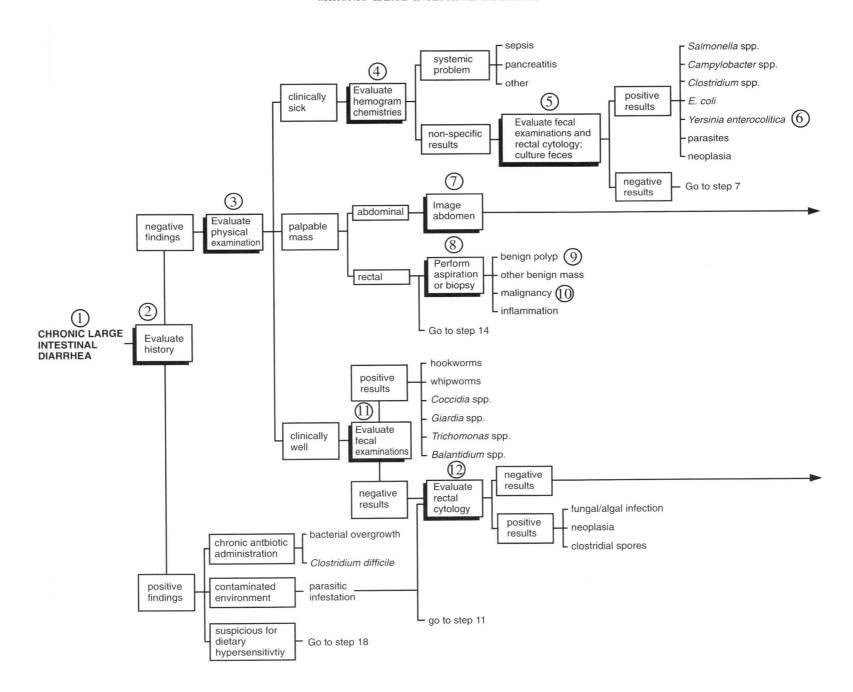

13 Megacolon (see the algorithm for constipation and tenesmus) can be identified radiographically. This condition may produce clinical signs that can be confused with those of LI diarrhea. Patients with colonic dilation and impaction or motility problems develop hard, impacted stool within the colon and hence generally present with signs of constipation. However, the presence of impacted stool can lead to colonic irritation. Fluid may be produced and excreted around the stool, giving the appearance of LI diarrhea.

14 Colonoscopy is the least invasive and most direct method of examining the colon. Unlike examination of the SI, where on occasion it may be more useful to perform full-thickness bowel biopsies, endoscopically performed biopsies of the colon are always best for disease processes that extend into the intestinal lumen. Colonoscopic biopsies reduce the risk of abdominal contamination, colonic perforation, and failure of the colon to heal postoperatively. However, if a mass lesion or intussusception is identified, it will be necessary to progress to exploratory surgery.

15 IBD affects the colon as well as the SI and can cause isolated signs of colitis. Once again, IBD is a histopathological diagnosis and does not necessarily define the underlying cause of the inflammatory infiltrates described. Lymphoplasmacytic colitis is the most frequently diagnosed form of IBD in dogs and cats, and the findings are similar to those for LPE. Eosinophilic colitis may represent a variant of IBD; may be a response to the presence of parasites, irritants, or other infectious organisms; or may be an allergic response to dietary constituents. Granulomatous eosinophilic colitis is rare and can cause mass lesions in the colon. Eosinophilic colitis also can be a manifestation of hypereosinophilic syndrome in cats. Chronic histiocytic ulcerative colitis, suppurative colitis, and granulomatous enterocolitis also are rare variants of IBD. Histiocytic ulcerative colitis is most frequently seen in young male boxer dogs and can be associated with clinical illness and weight loss. The prognosis is guarded to poor, unlike that of most other forms of IBD affecting the colon. Suppurative (neutrophilic) colitis is rare but occurs most commonly in cats. It may be associated with an enteric form of FIP, but otherwise the underlying causes are unknown.

16 Fiber-responsive diarrhea is LI diarrhea that is associated with no or only mild histopathological abnormalities that are insufficient to explain the clinical signs. Signs can be improved or cured by supplementation of dietary fiber. It should be noted that this condition probably represents a spectrum of disease and that individual patients respond to some fiber types (soluble versus insoluble) and not to others.

17 IBS is a diagnosis of exclusion. This is a motility disorder that can result in signs of LI diarrhea as well as vomiting and abdominal discomfort. Occasionally this condition may respond to increases in dietary fiber. There also is thought to be a psychological component to IBS. Antispasmodics or motility modifiers may provide a good response.

18 Dietary hypersensitivity can result in signs of colitis. Hypersensitivity usually develops as a result of chronic exposure to dietary protein. Therefore, it is rarely associated with a recent diet change unless the new diet contains proteins to which the patient already has become sensitized. The best way to diagnose dietary hypersensitivity is by a strict exclusion diet, followed by challenge testing as for chronic SI diarrhea.

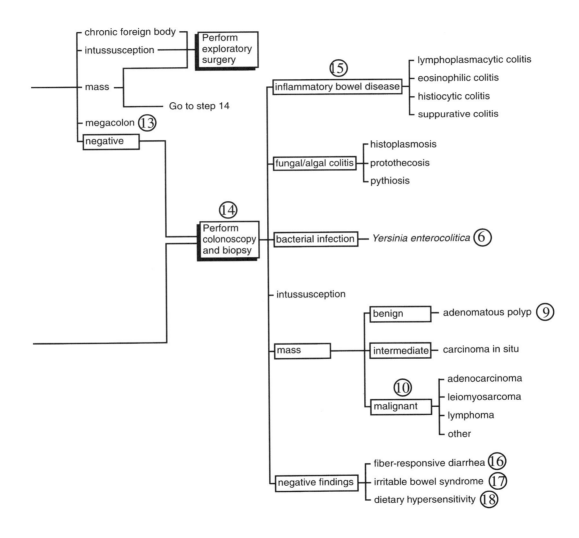

1 Hematochezia is fresh blood in stool with or without signs of LI or rectal irritation (tenesmus, diarrhea, mucus, perineal irritation). Acute hematochezia is due to trauma, foreign material, or parasitic, viral, or bacterial infection, or it is idiopathic (hemorrhagic gastroenteropathy [HGE]). It generally is self-limiting, but testing should be pursued in severe cases. Hematochezia is rare in cats.

2 Check the history for foreign body ingestion, trauma, drug therapy, preexisting conditions, and a description of the stool. Patients with liver and kidney failure can develop colonic ulcers, bleeding, and diarrhea due to failure of mucosal repair mechanisms. Congenital/acquired coagulopathies can cause colonic and rectal bleeding. Glucocorticoids affect colonic mucosal integrity, causing ulceration and bleeding. This may be particularly true in dogs with back trauma/disc disease. Ingested foreign bodies usually impact in the SI. Hair, bone, and rocks can cause LI irritation, bleeding, and impaction/obstipation, however. Stool consistency and the location of blood in relation to the stool are important guides for further testing. Normally formed stool with blood in or around it suggests a point source of colonic/rectal bleeding (foreign body trauma, colonic or rectal mass, perineal or anal sac disease). Normal stool consistency with shape changes suggests a constrictive colonic/rectal lesion (most likely a malignant neoplasm but possibly a stricture, perineal fistulation, or external structures such as the prostate impinging on the rectum). The last does not cause hematochezia. Changes in stool consistency as well as hematochezia suggest more diffuse colonic disease resulting in failure of water reabsorption or excessive fluid secretion. Causes may be infectious (bacterial, viral, or parasitic), inflammatory, or diffuse neoplasia.

3 Physical/rectal examination is the next step. The majority of patients with hematochezia are healthy apart from having LI signs. Exceptions occur when the problem also affects the SI or causes systemic debilitation (e.g., IBD, bacterial/mycotic infections, neoplasia).

A) Patients with a history of trauma or foreign body ingestion can have pelvic fractures impinging on or puncturing the rectum, impacted stool, or foreign material. Radiographs of the pelvis/abdomen also are warranted to determine the extent of the lesion and to plan therapy.

B) Patients with normally formed stool with changes in stool size or shape and hematochezia should be evaluated for colonic/rectal masses and anal sac lesions (impactions, masses). The perineum should be examined for masses, fistulas, and wounds.

C) Patients with diarrhea and hematochezia should be examined for bowel thickening and debilitation, fever, or shock suggesting sepsis, viral infection, or HGE.

4 Patients with a history of trauma, ingestion of foreign material, little stool production, constipation, or tenesmus should be radiographed for pelvic fractures, radiopaque foreign bodies, and constipation/obstipation. Radiographs may suggest ileocecocolic intussusception, masses, or stricture, but they are not as sensitive as colonoscopy. Abdominal ultrasound identifies masses or intussusceptions, but colonic gas can block the beam.

5 Any mass that is identified should be biopsied. Accessibility and the need for anesthesia will determine whether biopsy should be incisional or excisional. Colonic, rectal, and perineal masses can be benign or malignant. If they are malignant, patients should be screened for metastasis.

6 Anal sac impaction/infection is a common cause of hematochezia with normal stool. Sacs should be expressed and systemic antimicrobial administration initiated. Recurrent problems may require anal sacculectomy.

7 Perineal fistulas rarely cause hematochezia. The usual signs include pain, odor, discharge, tenesmus, stricture, and changes in stool consistency due to colitis/proctitis. Fistulas are common in German shepherds and also occur in other breeds (e.g., Irish setters). They may be related to conformation, tail carriage, and abnormal immune system responses.

8 Perineal hernias cause hematochezia with normal stool consistency. Stool impacts in the hernia, causing tenesmus and constipation. Patients usually present with unilateral or bilateral perineal swelling, but in some cases hernias are detected only on rectal examination. The condition is common in intact male dogs (testosterone affects pelvic diaphragm receptors and causes prostatomegaly

and tenesmus). It is also reported in neutered male and female dogs and in cats. In cats it may be due to tenesmus secondary to megacolon.

9 Perianal myiasis is infection of the perineum/anus with fly larvae. Eggs are laid in traumatized tissue, usually in debilitated patients or those with diarrhea or urine scald.

10 A few patients with hematochezia and diarrhea are systemically ill, with weight loss (due to diffuse neoplasia or SI involvement), fever (due to septicemia), or systemic disease. They may have coagulopathies, organ failure (hepatic, renal), or inflammation (hepatitis, pancreatitis). They may be in shock due to hypovolemia or endotoxemia. A minimum database (hemogram, chemistry profile, urinalysis) should be obtained early on. Those with renal failure, hepatic disease, or pancreatitis should undergo further testing to identify the cause of these conditions since hemorrhagic colitis is likely to be only a symptom of underlying disease. Patients that are septic/endotoxemic secondary to severe salmonellosis or those in which the disease process is diffuse (systemic histoplasmosis, prototheosis) can have a primary enteric problem with systemic signs including liver enzyme elevations and a degenerative left shift.

11 Severe hemoconcentration (PCV > 55%), vomiting, diarrhea, hematochezia, and hypovolemia suggest HGE. This relatively poorly defined disease commonly affects middle-aged, small-breed dogs. No underlying cause has been found. *C. perfringens* and certain strains of *Escherichia coli* have been postulated as sources of endotoxemia. Immune-mediated reactions against the enteric mucosa also are possible. Patients usually respond well to aggressive supportive care within 48 hours but occasionally die of shock or develop DIC. If clinical signs persist, patients should be evaluated further.

12 Dogs with low WBC counts should be tested for parvovirus if they are young, poorly vaccinated, or immunosuppressed, or if they have been exposed to a known case.

13 Thrombocytopenia can cause hematochezia with or without diarrhea. (If it is persistent, see the algorithm for thrombocytopenia.)

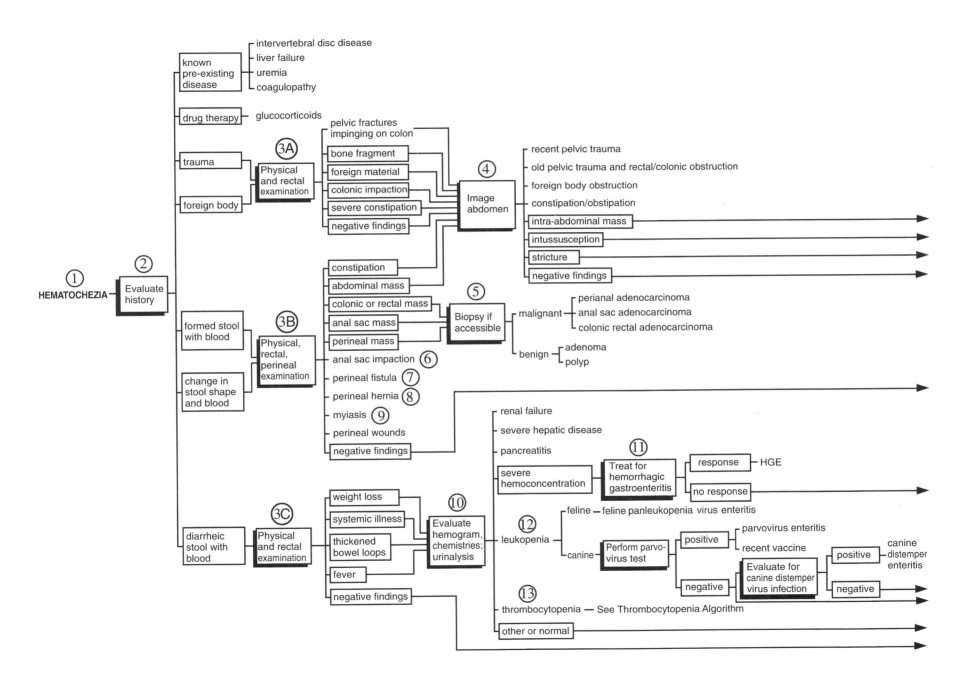

14 Patients with negative/nonspecific findings on the minimum database, physical examination, or abdominal imaging, and possibly those in which a mass lesion, stricture, or intussusception is suspected should undergo fecal examinations (three zinc sulfate fecal flotations and a wet preparation to look for *Giardia* spp. and *Campylobacter* spp.). This is done to look for underlying causes of undefined hematochezia or of already known conditions (e.g., intussusception may be secondary to parasitic infestation). Three fecal zinc sulfate flotations at least 24 hours apart are required to exclude *T. vulpis* infestation, since whipworms generally shed eggs intermittently.

15 When the fecal examination is negative, rectal cytology findings should be evaluated. These can reveal neoplastic cells (lymphoma or carcinoma) if the condition is rectal in origin or diffuse. This may be sufficient to make the diagnosis of neoplasia or it can be followed up by endoscopic evaluation and biopsy. Additionally, rectal cytology can find evidence of fungal or algal infection (*H. capsulatum, Pythium insidiosum, Prototheca* spp.). Mucosal biopsy may be required to diagnose these infections. Cytology may reveal spores of *C. perfringens*, an organism that may produce enterotoxin A (*C. perfringens* enterotoxin) when it sporulates. However, nontoxigenic *C. perfringens* also exists in the colon, and there is no real correlation between existence of spores and clinical signs of colitis. Fecal enterotoxin titers can be determined on fresh feces (step 18). Finally, an abnormal population of bacteria can be found on rectal cytology (if a fixed, stained sample is evaluated under oil immersion or a wet preparation of feces is examined). Motile spiral organisms (*sea gull wing* rods) on a wet preparation suggest *Campylobacter jejuni*. An abnormal population of bacteria (i.e., too many rods or cocci, a homogeneous bacterial population) also suggests overgrowth of a particular bacterium, indicating that fecal culture is appropriate.

16 Fecal culture is appropriate in systemically ill patients, when the history and clinical signs suggest a specific enteric bacterial infection, or when an unusual or uniform population of bacteria is seen on rectal cytology.

17 If patients exhibit signs of severe colonic bleeding, if there is evidence of bleeding elsewhere, or if there is a questionable history of anticoagulant ingestion, a coagulation profile (PT and PTT) should be evaluated.

18 Fecal enterotoxin titers (for *C. perfringens* enterotoxin) may be determined on fresh feces. This should be done if the presentation and clinical signs are appropriate even when spores are not seen on stained rectal cytology preparations.

19 In patients with hematochezia, when all previous tests are negative or equivocal or when further testing is needed, the next diagnostic step is colonoscopy. If this is not available, colonic contrast studies can be useful. Radiographic contrast studies with air and/or barium require colonic preparation (multiple enemas and possibly the use of a cathartic solution such as GoLYTELY) to cleanse the colon and reduce the likelihood of artifact due to residual stool. This makes contrast studies difficult to perform and interpret. Barium enemas may show obstruction of the lumen (e.g., by masses or strictures), but they do not allow annular neoplasms to be distinguished from strictures. They may also indicate colonic mucosal lesions/irregularities. However, contrast techniques do not allow a definitive diagnosis of the condition. Colonoscopy also requires colonic preparation with a cathartic solution and enemas to remove fecal material from the colon. This increases the clinician's ability to evaluate the walls of the colon endoscopically. Colonoscopy allows examination of the mucosal surface and lumen of the colon (although not the serosal layer) and allows biopsy specimens to be obtained for histopathology.

20 IBD may affect the colon (either on its own or in association with SI problems). It represents a spectrum of inflammatory conditions. The underlying causes are not always known. Probably the most common cause is an abnormal immune response to diet, colonic microflora, or enteric pathogens. Lymphoplasmacytic colitis is the most common form. Eosinophilic colitis may be a variant of this form or it may be a true allergic response to dietary allergens/parasites. Granulomatous eosinophilic colitis may respond less well to therapy than do other forms of IBD. Histiocytic ulcerative colitis is a severe form of IBD, diagnosed most commonly in young male boxer dogs. Unlike some other forms of colitis, patients often lose weight and have a guarded prognosis. Suppurative colitis includes inflammatory infiltrates with neutrophils as well as lymphocytes and plasma cells. The causes are unknown, but the condition is more common in cats than in dogs.

21 Ileocolic/cecocolic intussusceptions cause obstruction of the lumen of the colon at the level of the ascending colon as the ileum or cecum intussuscepts into the colon. Sometimes a mass lesion can be detected on physical examination, on radiographs, or on abdominal ultrasound scans. Occasionally, the lesion is so extensive that it protrudes from the rectum. Surgical reduction/removal is indicated.

22 Colonic/rectal neoplasia may be focal or diffuse. It is most commonly focal. Focal lesions may be benign or malignant, and range from adenomatous polyps and leiomyomas to carcinoma in situ and carcinomas. Polyps may be premalignant and transform over time if not removed.

23 When colonic biopsies are negative in patients with hematochezia, fiber-responsive diarrhea and IBS remain possible underlying conditions. Neither condition is associated with histological or clinicopathological abnormalities. Fiber-responsive diarrhea includes conditions that respond to different types of fiber, both soluble and insoluble. Patients with IBS have no histological abnormalities and often show little or no response to fiber supplementation. They may be high-strung or excitable. Some response may be seen to intestinal motility modifiers and environmental changes. Therapy for both fiber-responsive diarrhea and IBS may need to be lifelong.

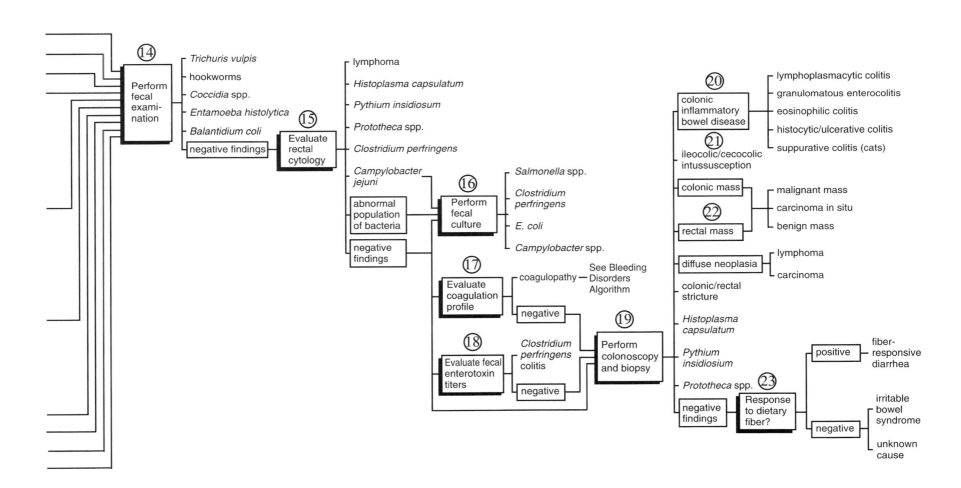

1 Tenesmus is straining to defecate. It may be caused by excessively hard, dry stool (constipation), physical obstruction of the colon or rectum, irritation of the colon or rectum, or colonic motility disorders that result in excessive stool accumulation. Irritation leads to the sensation that stool is still present in the terminal portions of the colon and rectum (colitis or proctitis), hence the continued straining. Unlike most other causes of tenesmus, colitis and sometimes proctitis are associated with soft stool or diarrhea. Tenesmus may be the result of constipation. However, conditions that cause tenesmus also may cause constipation (e.g., if there are anal, terminal rectal, orthopedic, or neurological problems that make it difficult or painful for the patient to defecate).

2 The history is important. If the patient has soft or poorly formed stool, diarrhea, or evidence of mucus or blood in the stool, pursue colitis or proctitis. If the stool is normal to hard, then obstructive conditions or constipation are likely underlying causes. A complicating factor in making this assessment is that obstructive conditions cause most of the stool to be retained in the colon and rectum, but a small amount of liquid feces is produced as a result of mucosal irritation. Therefore, it also is important to determine whether the patient is producing normal or decreased quantities of fecal material. Stool shape also should be evaluated. Patients with intra- or extraluminal obstructions of the colon may produce narrow or distorted stool (flattened and "ribbon-like"). However, patients with colitis and proctitis also may produce smaller or narrow stools because of an increased rate of passage of fecal material through the colon. Single foreign bodies such as rocks or bones are unlikely to impact in the colon if they have already passed through the rest of the gastrointestinal tract without problems. However, large numbers of small rocks or bones, along with hair, cat litter, or plastic, may lead to fecal impaction, obstipation, or mucosal irritation, diarrhea, and tenesmus.

3 The drug history should be evaluated since many drugs result in constipation by causing dehydration, increasing fluid reabsorption from feces, slowing colonic transit of feces, altering intestinal motility, or acting by undetermined mechanisms.

4 Prior trauma may lead to rectal or colonic obstruction (e.g., due to malunion of pelvic fractures), constipation due to patient inactivity, or inability to posture to defecate.

5 Straining to urinate is commonly mistaken for tenesmus. Therefore, it is important to ensure that the patient can urinate normally, has a good urine stream, and has no urgency to urinate that would suggest bladder or urethral irritation.

6 Lifestyle factors or changes may predispose to constipation or reluctance to defecate. For example, some cats will not use the litter box unless it is completely clean. Additionally, some dogs and cats have a routine that culminates in defecation, and if that routine is disrupted, constipation may ensue. Patients that are undergoing enforced inactivity, due either to hospitalization or to restriction after orthopedic or neurological problems, also may develop constipation and exhibit tenesmus.

7 Detailed physical examination, including rectal and in some cases vaginal palpation, may help to refine the differential diagnosis list in a patient presenting with tenesmus. It can answer questions regarding stool consistency if the client is not sure. If stool is soft or diarrheic and present in normal or increased amounts, tenesmus is due to colitis or proctitis. The perineum and anus should be examined for lesions causing obstruction or discomfort when defecating (e.g., masses and fistulas), resulting in either tenesmus or reluctance to defecate and secondary constipation.

8 Perineal hernias result from the breakdown of the pelvic diaphragm. They may be unilateral or bilateral and most commonly are bilateral but worse on one side than the other. Perineal hernias cause tenesmus because of diversion of feces into the part of the rectum within the hernia sac. However, perineal hernias also may result from tenesmus. Therefore, other causes of clinical signs must be excluded from the differential list once the diagnosis of perineal hernia is made. In intact male dogs, perineal hernias may be due to the influence of testos-

terone on muscles of the pelvic diaphragm, leading to breakdown. In older neutered male and female dogs, other causes of muscle wastage, such as hyperadrenocorticism, should be sought. Perineal herniation is uncommon in cats but may occur secondary to colonic motility disorders.

9 Anal strictures may be congenital (atresia ani), in which case they manifest during the neonatal period. They also may be acquired secondary to trauma, surgery of the perineum, or chronic fistulation and secondary fibrosis.

10 In German shepherd dogs, perineal fistulation is suspected to be an autoimmune condition that results in formation of draining fistulas around the perineum, secondary fibrosis, and scarring. In other breeds, perineal fistulation most commonly is associated with anal sac disease. Biopsy may be required for confirmation, although usually the diagnosis is based on the appearance of the lesion. Colonoscopy or proctoscopy is necessary in some instances, as IBD can occur coincidentally in patients with perineal fistulas.

11 Dehydration can lead to hard stools and constipation. Correction of dehydration resolves the problem.

12 Orthopedic abnormalities of the pelvic limbs result in inability of the patient to posture to defecate. This produces the appearance of tenesmus since the patient has to posture repeatedly or suffers stool retention and develops constipation.

13 Neurological abnormalities of the rear limbs have an effect similar to that of orthopedic abnormalities, resulting in tenesmus or constipation. In addition, certain neurological abnormalities may result in segmental colonic dysfunction and stool retention.

14 In female animals, vaginal and possibly uterine conditions (irritation, cysts, or masses) should be considered. Rectal or vaginal examination will detect these conditions.

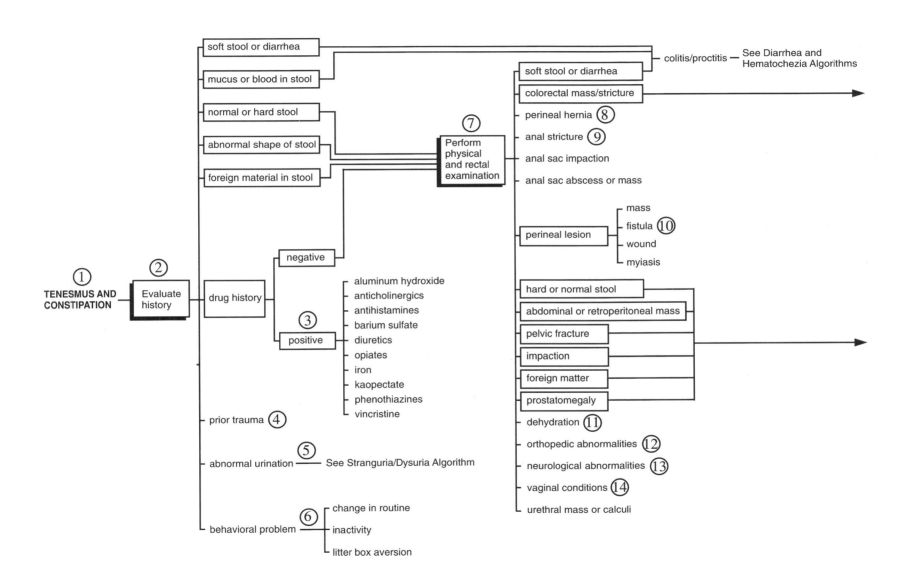

15 Patients with normal to hard stool, masses, pelvic fractures, prostatomegaly, suspected foreign bodies, or normal physical examination should undergo abdominal imaging. Radiographs are most useful for radiodense foreign material (bones, rocks) and to diagnose megacolon. Patients with pelvic fractures should have two-view radiographs to determine the extent to which fracture displacement impinges on the pelvic canal and whether the patient has secondary megacolon. Contrast radiographs may be useful, although barium enemas are difficult to interpret and stool in the colon may cause artifacts. They are useful for outlining radiolucent foreign bodies, strictures, and intussusceptions. Abdominal ultrasound shows abdominal, retroperitoneal, or intrapelvic mass lesions effectively unless they are associated with gas-filled bowel. Ultrasound also allows the structure of mass lesions to be determined (e.g., cavitated, homogeneous, impinging on blood vessels). Most lesions can be aspirated under ultrasound guidance. In patients with prostatic enlargement, ultrasound may allow the clinician to determine whether there is a mass, abscess, or intra- or paraprostatic cyst, or whether the appearance is more consistent with prostatitis or benign prostatic hyperplasia. Intact males with benign prostatic hypertrophy do not generally have tenesmus.

16 Megacolon (generalized, extreme colonic distention accompanied by flaccidity) occurs in both cats and dogs. Typically, the LI is more than twice its normal diameter, with little or no muscle tone. As an idiopathic condition thought to result from undetermined neurological abnormalities leading to disruption of segmental smooth muscle function in the colon, megacolon is much more common in cats than in dogs. It may be congenital, particularly in Manx cats. More generalized, severe neurological problems such as dysautonomia also result in colonic motility problems and megacolon in both dogs and cats. Obstructive conditions of the colon and rectum, if left untreated, result in progressive colonic distention, motility abnormalities, and eventually megacolon.

17 Patients with constipation or obstipation most commonly have ingested an inappropriate diet (e.g., bones or fur in dogs). However, there also may be underlying metabolic or hormonal abnormalities such as dehydration, hypokalemia, or hypercalcemia. Routine laboratory work (hemogram, chemistry profile, and urinalysis) helps diagnose many of these conditions.

18 Canine patients with recurrent constipation/obstipation, other appropriate clinical signs, mild nonregenerative anemia, hypercholesterolemia, and so on should be tested for hypothyroidism as a potential underlying cause. Hypothyroidism is thought to diminish colonic motility, resulting in constipation.

19 Patients with LI mass lesions, focal colonic distention suggestive of obstruction, or an obvious foreign body are candidates for colonoscopy. Other patients also may need to be evaluated this way, including those with recurrent constipation and generalized colonic distention with no obvious source of obstruction. Colonoscopy is definitely indicated in patients with tenesmus and hematochezia in case there is a focal lesion. Colonoscopy requires correct preparation of the LI to allow visualization of mucosal lesions. Patients should be fasted for 24 hours and receive an oral cathartic (such as GoLYTELY) and multiple warm water enemas. If available and appropriate, colonoscopy is preferable to surgery for obtaining colonic biopsy specimens, as it is less invasive and carries little risk of colonic disruption and peritonitis.

20 Most intraluminal masses can be diagnosed via colonoscopy and biopsy. Colonoscopy also allows removal of benign polypoid lesions by means of a snare device passed through the endoscope. It is more difficult to biopsy masses that arise in submucosa or muscularis layers of the intestine (e.g., leiomyomas and leiomyosarcomas).

21 Ileocecocolic intussusceptions actually are ileocolic (more common) or cecocolic. Both are common in young dogs and rare in cats. They usually are secondary to conditions that affect motility of the ileocecocolic junction, including enteritis, colitis, intestinal parasites, parvovirus infection, and intraluminal masses. Patients may have tenesmus, hematochezia, and intussuscepted bowel protruding from the rectum mimicking rectal prolapse, abdominal pain, or vomiting. The lesion may be palpable in the midabdomen. Radiographs suggest a mass lesion. Ultrasound highlights the classical appearance of intussuscepted bowel, with one loop seen within the other (an "onion skin" appearance). Colonoscopy will reveal intussuscepted bowel within the colonic lumen. Surgical resection is the treatment of choice, and the underlying cause of the intussusception should be identified to help treatment and prevent recurrence.

22 Colonic or rectal strictures result from fibrosis/scarring of the colon, causing concentric luminal narrowing. Strictures are unusual in cats and dogs unless there is a prior history of trauma, foreign body impaction, or surgery at the site. If no such history exists, the tissue around the stricture should be biopsied and exploratory surgery should be considered, since many colorectal neoplasms present as concentric or asymmetric bowel lesions, luminal narrowing, and the appearance of a stricture. True strictures may be dilated (like esophageal lesions), but generally surgery is required to resect the area. Samples should be submitted for histopathology.

23 Exploratory celiotomy may be needed to investigate lesions that cannot be diagnosed by other techniques, to exclude the possibility of neoplasia as a cause of stricturing or extraluminal bowel obstruction, and, in some instances, to treat the underlying condition. Surgical biopsy or colonic resection carries some risks, including peritoneal contamination and wound breakdown following surgery.

24 Colonic and rectal masses are most commonly malignant in dogs and cats. Adenocarcinoma and lymphoma of the colon and rectum are most frequently diagnosed, followed by leiomyosarcoma. Mast cell tumors are seen in cats and occasionally in dogs. Benign adenomatous polypoid lesions are not as common as in human beings, and dogs and cats rarely present with multiple polyps, each with the potential to transform into a malignant neoplasm. Benign leiomyomas occur occasionally. Some malignant lesions are diagnosed as carcinoma in situ (i.e., malignant but with no evidence of extension through the mucosal/submucosal layer). These carry a less guarded prognosis than adenocarcinoma, with a better chance of cure if resection is complete. All colonic and rectal mass lesions should be assumed to have the potential to transform into malignant lesions and should be completely excised. Benign lesions may recur if incompletely resected.

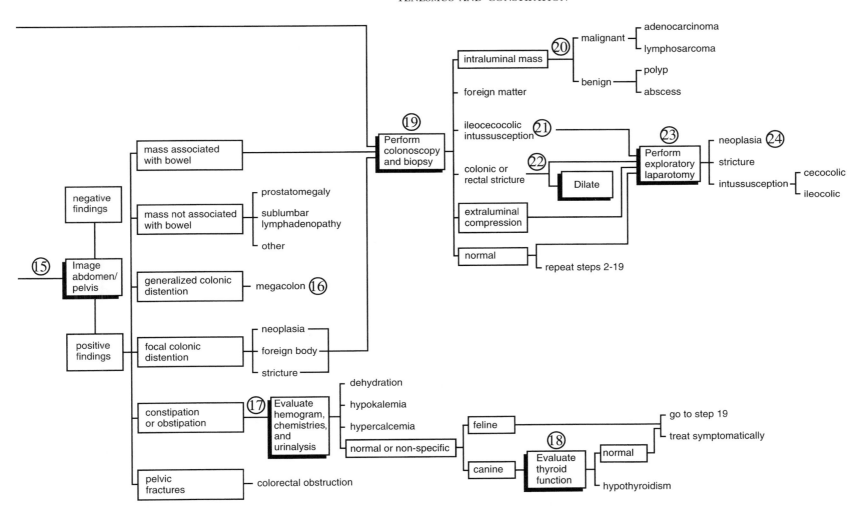

1 Fecal incontinence is inability to retain feces, resulting in involuntary passage of fecal material. There are two types of incontinence. Reservoir fecal incontinence occurs when disease processes reduce the capacity or compliance of the rectum. Sphincter incontinence develops when the external anal sphincter is anatomically disrupted (nonneurogenic sphincter incontinence) or denervated (neurogenic sphincter incontinence). Neurogenic sphincter incontinence is most often caused by damage to the pudendal nerve or sacral spinal cord. Damage to the levator ani and coccygeal muscles can also contribute to fecal incontinence.

2 If the patient is young, clients should be questioned about house training and deworming. Determine if there have been previous or recent neurological signs, anorectal or perirectal surgery, or trauma. To distinguish fecal incontinence from diarrhea, a description of the event and characterization of the feces are helpful. Increased frequency of defecation, the presence of blood or mucus in stool, and tenesmus suggest LI diarrhea (see the LI diarrhea algorithms). Concurrent urinary incontinence is most suggestive of neurological sphincter incontinence.

3 Reservoir fecal incontinence causes an urge to defecate. Signs include frequent, conscious defecation, often associated with tenesmus, dyschezia, or hematochezia. Causes of reservoir fecal incontinence include colitis or colorectal neoplasia. Rectoanal sensitivity or pain is found on digital rectal examination. This type of incontinence also can occur in patients that have had a total or subtotal colectomy for treatment of megacolon.

4 Improper house training usually is seen in young dogs and cats or those recently introduced to an indoor environment. Separation anxiety causes inappropriate defecation when owners leave the house, and it is often associated with destructive activity and vocalization.

5 Because signs of fecal incontinence can be misinterpreted as constipation, diarrhea, or colitis, observing the patient during the act of defecation is an important part of the physical examination. Visually inspect the perineum for inflammation, masses, herniation, rectoanal prolapse, and fistulas prior to rectoanal palpation. Digitally palpate the anorectum to determine the dimensions and texture of anal sacs, anal sphincter tone integrity of the pelvic diaphragmatic musculature, diameter of the rectal lumen, and texture and regularity of the rectoanal mucosa. Causes of reservoir incontinence found on visual, digital, and rectal examinations include anal gland impaction, anal gland masses or abscesses, perianal fistulas or lacerations, scar tissue from previous surgery, and rectal masses or thickening of the rectal mucosa. Also, evaluate anal tone and reflexes. These often are reduced or absent with neurogenic sphincter incontinence.

6 If the patient is a young, tailless cat (Manx and Manx crosses) or a brachycephalic breed of dog, fecal incontinence is probably caused by a malformation of the sacrocaudal spinal cord, nerve roots, and vertebrae (sacrocaudal dysgenesis). Anal tone and reflexes are often decreased or absent.

7 Finding urinary incontinence and/or decreased tail tone or movement increases the suspicion of neurogenic fecal incontinence.

8 Perform a complete neurological examination in patients that do not have obvious anatomical reasons for fecal incontinence. The most common site of neurological disease causing fecal incontinence is the lumbosacral area. Signs associated with disease at this site include decreased voluntary movement of the pelvic limbs and tail, lumbosacral pain, and hyporeflexic myotatic reflexes to the pelvic limbs (LMN signs). Occasionally, lesions above the fourth lumbar vertebra produce fecal incontinence in conjunction with limb weakness and hyperreflexic myotatic reflexes (UMN signs) to the pelvic limbs. If LMN signs are found, radiograph the lumbosacral spine. If UMN signs are found and lumbosacral spinal radiographs are normal, radiograph the thoracic and lumbar spines. If the neurological examination is normal, repeat the algorithm, beginning at step 2, or radiograph the lumbosacral spine since some cases of lumbosacral disease start with fecal incontinence.

9 Lateral and ventrodorsal survey radiography of the lumbosacral spine may show evidence of intervertebral disc herniation, discospondylitis, vertebral neoplasia, spina bifida, lumbosacral trauma, and vertebral malformation.

10 Lumbosacral instability can be congenital or acquired. Congenital stenosis tends to occur in small to medium-sized dogs, while acquired stenosis is seen in large-breed dogs, especially German shepherd dogs. Signs depend on the extent of compression of L7, sacral, and caudal nerve roots. Pudendal nerve root involvement causes fecal or urinary incontinence, while caudal nerve root involvement causes a weak or paralyzed tail. Sciatic nerve root involvement causes lameness, pelvic limb weakness, proprioceptive deficits, and muscle wasting. Radiographic changes at L7-S1 include spondylosis deformans, a narrowed L7-S1 disc space, and ventral displacement of the sacrum relative to the lumbar vertebrae. Interpret these changes with caution since all of them can be found in clinically normal animals. Epidurography and CT or MRI scans of the area often yield more evidence of nerve root compression. Surgical decompression of the area is the treatment of choice.

11 Needle EMG evaluates the electrical activity of muscle. This becomes abnormal if the nerve supply to the muscle is damaged or if the muscle itself is injured. Needle EMG changes found in numerous muscle groups of both front and rear limbs suggest a generalized myopathy or neuropathy. Autonomic dysfunction and generalized peripheral neuropathies or myopathies rarely cause neurogenic sphincter incontinence. Needle EMG changes localized to the muscles of the tail, perineum, and lower lumbar paraspinal muscles indicate lumbosacral disease.

12 If survey spinal radiographs are not diagnostic and neurogenic sphincter incontinence is suspected, spinal fluid analysis and advanced radiographic procedures should be considered. Some cases of lumbosacral instability are difficult to diagnose without epidurography or CT or MRI imaging. If UMN signs are present, a myelogram may be required to diagnose compressive lesions.

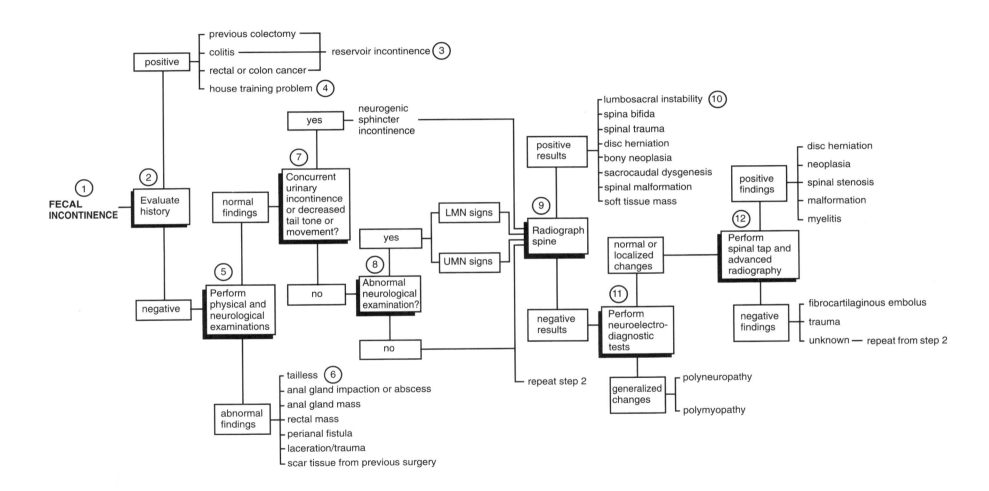

Urinary Disorders

1 Anuria is defined as no urine production by the kidneys. Oliguria is production of insufficient urine. Minimal daily urine production in dogs is about 40 ml/kg (1–2 ml/kg/hr). Patients may present with failure to urinate or decreased urination, but often these signs are not noticed unless there is concurrent stranguria, or dysuria. Patients generally develop systemic signs secondary to anuria/oliguria (anorexia, vomiting, diarrhea, weight loss, weight gain, peripheral edema, CNS depression). Problems with urine production often are detected only after azotemia is identified on a serum chemistry profile, and owners are questioned about urination or urine production is monitored after initiation of therapy. As a result, anuria/oliguria can be well established when detected.

2 The history is important in detecting toxins and factors that lead to acute renal failure (ARF). Nephrotoxic drugs include aminoglycosides, some chemotherapeutics, NSAIDs, and ACE inhibitors. Toxins include calcium oxalate–containing plants and ethylene glycol. Other factors causing ARF include anesthesia, severe systemic illness, fever, trauma, anaphylaxis, and other conditions causing hypotension and hypovolemia. Preexisting renal disease (calculi, infection), old age, and potential exposure to *Leptospira* spp. also are important. Therapy can be directed toward specific causes (antidotes to ethylene glycol, ampicillin for leptospirosis) or precipitating factors can be removed.

3 The size of the urinary bladder should be evaluated. If the bladder is large and the patient is not paralyzed, wait 30–60 minutes and give the patient the opportunity to urinate (by taking dogs outside or providing cats with a litter box and a quiet environment). Voiding should be observed if possible.

4 If the patient tries to void or does not void, a urinary catheter should be placed to determine whether urethral obstruction is present. If a soft red rubber or Foley catheter cannot be passed, it may be appropriate to try a more rigid polypropylene catheter. This may pass partially obstructed areas and it may be easier to feel "grating," suggesting the presence of stones or crystalline material. Care should be taken not to use excessive force and rupture the urethra.

5 If the bladder is small, cannot be palpated, or is large but not obstructed, check a chemistry profile and urinalysis. Note that the presence of urine in the bladder does not necessarily mean that urine is still being produced. The patient could have become anuric/oliguric but has not urinated recently. The chemistry profile identifies hyperphosphatemia and azotemia (elevated BUN and creatinine). If the patient is not azotemic, anuria/oliguria is unlikely or laboratory tests have been assessed so early that the values have not increased. In the latter case, the patient is unlikely to have been taken to the veterinarian except for another illness that could precipitate anuria/oliguria (shock, trauma, etc.). The chemistry profile also identifies potential causes of ARF such as hypercalcemia (a concern if the calcium-phosphorus product exceeds 70, predisposing the patient to dystrophic renal mineralization). Hypercalcemia can both cause and result from ARF. An anion gap greater than 30 is suspicious for ethylene glycol intoxication.

6 Azotemia with dilute urine (urine specific gravity [USG] <1.035 for dogs and <1.045 for cats) is diagnostic of renal failure. In these patients, the signalment, history, and physical examination should be reviewed. Even if there is no history of ethylene glycol ingestion, patients with ARF need be tested since those who are azotemic have a poor prognosis without dialysis. Patients also should also be evaluated for more chronic renal problems (e.g., a history of weight loss, PU, PD, nonregenerative anemia, and small, misshapen kidneys). The prognosis is worse for these patients if they develop anuria/oliguria since this probably represents end-stage renal failure. Patients with ARF have some capacity to recover with supportive care. Canine patients should be placed on injectable ampicillin (once culture samples have been obtained) to cover them for *Leptospira* spp. infection.

7 If there is concentrated urine in the bladder, then either the patient is dehydrated (causing azotemia and reduced urine production) or urine production is normal and the patient has postrenal obstruction. Postrenal obstruction is most likely to be urethral because unilateral ureteral/renal pelvis obstruction may not obviously affect urine production initially. Bilateral ureteral obstruction causes renal failure and oliguria/anuria.

8 If no urine is present, then there is anuric/oliguric renal failure, the patient has urinated recently, or is dehydrated and producing little urine. A urinary catheter should be passed or the bladder scanned by ultrasound to see whether there is any urine. If urine is present, maximal effort should be made to obtain it prior to rehydration for the USG to differentiate renal failure definitively from dehydration. The client also should be questioned about recent urination.

9 It is vital to exclude other causes of apparent anuria/oliguria. These include severe dehydration, which reduces renal blood flow, glomerular filtration rate (GFR), and urine production. Even severe dehydration is unlikely to result in anuria since some renal function has to continue. It can cause oliguria, however. Dehydration in addition to preexisting renal dysfunction may produce renal failure. Patients should be assessed for signs of dehydration (sunken eyes, skin tenting, elevated serum protein and hematocrit). Note that debilitated patients have loss of subcutaneous fat, poor body condition, and loss of muscle and thus may appear dehydrated when they are not. If the patient is clinically dehydrated, rehydrate and verify that urine production is adequate before diagnosing dehydration. In very sick or obviously dehydrated patients, rehydrate quickly to ensure that early renal problems do not progress. If the patient is not clinically dehydrated and urine can be obtained, the sediment should be assessed.

10 If there is little or no urine production, evaluate an ethylene glycol test (commercial kit). Perform test as soon as possible (preferably within 24–36 hours of potential ingestion). Urine, if available, can be assessed under ultraviolet light (a Wood's lamp) for the fluorescent dye added to commercial products. Calcium oxalate crystalluria develops within 3–6 hours of ingestion of ethylene glycol.

11 Patients that are oliguric/anuric but adequately hydrated are in renal failure and require immediate therapy. The mainstay of therapy is aggressive diuresis with close monitoring of body weight and urine production, and if necessary, central venous pressure (CVP). If, after appropriate rehydration, there is inadequate urine production, either dehydration was underestimated or more aggressive therapy (low-dose dopamine infusion, furosemide, mannitol, or a combination of these therapies) needs to be initiated.

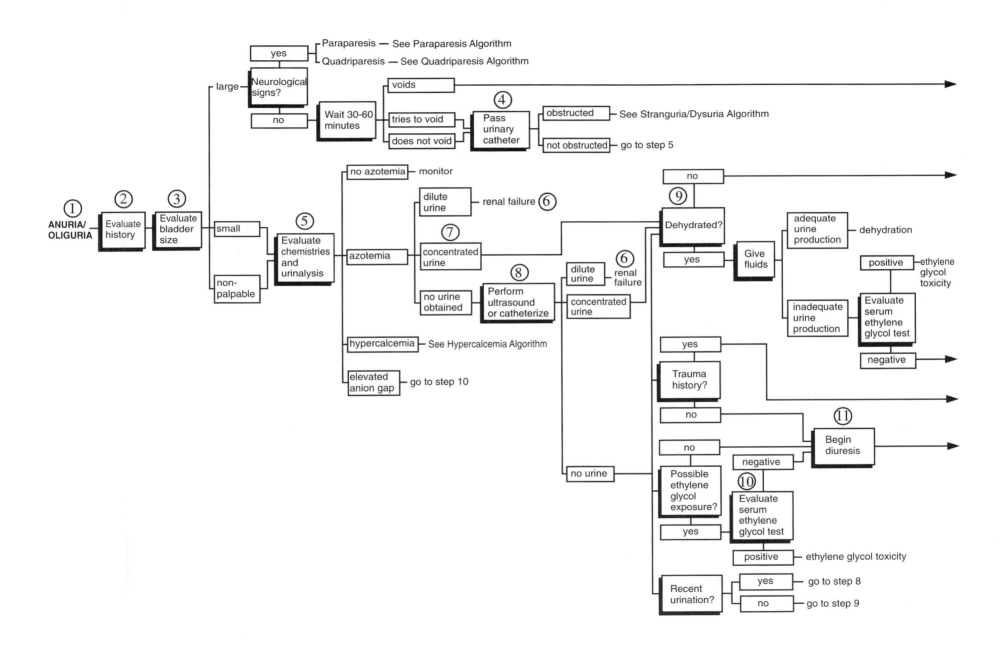

12 In apparently anuric/oliguric or dysuric patients, especially those with concentrated urine, a urinalysis should be evaluated if possible. Sediment should be examined for casts (suggesting renal tubular damage or pyelonephritis), crystals (suggesting potential for calculus formation and renal or urethral obstruction, ethylene glycol or other intoxication if the crystals are calcium oxalate, or bacterial infection if the crystals are struvite), and bacteria. If the sediment is active, this guides further evaluation (e.g., for pyelonephritis, ureteral obstruction). All samples probably should be cultured, regardless of the sediment, since patients with pyelonephritis may not have obvious bacteriuria and patients with hyperadrenocorticism and diabetes mellitus may have bacterial infections with an inactive urine sediment.

13 If the urine sediment is inactive and the culture is negative, urine should be checked for protein and the urine protein/creatinine ratio should be measured. This should be done even if only trace protein is present on the urine dipstick, especially if urine is dilute. Proteinuria indicates glomerulonephritis or amyloidosis, both of which can lead to anuric/oliguric renal failure.

14 Dark ground examination of urine may be done for *Leptospira* spp. Organisms are seen only in acute infection. Given the relative rarity of leptospirosis in dogs, this a relatively low-yield test. It should be done in patients with ARF that were previously healthy, and that have access to slow-moving water or other locations where they could be exposed to the bacterium, or that have both renal failure and hepatic disease. Note that both organ systems do not necessarily have to be involved in the infection.

15 In patients with no factors predisposing to renal failure, an active urine sediment, an inactive sediment but no proteinuria, or no urine for analysis, the urinary tract should be imaged for correctable causes of anuria/oliguria. Plain abdominal radiographs allow estimation of renal size and outline. Small kidneys are found in end-stage renal disease/CRF when patients have decompensated into anuric/oliguric ARF. Large kidneys occur with pyelonephritis, ureteral obstruction and hydronephrosis, renal cysts, lymphoma, and other renal neoplasms. Plain radiographs show increased renal parenchymal density (with hypercalcemic renal failure and ethylene glycol toxicosis). They are best for imaging radiodense calculi,

especially in the ureters, if evaluated carefully. Abdominal ultrasound is probably the highest-yield, least risky technique, allowing assessment of changes in renal parenchymal structure (loss of normal corticomedullary definition, nonspecific changes in renal parenchymal detail that suggest inflammation), renal size, masses, and renal pelvic and proximal ureteral dilation. It also allows ultrasound-guided needle aspiration of the renal parenchyma for cytology and ultrasound-guided renal biopsy. Ultrasound evaluates the bladder wall for potential rupture and diagnoses abdominal fluid. Renal contrast studies (intravenous urography [IVU]) may be used to diagnose radiolucent ureteral obstruction (blood clots, strictures, purulent debris) and can outline abnormal areas of renal parenchyma. However, these studies require some residual renal function for the contrast to pass into the urinary tract from the blood, and iodine-based contrast agents may precipitate or worsen ARF. Therefore, consider whether an IVU is needed in oliguric or anuric patients. Almost the only indication in ARF would be to highlight bilateral radiolucent ureteral obstruction.

16 Urinary bladder rupture occurs with trauma, excessive palpation, damage by catheterization, obstruction and overdistention, and secondary to underlying pathology (tumors, severe sterile hemorrhagic cystitis, etc.). Urine will pass into the abdomen, leading to ascites. Patients may produce some urine or may fail to void urine altogether (appearing anuric/oliguria) and become progressively azotemic. Clinical signs do not usually develop for 4–5 days after rupture unless urine is infected.

17 Polycystic renal disease occurs particularly in Persian and other longhaired breeds of cat (e.g., Himalayans). Young animals have multiple fluid-filled cysts in the renal and sometimes hepatic parenchyma. Not all patients progress to renal failure. Sometimes quite large cysts and renomegaly are found in older patients with no sign of renal dysfunction. However, in patients with ARF or CRF, the cysts are likely to be the underlying cause, and further diagnostic testing may not be required.

18 Renal pelvis dilation can be due to fluid diuresis, renal pelvis or ureteral obstruction (by calculi, strictures, blood clots, or debris), or infection. To produce oliguric/anuric

renal failure, these conditions have to affect both kidneys or preexisting renal disease must be present.

19 In patients with focal renal masses or unilateral/bilateral renomegaly (especially with loss of normal renal structure on ultrasound) the abnormal kidney(s) should be aspirated. Tumors such as renal carcinoma occasionally exfoliate. However, the main reason to aspirate enlarged kidneys is to look for lymphoma since this can cause anuric/oliguric renal failure in cats and dogs.

20 If aspirates are negative, renal structure is relatively normal on ultrasound, and kidneys are normally sized or enlarged, and especially if they are painful on palpation, there is concurrent hepatic disease, or patients are febrile, leptospirosis should become more of a consideration in dogs. Blood samples should be obtained for titers, including those for serovars other than icterohemorrhagia and canicola. In the interim, patients should be treated with injectable penicillins. This specifically treats acute leptospirosis but also helps many renal bacterial infections.

21 In cats, blood should be tested for titers to FeLV, FIV (there is an FIV-associated glomerulonephropathy), and FIP (which causes granulomatous nephritis).

22 If testing to this point is negative or nonspecific, renal biopsy should be considered to determine the underlying cause and potential reversibility of anuric/oliguric renal failure. Reversibility can be assessed by determining the amount of normal tissue remaining in the sample. Other conditions causing some renal structural changes can result from congenital dysplasia in dogs and cats, renal amyloidosis in shar-peis and Abyssinian cats, and renal/hepatic telangiectasia in corgis. Structural abnormalities can be identified ultrasonographically, but biopsy is required for definitive diagnosis. In critically ill and completely anuric patients, the risks of anesthesia and renal biopsy should be weighed against the potential benefits. If hemodialysis is to be performed, renal biopsy is required for the prognosis and suitability for therapy (since long-term dialysis is not available for veterinary patients). Biopsy also is required in feline patients to assess suitability for renal transplantation.

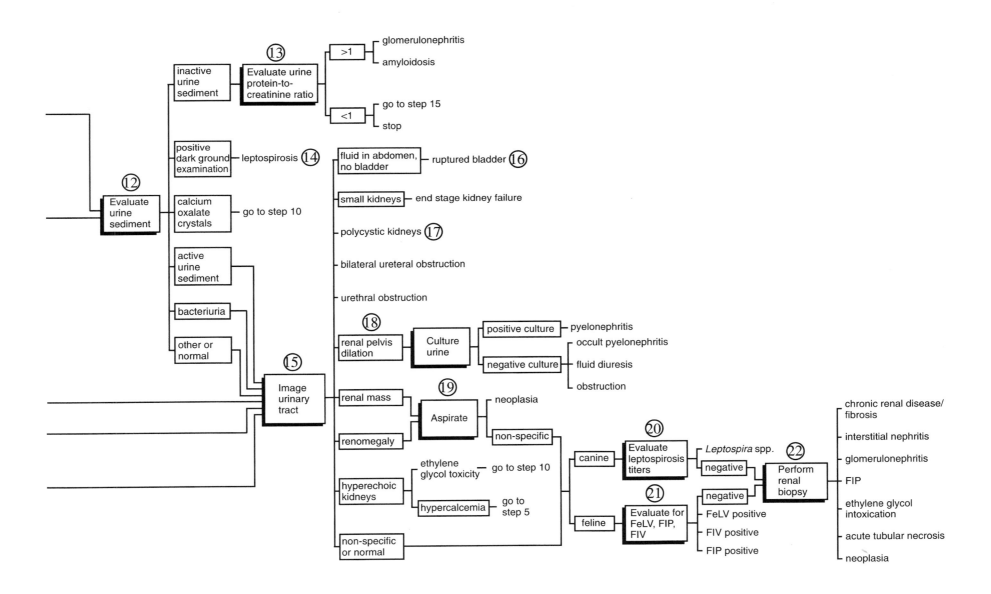

1 Azotemia is an increased concentration of nitrogenous compounds in blood (BUN and creatinine). It results from an increased rate of production of these compounds, a decreased rate of excretion, or both. A decreased rate of excretion usually is associated with a decreased glomerular filtration rate(GFR) caused by prerenal, renal, or postrenal disorders.

2 Increased production of urea (BUN) occurs with various catabolic states, consumption of a high-protein diet, or gastrointestinal hemorrhage. Such conditions usually result in mild increases in BUN (<40–50 mg/dl) with no concurrent increase in creatinine.

3 Evaluate patients for signs of dehydration, hypovolemia, or cardiac disease since these are likely to cause decreased renal perfusion and prerenal azotemia. Urine specific gravity in these patients should be greater than 1.035 (dogs) or 1.045 (cats). Fluid therapy improves renal perfusion and BUN, and creatinine should return to normal.

4 Rupture anywhere in the urinary tract should be suspected if the patient has a history of recent trauma and particularly if urination has not been observed after trauma. Such cases need further evaluation via abdominal radiographs/ultrasonography. Abdominal radiographs also may show an enlarged urinary bladder or mineralized densities within the urinary tract. Intravenous urography (IVU) or cystourethrography may be necessary to show rupture or obstruction of the urinary tract. Ultrasonography is useful for detecting uroliths, masses, intra-abdominal fluid accumulation from urinary tract rupture and distention anywhere in the urine-collecting system. Peritoneal fluid with a creatinine concentration greater than the serum creatinine concentration supports the diagnosis of urine leakage into the abdominal cavity.

5 A history of PU/PD producing dilute urine in conjunction with elevated BUN and creatinine suggests renal failure. Progressive weight loss, small kidney size, mucous membrane pallor, and uremic stomatitis may be present in patients with CRF. However, since other diseases (pyometra, hypoadrenocorticism, diabetes mellitus) can cause PU/PD and azotemia, it is important to evaluate a complete serum chemistry profile to identify nonrenal disease.

6 If there are signs of stranguria or dysuria, suspect obstruction of the urinary tract. The bladder often will be enlarged on palpation. A urinary catheter should be passed to relieve the obstruction if possible and to obtain urine for urinalysis.

7 Palpate the bladder if possible and note its size, tone, and wall thickness. An enlarged, firm bladder is suspicious for urinary tract obstruction. A urinary catheter should be passed to confirm this potential problem. A small bladder in a patient with azotemia should make one suspicious of ARF or urinary tract rupture, especially if the kidneys are normal or large or if urine output is diminished. Exposure to ethylene glycol should be considered in any patient that roams or is not supervised when outside, or in any patient kept in an outside area accessible to the public (malicious poisoning). Ethylene glycol intoxication can be documented by chemical analysis of blood (12–24 hours) or urine (24–48 hours) after exposure. Laboratory diagnosis of ethylene glycol intoxication can be made presumptively by the presence of increased serum osmolality, an increased anion gap, profound metabolic acidosis, and the presence of calcium oxalate crystalluria. Exposure to other common nephrotoxicants such as gentamicin, amphotericin B, thiacetarsamide, and NSAIDs (flunixin meglumine, ibuprofen) usually can be determined from the history and the medical record. Acute ischemic renal injuries also cause ARF. Potential ischemic events include shock, decreased cardiac output, deep anesthesia/extensive surgery, trauma, hyperthermia, hypothermia, extensive cutaneous burns, DIC, and hypotension.

8 Postrenal azotemia occurs when there is impaired urine elimination from the body, as occurs with urinary tract obstruction by uroliths, mucous plugs, blood clots, or masses, or rupture of the tract. Rupture of the urinary tract diverts urine into the retroperitoneal space (ureteral rupture), peritoneal cavity (ureteral, bladder rupture), or pelvic interstitium (urethral rupture) and causes oliguria/anuria and uremia. However, with early recognition and treatment, azotemia resolves quickly, without permanent morphological damage to the kidneys.

9 Azotemia can be classified into prerenal, renal, and postrenal in origin if the usg is evaluated at the same time that azotemia is diagnosed. A usg of 1.035 or more in a dog and 1.045 or more in a cat is compatible with prerenal azotemia (see step 3). A usg of 1.008 to 1.013 indicates renal azotemia or possibly prerenal azotemia with a concurrent concentrating defect due to underlying disease (diabetes mellitus, pyometra, liver disease) or drug administration (diuretics, glucocorticoids, fluid therapy, anticonvulsants). A usg between 1.013 and 1.030 is suggestive of prerenal azotemia with a concurrent concentrating deficit that could be caused by many different diseases. A usg of less than 1.008 (hyposthenuria) is caused by damage to renal tubules, altered tonicity of the medullary interstitium (medullary washout), or interference with the synthesis, release, or action of ADH.

10 With prerenal azotemia there is decreased renal perfusion. Normal renal function will return if the prerenal insult is corrected before permanent renal damage occurs.

11 Renal azotemia occurs when 75% or more of the nephrons are nonfunctional. Thus, disorders of renal glomeruli, tubules, interstitium, or vasculature can result in renal azotemia. There are many intrinsic renal diseases as well as systemic diseases that result in renal azotemia. Infectious causes include leptospirosis, pyelonephritis, FIP, borreliosis, leishmaniasis, babesiosis, and septicemia. Systemic diseases that are associated with renal azotemia include DIC, pancreatitis, hypoadrenocorticism, hepatic failure, vasculitis, glomerulonephritis, renal artery or vein thrombosis, SLE, neoplasia, hypercalcemia, malignant hypertension, and polycythemia. Numerous nephrotoxins and various causes of shock and hypotension (e.g., burns, heat stroke, septic shock, hemorrhage) also result in renal azotemia. Many of these causes of azotemia are found by evaluating the history, physical examination findings, and routine blood chemistries and urinalysis.

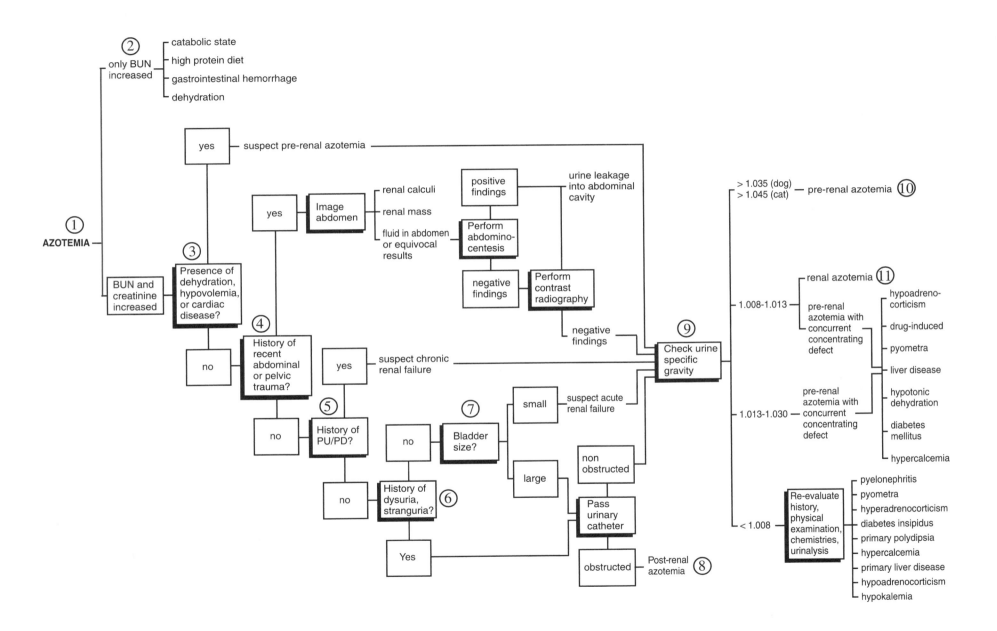

① **AZOTEMIA**

② only BUN increased
- catabolic state
- high protein diet
- gastrointestinal hemorrhage
- dehydration

BUN and creatinine increased

③ Presence of dehydration, hypovolemia, or cardiac disease?

yes — suspect pre-renal azotemia

no

④ History of recent abdominal or pelvic trauma?

yes — Image abdomen
- renal calculi
- renal mass
- fluid in abdomen or equivocal results

no

positive findings — urine leakage into abdominal cavity

Perform abdomino-centesis

negative findings — Perform contrast radiography

negative findings

⑤ History of PU/PD?

yes — suspect chronic renal failure

no

⑥ History of dysuria, stranguria?

no — ⑦ Bladder size?

small — suspect acute renal failure

large

Yes

non obstructed

Pass urinary catheter

obstructed — Post-renal azotemia ⑧

⑨ Check urine specific gravity

> 1.035 (dog)
> 1.045 (cat) — pre-renal azotemia ⑩

1.008-1.013
- renal azotemia ⑪
- pre-renal azotemia with concurrent concentrating defect

1.013-1.030
- pre-renal azotemia with concurrent concentrating defect
  - hypoadreno-corticism
  - drug-induced
  - pyometra
  - liver disease
  - hypotonic dehydration
  - diabetes mellitus
  - hypercalcemia

< 1.008 — Re-evaluate history, physical examination, chemistries, urinalysis
- pyelonephritis
- pyometra
- hyperadrenocorticism
- diabetes insipidus
- primary polydipsia
- hypercalcemia
- primary liver disease
- hypoadrenocorticism
- hypokalemia

1 Small amounts of protein (up to 50 mg/dl) are normal in concentrated urine (>1.030 for dogs, >1.040 for cats). Normal daily urinary protein loss is <20 mg/kg/24 hr in dogs. Proteinuria is identified on dipstick evaluation and is unlikely to be the problem for which a patient is presented. Proteinuria should be checked for in patients with persistently dilute urine, PD, PU, renal failure, hypoalbuminemia, or ascites. It also should be evaluated for in patients with neoplasia, chronic systemic immune-mediated disease, or chronic infections (otitis, granulomas, leishmaniasis) since proteinuria can be an early indicator of renal dysfunction. It is important to determine the source of urine protein. Proteinuria can indicate infection anywhere in the urinary tract, mechanical irritation of the urinary tract epithelium lining by calculi and crystals, idiopathic irritation (feline idiopathic cystitis), and neoplasia. Proteinuria also can be due to renal protein losses with glomerulonephritis or amyloidosis. Persistent renal proteinuria causes glomerular inflammation and damage, protein accumulation in renal stroma, glomerulosclerosis, and eventually renal failure. Urine dipsticks are most sensitive for albumin. Certain types of protein (Bence Jones/immunoglobulin light chain proteins) are not detected on the urine dipstick and require urine protein electrophoresis or heat precipitation to be measured. This type of proteinuria often is unsuspected and is diagnosed only when it is assessed to fulfill the criteria for the diagnosis of plasma cell myeloma.

2 Once proteinuria is detected, it is important to evaluate the urine sediment for inflammation, infection, or blood loss as a source of protein. The initial urine sample should be obtained by cystocentesis to allow determination of the significance of an inflammatory sediment. RBCs (zero to five per high-power field [hpf]), WBCs (zero to three per hpf), or bacteria should lead the clinician to investigate for infection, sterile inflammation, irritation, or neoplasia anywhere in the urinary tract. Crystalluria alone is unlikely to cause proteinuria unless there is hematuria or pyuria suggesting infection or inflammation.

3 Active urine sediments should be evaluated further based on the cell type present. Patient signalment can be important because although it does not indicate a specific diagnosis, it can focus the investigation on specific areas of the urogenital tract (e.g., prostate in intact or recently neutered males). Investigation of an active urine sediment takes a somewhat different course in cats because the incidence of UTI is low.

4 If the urine sediment is inactive, the kidneys are the likely source of protein loss (causes include glomerulonephritis and amyloidosis). Before pursuing this, it is advisable to culture a cystocentesis urine sample to ensure that no occult infection is present. Infection with no inflammatory sediment is relatively common in patients with diabetes mellitus, hyperadrenocorticism, and, rarely, pyelonephritis.

5 Hematuria found on a cystocentesis urine sample should be evaluated further via a free catch urinalysis to exclude iatrogenic contamination. If hematuria is present on a free catch sample, follow the algorithm for discolored urine.

6 Pyuria results from inflammation and can be due to infection (bacterial, fungal, possibly viral in cats), mechanical irritation of the urinary tract (calculi, crystals, foreign material), or neoplasia.

7 Bacteriuria is significant in a cystocentesis sample and suggests infection, provided that the sample has been obtained and handled correctly. The significance of bacteriuria in any sample can be determined via quantitative urine culture that takes account of the likely amount of contamination.

8 Other rare urine sediment abnormalities include fungi (mycelia/budding forms), nonspecific debris, and tubular casts, all of which contribute to proteinuria. Casts suggest renal disease. Debris represents infection/inflammation anywhere in the urinary tract and should be pursued via specialized cultures or urinary tract imaging.

9 The first episode of pyuria/bacteriuria in a dog (especially a young or female patient or one with predisposing factors) can be assumed to indicate infection. An empirical course of antimicrobial therapy, using a broad-spectrum agent that concentrates well in urine, can be elected. If problems continue or recur, further investigation is necessary. Pyuria is less likely to indicate UTI in cats because true infections are rare in this species. It is more likely to be due to sterile irritation by calculi or crystals or to result from idiopathic irritation or interstitial cystitis. Attention should be paid to urine pH, crystalluria, and the duration of the problem since cases are often self-limiting, although they can be recurrent. In cats, the investigation of pyuria should progress more quickly to urinary tract imaging.

10 Recurrent pyuria or bacteriuria, especially in older animals or if accompanied by stranguria or dysuria, should be investigated further, initially via urine culture and sensitivity testing of urine. If cultures are positive, the infection should be treated on the basis of sensitivity test results with appropriate doses/dose frequency of antibiotics. A 10-day course of antibiotics is sufficient for most infections. However, if the problem is recurrent, it is advisable to treat for a longer period (3 to 4 weeks), especially if a predisposing cause is identified.

11 Determining the urine protein/creatinine ratio is important for measuring the extent of urinary protein loss. Where protein is present on the urine dipstick and no obvious cause (hematuria, pyuria) is identified, it is important to assess the severity of proteinuria in a way that is not influenced by urine concentration. Determination of the urine protein/creatinine ratio requires a single sample and correlates well with 24-hour urine protein excretion. The urine sediment *must* be examined on the sample submitted to ensure that it remains inactive. Ranges for urine protein vary among laboratories, but normal values are usually <1. Very high creatinine ratios have been associated with amyloidosis but there is considerable overlap with glomerulonephritis, and renal biopsy is required to differentiate between the two conditions.

12 If urine culture is negative or active sediments recur despite appropriate therapy, further investigation is needed. This may require culturing for unusual infections (*Mycoplasma* spp., fungi). Alternatively, the next step is urinary tract imaging. Abdominal radiographs identify mineralization and are particularly important for identifying radiodense calculi in the ureters and urethra, neither of which is easily identified with ultrasound. Special positioning and preparation may be needed for assessment of these areas, and contrast administration may be necessary to outline lesions (masses, radiolucent calculi). Ultrasound is best for soft tissue abnormalities, including masses in the prostate, bladder, proximal urethra, and renal parenchyma, renal pelvis dilation with obstruction or pyelonephritis, and radiolucent calculi. It can be too sensitive for cystic calculi.

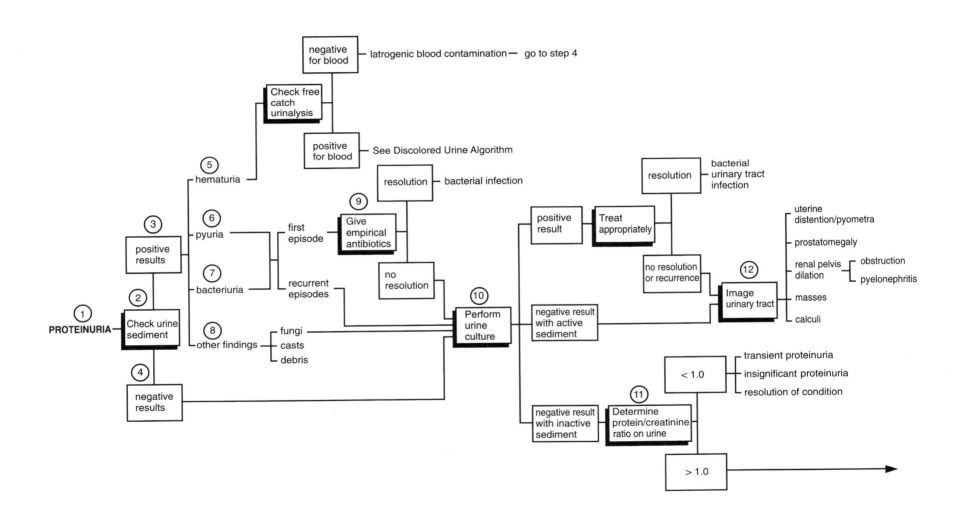

13 Signalment can be an important factor in directing the further evaluation of patients with significant proteinuria and inactive urine sediments. Systemic reactive amyloidosis has been reported as a familial problem in Chinese shar-pei dogs and Abyssinian cats. Patients are generally young to middle-aged. In these breeds it might be advisable to progress directly to renal biopsy (step 16) to identify the condition. It should be noted that in Abyssinian and Chinese shar-peis, amyloid accumulation is medullary and not cortical. This must be taken into account when obtaining renal biopsy specimens, since most Tru-cut biopsies sample cortex and not medulla. A wedge biopsy might be needed to sample the renal medulla. Amyloid also has been reported in other breeds, but not with the same reported predisposition. It tends to be distributed within the renal cortex, and prior evaluation of these other breeds should follow the rest of this algorithm.

14 There is considerable overlap among the underlying causes of glomerulonephritis and amyloidosis. In immune-mediated glomerulonephritis, antibody-antigen complexes resulting from chronic antigenic stimulation either form in the glomerulus itself or circulating complexes are filtered out at the glomerulus. The antibody-antigen complexes activate complement and initiate an inflammatory response, leading to structural damage to the glomerulus and loss of small proteins (albumin, antithrombin III) through the pores in that structure. In amyloidosis, a likely familial predisposition to laying down amyloid chains in the kidney combines with a similar catalog of chronic conditions that lead to inappropriate or excessive stimulation of the immune system. Additionally, systemic inflammation can cause a reactive form of amyloidosis. A good history is needed to obtain information about previously diagnosed conditions that might predispose the patient to immune complex formation or cause generalized systemic inflammation. A complete physical examination identifies potential causes of chronic immune system overstimulation (e.g., chronic otitis externa, skin disease, masses, a swollen and painful prostate, fever, joint pain).

15 If the history and physical examination do not provide further direction, a relative barrage of diagnostic tests is indicated to try to determine the underlying problem causing proteinuria. The list of tests presented here is not exhaustive, and the order in which tests are performed is influenced by the patient's environment, clinical presentation, and stability. Useful tests include thoracic radiographs for masses, abscesses, or pneumonia and abdominal radiographs or ultrasound. A minimum database of laboratory work (hemogram, serum chemistry profile), appropriate testing for *Dirofilaria immitis* (depending on whether the patient is a cat or a dog), and the FeLV/FIV status of cats should be determined. More specific tests are then determined by the results of this baseline evaluation (e.g., titers for specific infectious diseases, ACTH stimulation testing, echocardiography, arthrocentesis, tissue biopsy or aspiration for histopathology, cytology, and culture, blood pressure monitoring, ANA titers). It is very important to determine the underlying causes of glomerular protein loss when possible because if the underlying condition can be treated or removed, proteinuria may be reduced and progression to renal failure slowed.

16 Glucocorticoid use can predispose patients to renal protein loss, probably as a result of changes in blood pressure within the glomerulus.

17 Chronic sterile inflammatory conditions such as pancreatitis and hepatitis can cause proteinuria secondary to immune system overstimulation.

18 Chronic infections of the skin, ears, prostate, kidneys (pyelonephritis), and heart (endocarditis, myocarditis) also can result in proteinuria by the same mechanisms. Acute, overwhelming infection and inflammation secondary to pyometra, prostatic abscessation, and sepsis can have similar effects. Specific diseases that can induce renal damage due to chronic proteinuria include FIV (cats), FeLV (cats), FIP (cats), *Mycoplasma* spp., brucellosis (dogs), ehrlichiosis (mainly dogs), Rocky Mountain spotted fever (dogs), leishmaniasis, and bacterial septicemia.

19 A variety of neoplasms may cause renal proteinuria either by immune complex formation and glomerulonephritis or by stimulating amyloid deposition. Plasma cell myeloma of the bone marrow and occasionally of other tissues and, rarely, lymphoma cause proteinuria by a different mechanism. Immunoglobulin light chains are formed by neoplastic cells and are lost through the relatively normal glomerulus because they are small proteins compared to the entire immunoglobulin molecule.

20 Primary immune-mediated diseases such as SLE and secondary immune-mediated diseases such as polyarthritis and IBD may lead to glomerulonephritis and proteinuria.

21 Other conditions that can cause either transient or more sustained proteinuria include fever, hypertension, diabetes mellitus, and hyperadrenocorticism. In the last two conditions, proteinuria is likely the result of a combination of immune system overstimulation and glomerular hypertension.

22 At some stage in the diagnostic process, it will be necessary to perform a renal biopsy to definitively diagnose the underlying condition, allow differentiation of amyloidosis and glomerulonephritis, and assess the severity and distribution of renal lesions. Less work has been done on glomerulonephritis in dogs and cats than in human beings to identify the different types and to assess efficacy of therapy and the prognosis associated with different forms of the condition. Therefore, at this stage, the main reason for a biopsy is to differentiate amyloidosis and glomerulonephritis because of different therapeutic recommendations for these two conditions and the poorer prognosis for patients with amyloidosis. If more renal biopsies are performed in proteinuric patients, it may become possible to categorize different forms of glomerulonephritis and determine the response to different types of immunosuppressive agents and modulation of glomerular filtration pressures. However, the prognosis is guarded to poor in any proteinuric patient presenting with established renal failure.

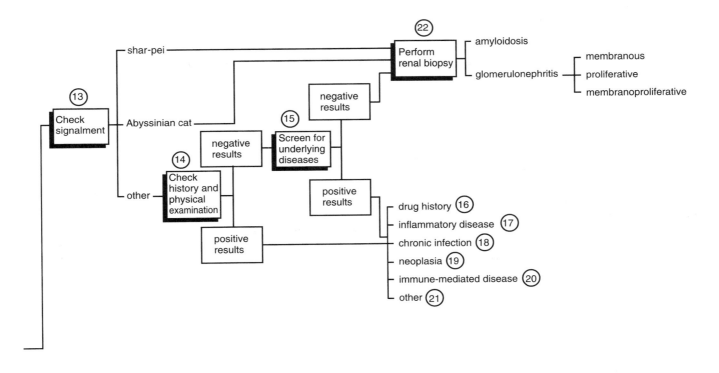

1 The normal color of urine is yellow to amber. The depth of color is related in part to the volume collected and the concentration of the sample. Discolored urine can vary in color from yellow-orange to red to green. The most common causes of discolored urine are hematuria, hemoglobinuria, and bilirubinuria.

2 Since certain chemicals, dyes, antibiotics, drugs, and toxins can cause discolored urine, inquire about possible exposure to such substances. Also ask about the possibility of trauma, pollakiuria, stranguria, liver disease, muscle damage, and hyperthermia since all of these disorders can give the urine an abnormal color.

3 To begin evaluation of discolored urine, collect a urine sample during midstream voiding or via cystocentesis. Evaluation of the sample includes a dipstick analysis, specific gravity determination, and sedimentation cytology.

4 A cloudy or milky urine color is likely related to pyuria. This can be diagnosed by urine sediment examination. Ideally, a cystocentesis sample should be analyzed and a portion saved for culture if bacteria, excessive numbers of WBCs, or crystals are observed. Large amounts of lipid also can give urine a milky appearance.

5 Red, brown, orange, or dark yellow urine is most commonly caused by hematuria, hemoglobinuria, or bilirubinuria. To distinguish these conditions, examine the urine dipstick for positive values on the hemoglobin or whole blood pad areas and then evaluate the urine sediment.

6 If the hemoglobin and/or the whole blood pad on the dipstick are positive, check the urine sediment. If RBCs are present, hematuria is the cause of the discolored urine. If RBCs are absent, hemoglobinuria or myoglobinuria is potentially responsible for the color change.

7 If RBCs are not observed in the sediment, evaluate the color of the patient's plasma. If the plasma is pink, the urine discoloration likely is due to hemoglobinuria. If the plasma is clear, then myoglobinuria is likely. Plasma is clear because myoglobin in plasma is not bound significantly to a carrying protein, resulting in prompt filtration of myoglobin at the glomerulus. Myoglobinuria is caused by muscle damage.

8 If the hemoglobin and/or the whole blood pad on the dipstick are negative in a patient with discolored urine, evaluate the bilirubin pad or the dipstick and usg. The significance of bilirubinuria is somewhat dependent upon the species (cat versus dog), gender (1+ bilirubin is normal for male dogs), and usg.

9 Any amount of bilirubin in feline urine is significant. Hepatic and posthepatic biliary obstruction should be considered and investigated via a serum chemistry profile and abdominal imaging. Hemolysis often is accompanied by weakness and pale mucous membranes. Evaluation of the hemogram, with a reticulocyte count, should show RA if hemolysis is present.

10 In the female dog, a urine bilirubin greater than 1+ in conjunction with a usg of 1.020 or less is significant bilirubinuria. Differential diagnoses include hepatic and posthepatic biliary obstruction and hemolysis.

11 If urine bilirubin is 1+ in conjunction with a usg of more than 1.020, the dog may be dehydrated or have concentrated urine unrelated to hydration status. In such cases, make sure the dog is hydrated and repeat the urinalysis at a later date. 1+ bilirubinuria is normal in male dogs.

12 If the urine bilirubin is less than 1+ and the specific gravity is more than 1.020, the test is normal for the dog.

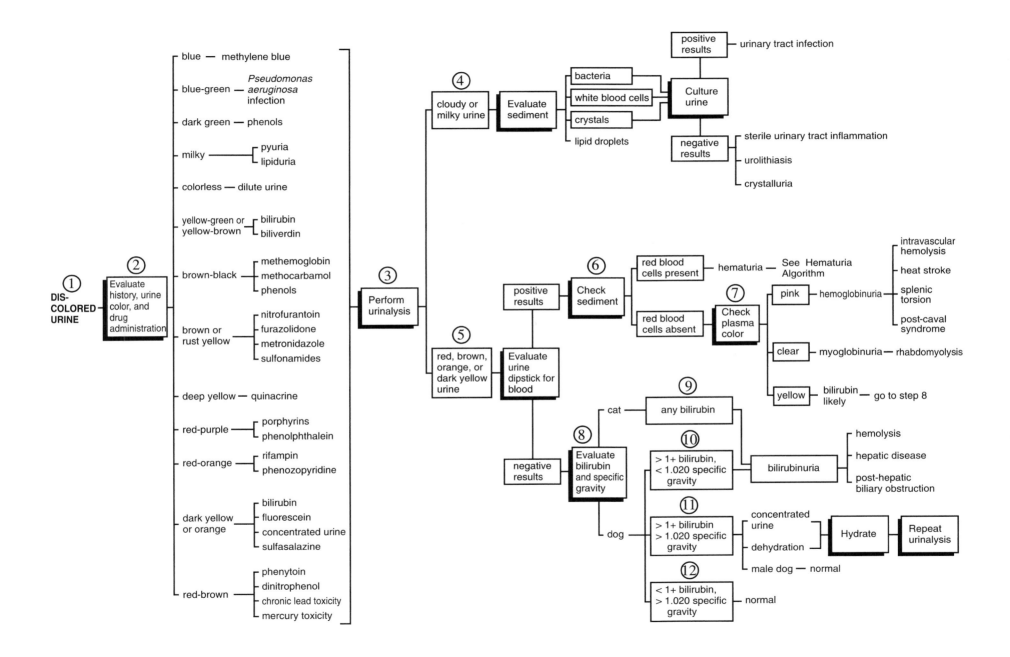

1 Hematuria means that RBCs are present in the urine. Most often it is secondary to diseases of the lower urinary tract and usually is accompanied by other signs such as pollakiuria, stranguria, and dysuria. Sometimes hematuria results from disorders of the kidneys and ureters, in which case patients are usually asymptomatic.

2 Based on the history, determine the stage of urination at which hematuria occurs. Also determine the presence or absence of stranguria, pollakiuria, and increased frequency of urination. Hematuria at the beginning of urination suggests disease of the prostate, urethra, penis, uterus, or vagina. Hematuria at the end of urination is more typical of prostatic or especially urinary bladder disorders. Hematuria that persists for the duration of urination suggests disease of the kidneys, ureters, sometimes the urinary bladder, or the prostate gland. The physical examination should include visualization of vaginal/penile areas, palpation of kidneys, bladder, and prostate, and observation of skin and mucous membranes for evidence of bleeding, petechiation, or bruising.

3 Prolapse of the urethral mucosa appears as a red mass at the end of the penis. English bulldogs are predisposed to this condition.

4 If petechiae, ecchymoses, or hematomas are found on the physical examination, suspect a systemic coagulopathy and evaluate a coagulation profile.

5 If there is no evidence of coagulopathy, urine should be collected via cystocentesis and analyzed. If hematuria is present in a voided urine sample but absent in a cystocentesis sample, hemorrhage from the urethra or genital tract is likely. In males, prostatic hemorrhage may result in hematuria on a cystocentesis sample because prostatic fluid can reflux into the urinary bladder.

6 If a kidney of abnormal size or shape is found on physical examination or if RBC casts are found in the urine sediment, proceed with renal ultrasound.

7 Urine should be cultured if bacteria, WBCs, yeast, hyphae, or crystals are observed in urine sediment.

8 Finding struvite crystals in a cat with hematuria is common and is often associated with FLUTDs. Urethral plugs, composed of struvite crystals and mucus, are a common cause of urethral obstruction. Urine culture is indicated to exclude UTI, but the results usually are negative since bacterial and other UTIs are rare in cats. Cats also can have calcium oxalate and less commonly observed crystals. If there is no response to medical treatment in unobstructed cats, abdominal radiographs should be evaluated for radiopaque uroliths.

9 Crystalluria in dogs indicates an increased risk of urolith formation; however, the presence of crystalluria is not diagnostic for urolithiasis. Urine culture is recommended because UTIs may predispose to crystalluria or urolith formation (especially struvites).

10 *Dioctophyma renale*, the canine kidney worm, is a rare condition. Dogs become infected by ingesting larvae directly or fish that contain encysted larvae.

11 If urine is red or brown and positive for blood on the urine dipstick but does not have RBCs on sedimentation cytology, the diagnosis is hemoglobinuria or myoglobinuria. To distinguish between the two disorders, check the color of the plasma. If the plasma is red or pink, hemoglobinuria is more likely than myoglobinuria.

12 Survey abdominal radiographs show radiopaque uroliths, but most other disorders require contrast procedures or ultrasound to make the diagnosis.

13 If the animal has a recent history of trauma concurrent with hematuria, damage anywhere along the urinary tract should be suspected.

14 Fast the patient for 12–24 hours prior to performing contrast procedures of the urinary bladder. Give an enema 2 hours before the procedure to remove fecal material that could obscure radiographic changes in the caudal abdomen. Sedation is helpful, especially for catheterization and removal of all urine from the bladder. Attach a three-way stopcock to the urinary catheter and inject an organic iodide solution diluted with sterile water or saline to a final concentration of 20% iodide. Use about 10 ml/kg body weight contrast. Discontinue the injection if the bladder is adequately distended, if there is reflux around the catheter, or if back pressure is felt on the plunger of the syringe.

15 If a space-occupying mass is identified at the urinary bladder trigone, excretory urography is indicated to determine the presence and extent of urethral involvement. Ultrasound imaging also may be diagnostic.

16 Excretory urography (an IVU) evaluates the upper urinary tract. The animal should be fasted for 12–24 hours prior to the procedure. An enema is administered the night before and again 2 hours before the procedure. A bolus of water-soluble iodinated contrast medium (180 mg of iodine per kilogram of body weight) is administered via an intravenous catheter. Ventrodorsal and lateral films are taken immediately and at 5–10, 10–20, and 30–40 minutes post contrast injection.

17 If hematuria persists and a diagnosis has not been made at this point, exploratory surgery to look for primary renal hematuria should be considered. This diagnosis requires catheterization of both ureters, to allow urine collection and its gross and microscopic evaluation. This permits identification of the kidney from which blood loss is occurring.

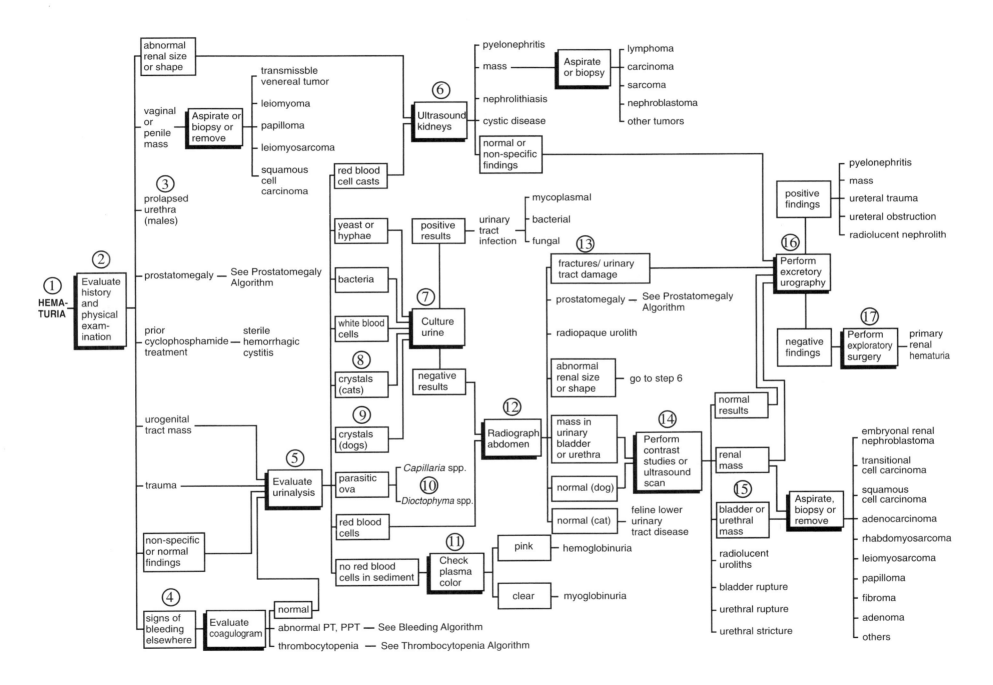

1 Stranguria is slow and/or painful urination characterized by straining. Dysuria is painful or difficult urination. Pollakiuria is frequent passage of small amounts of urine. Such clinical signs are most commonly associated with diseases of the urinary bladder and urethra that result in irritation and/or obstruction.

2 Signs associated with stranguria, dysuria, and/or pollakiuria include frequent attempts to urinate, inability to pass urine after repeated attempts, and urination in inappropriate places. Cats with feline lower urinary tract disease (FLUTD) present with frequent attempts to urinate, often associated with discolored urine. Behavioral problems in cats can lead to urination in inappropriate places but do not cause straining or discolored urine. With complete urethral obstruction postrenal azotemia develops, resulting in depression, inappetence, and/or vomiting.

3 Physical examination findings may be normal in patients with stranguria, dysuria, and pollakiuria. If complete urethral obstruction is present, expect signs of postrenal azotemia (depression, dehydration, bladder enlargement). A thickened bladder wall may be palpated in some cases of FLUTD, chronic urinary tract infections (UTIs), or urolithiasis. Caudal abdominal mass(es) can be found on abdominal palpation and rectal examination. This finding should be investigated further with abdominal imaging. In male dogs, caudal abdominal masses may represent prostatomegaly. However, this more commonly causes tenesmus rather than dysuria. Findings on rectal palpation include prostatomegaly, urethral masses, or generalized urethral thickening. Prolapse of the urethral mucosa appears as a red mass at the end of the penis. It can result in stranguria or pollakiuria. English bulldogs may be predisposed to this condition.

4 Complete lower urinary tract obstruction can cause rapid patient deterioration; therefore, it must be ruled out promptly in patients with stranguria or dysuria. The easiest and quickest method of diagnosing obstruction is by attempting to pass a urinary catheter.

5 If a urinary catheter cannot be passed or is passed only with difficulty, mechanical obstruction of the urethra or bladder neck is likely. Common causes include urethral masses, strictures, uroliths, and urethral plugs. If a catheter cannot be passed and the bladder is enlarged, cystocentesis provides temporary relief and reduces azotemia.

6 In obstructed patients, a serum chemistry profile should be evaluated to detect the extent of metabolic disturbances (uremia, hyperkalemia, metabolic acidosis). These may be life-threatening and require immediate treatment. Any urine sampled should be assessed via urinalysis and culture to attempt to identify the underlying causes of the problem.

7 If a urinary catheter can be passed without difficulty, the patient was either not obstructed or catheterization relieved the obstruction. Collect a urine sample for analysis and bacterial culture because most nonobstructed dogs with dysuria or pollakiuria have a UTI. Cats tend to have clinical signs as a result of crystalluria or sterile inflammation resulting from FLUTD. Cystocentesis is the preferred method of urine collection for analysis and culture.

8 Finding crystalluria or hematuria in feline urine is suspicious for FLUTD. In such cases, a dietary and therapeutic trial can be attempted to resolve clinical signs prior to performing other tests. The condition known as FLUTD may represent a self-limiting bladder irritation and may not require therapy at all unless recurrent or more persistent.

9 Finding crystalluria or hematuria in canine urine is an indication for abdominal imaging, especially if the problem is recurrent, since dogs are more likely than cats to have uroliths or masses.

10 Finding pyuria or bacteriuria in the urine of either dogs or cats suggests inflammation or infection. A urine culture and appropriate antibiotic treatment are recommended. If there is no response to treatment or if signs recur, perform radiography or obtain ultrasound scans of the caudal abdomen to look for underlying causes. Cats are relatively unlikely to have infectious cystitis (less than 10% of cats with signs of cystitis have a bacterial infection).

11 Finding neoplastic cells or parasitic fungal organisms in urine is rare. Depending on the situation, diagnostic tests can stop at this point or continue with abdominal imaging.

12 If the urinalysis and culture are negative, perform a neurological examination to exclude neurological problems. If pelvic limb reflexes are abnormal in conjunction with ataxia, weakness, or proprioceptive deficits, a neurological cause of dysuria/stranguria (e.g., reflex dysynergia, UMN bladder) is likely. Spinal radiographs may be helpful (see the algorithms for paraparesis and urinary incontinence). If the neurological examination is normal in a dog, proceed to abdominal imaging. If the neurological examination is normal in a cat, FLUTD still should be considered even though the urinalysis is normal. A dietary and therapeutic trial is recommended prior to imaging the abdomen because of the high incidence of FLUTD in this species.

13 Plain abdominal radiographs can detect radiodense uroliths and some caudal abdominal masses. Ultrasonography detects most uroliths, urinary bladder masses, and proximal urethral masses. If a diagnosis is not readily made, contrast studies of the urinary tract may be required.

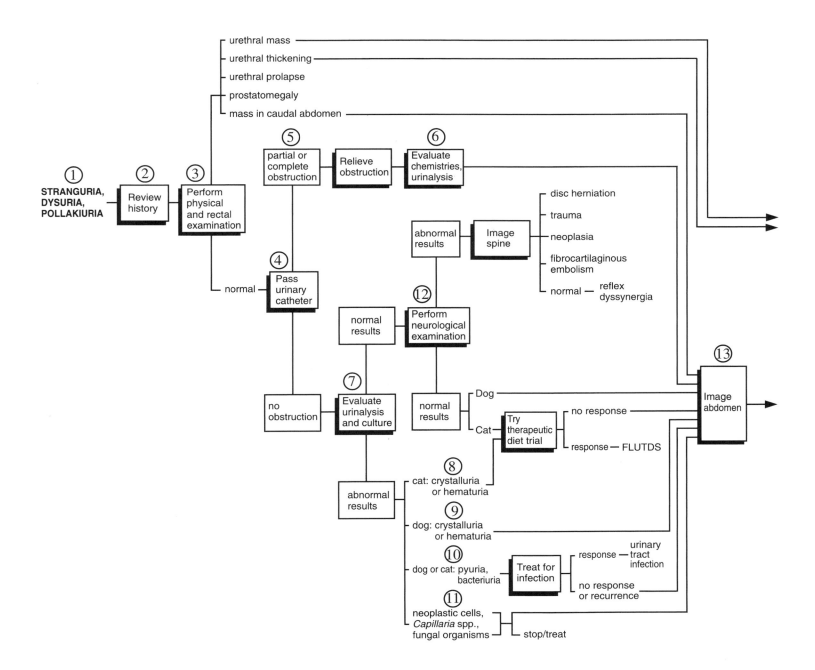

14 Contrast urethrography can identify luminal filling defects, strictures, and ruptures. Double-contrast cystography identifies urinary bladder rupture, radiolucent uroliths, neoplasia, or bladder herniation. If a space-occupying mass is identified at the urinary bladder trigone, excretory urography may be needed to determine the presence and extent of ureteral involvement. Ureteral/ renal pelvis dilation also can be identified on abdominal ultrasound.

15 Cytological evaluation of material obtained from fine-needle aspirates, traumatic urethral flushes, or histopathology on biopsy specimens of abnormal tissue helps in a diagnosis of neoplasia or inflammatory tissue. Bladder tumor antigen testing can be performed on urine to assess the likelihood of occult neoplasia or neoplasia of the masses. False positives may occur with hematuria.

16 If lower urinary tract contrast studies are normal, then there is likely a physiological rather than an anatomical reason for dysuria/stranguria. Urodynamic studies, such as a urethral pressure profile and cystometry, might be needed for confirmation. These tests are not widely available, and referral to a teaching hospital or specialty center is likely to be needed.

17 Reflex dyssynergia is the inability of the urethra to dilate in conjunction with bladder contractions, resulting in a functional, rather than a mechanical, outflow obstruction. Underlying spinal cord diseases, such as trauma, fibrocartilaginous embolism, intervertebral disc herniation, and neoplasia, are possible causes. In many cases, there are no other neurological deficits and the onset is usually sudden. If mechanical obstruction is eliminated, as outlined above, reflex dyssynergia becomes the diagnosis of exclusion. Some patients can improve over time.

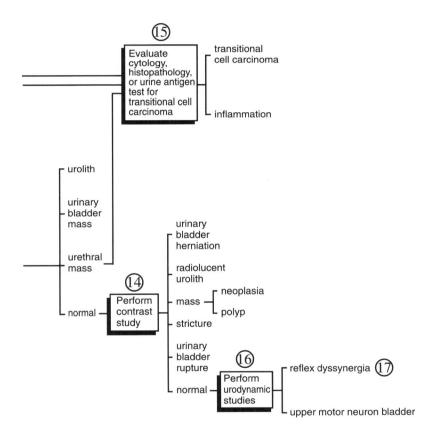

1 Prostatomegaly is enlargement of the prostate gland. The condition may be one of benign hypertrophy (BPH), which is physiological enlargement of the prostate in an intact male, premalignant, malignant, or due to abscessation or intraprostatic/paraprostatic cyst formation. Patients with prostatic enlargement generally present with signs of tenesmus, pain on defecation, and changes in the size and shape of the stool ("ribbon-like" stool). They also may present with signs related to the lower urinary tract (hematuria, dripping blood at the end of urination or between urinations). Urethral obstruction generally does not occur as a result of prostatic enlargement in dogs since enlargement of the gland tends to occur outward, leading to compression of surrounding structures rather than of the urethra. Nonphysiological prostatomegaly is extremely rare in cats.

2 Physical examination and consideration of patient signalment are important in patients with prostatomegaly in helping to determine an underlying cause. An enlarged prostate often will move forward, out of the pelvic canal and into the abdomen. Therefore, it may not be possible to assess the prostate per rectum, especially in a large dog. A combination of abdominal palpation and various imaging techniques may be required to detect prostatomegaly in these circumstances. Sometimes only the tail of the prostate may be palpated per rectum. A smooth, symmetrical, nonpainful prostate suggests either a normal gland or BPH in an intact male. Even minor prostatic enlargement should be viewed with suspicion in a male that has been neutered for more than 6 to 12 months. If a patient had clinical signs of lower urinary tract disease or prostatitis when neutered, it is still possible to have chronic prostatic abscessation up to 6 months later. Beyond 6 months however, prostatic neoplasia should be at the top of the differential list. Irregular enlargement of the prostate is very suggestive of neoplasia or cyst formation. Cysts tend to be softer and more fluctuant than prostatic masses. A painful prostate, especially in a sick or febrile patient, points toward infection, either acute prostatitis or prostatic abscessation. Patients with chronic prostatitis may not have pain or fever.

3 If the prostate is only slightly enlarged and is not painful, and the patient is an intact, asymptomatic male, the diagnosis is BPH and no further evaluation is required.

4 Prostatic enlargement with associated clinical signs in any patient that has been neutered for over 6 months is highly suggestive of prostatic neoplasia. If the prostate is palpable per rectum and feels enlarged or irregular, neoplasia is likely. However, if the prostate is palpable through the caudal abdomen or if prostatomegaly has been picked up as an incidental finding on an abdominal radiograph, a paraprostatic cyst or some other caudal abdominal mass remain possibilities. Some of the diagnostic tests indicated for intact male dogs may be performed (e.g., urinalysis and prostatic massage) in an attempt to retrieve neoplastic or inflammatory cells. However, further imaging of the prostate and caudal abdomen, and probably fine-needle aspiration of prostatic tissue for cytology, are indicated fairly quickly after finding prostatomegaly in a neutered male dog.

5 A urine sample obtained by cystocentesis allows the significance of any WBCs or bacteria in the sample to be accurately assessed, without the possibility of contamination from the urethra or external urethral orifice. However, not all patients with prostatitis will have bacteria in urine obtained from the urinary bladder. Passage of a sterile urinary catheter, combined with quantitative urine culture, will allow assessment of the clinical significance of any bacteria seen in the sample. Note that patients with prostatitis do not always have bacteria, regardless of the route by which urine is obtained. This is especially true of patients with chronic prostatitis and/or abscessation, in which bacteria are confined to the prostatic tissue. In addition to assessment for bacteria and pyuria, some patients with prostatic neoplasia will shed neoplastic cells into the urinary tract, making this a relatively quick and easy diagnostic test for cancer. If clumps of abnormal cells are seen in the urine sediment, the sample should be submitted for cytological evaluation because inflamed and irritated cells from the lining of the urinary tract may have dysplastic/metaplastic features, making it difficult to diagnose neoplasia definitively.

6 Identification of bacteria in a sample from an intact male, especially one with clinical signs of fever, hematuria, pain on palpation of the prostate, and leukocytosis or a history of recurrent UTIs, is diagnostic for bacterial prostatitis or a prostatic abscess. Patients with prostatic abscesses may be less likely to shed bacteria into the urine and may require prostatic massage, ejaculation, or even fine-needle aspiration/surgical exploration of a cavitated prostate to make the diagnosis. Patients with acute prostatitis and prostatic abscesses may experience too much pain to perform prostatic massage or obtain an ejaculate.

7 In patients with prostatitis, urine or a prostatic wash sample should be cultured for identification of bacteria and for antimicrobial sensitivity. This is particularly important if the patient is not going to be neutered, as only long-term therapy with appropriate antimicrobials will permit eradication of infection from the relatively sequestered site of the prostate in intact males.

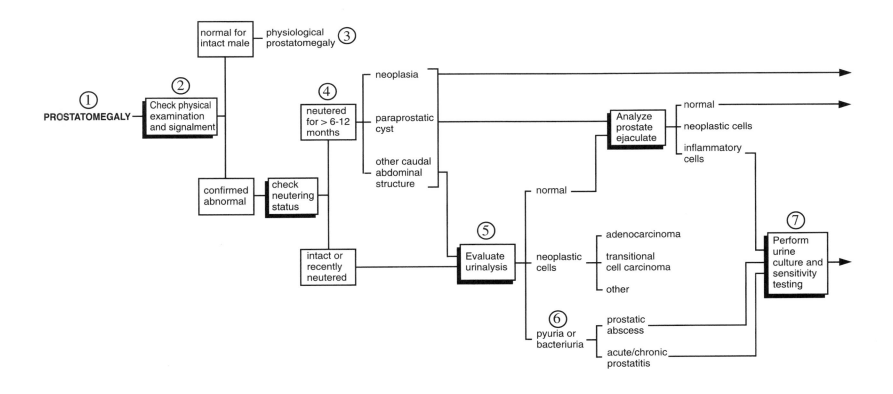

8 If urine cultures are negative but the patient is intact, febrile or painful, or has a history of recurrent signs of UTI or urethral discharge, the breeding history should be investigated. If the patient has not been bred within the last few months, either empirical antimicrobial therapy may be attempted using high doses of antibiotics known to penetrate the prostate (e.g., fluoroquinolones, trimethoprim sulfa) or further imaging is required to assess for a walled-off prostatic abscess.

9 If the patient is a stud dog or has been bred recently, testing for *Brucella canis* should be performed. Most male dogs with *B. canis* have low-grade fever, orchitis, epididymitis, or lymphadenopathy. The incidence of prostatitis alone is relatively low. However, the organism is unlikely to be found on a urinalysis sample and is only slightly more likely to be seen in an ejaculate, so further testing (rapid slide agglutination, tube agglutination, or agar gel immunodiffusion) is advised.

10 If the patient is a neutered male with prostatic enlargement or a caudal abdominal mass, or is an intact male suspected of having any condition other than acute bacterial prostatitis, the next step is to image to the bladder, prostate, caudal abdomen, and retroperitoneum. Abdominal radiographs will identify soft tissue masses in the caudal abdomen and determine their location relative to the urinary bladder. If mineralization is present in the abnormal area, this should be seen on radiographs and is suggestive of neoplasia, although prostatic cysts also have been reported to develop mineralized areas within the epithelial lining. Contrast radiography may be used to outline the bladder and urethra and thus determine the location of any abnormal tissue relative to these areas. Contrast studies are most useful to define a prostatic mass, abscess, or cyst versus a paraprostatic cyst. The last rarely will communicate with the urethra and might, therefore, fill with contrast if a urethrogram is performed. The most useful, commonly available imaging technique for an enlarged prostate is abdominal ultrasound. It quickly allows definition of prostatic size and shape, and occasionally is able to differentiate between a mass lesion and BPH. Ultrasound also will identify cavitations within the prostate that represent cysts or abscesses, and may allow distinction between large cysts arising from within the prostate and paraprostatic cysts that are visible away from or around the prostate, with no obvious connection to that structure. Abdominal ultrasound also allows evaluation of the draining lymph nodes (sublumbar lymph nodes) and more distant organs for evidence of metastasis if prostatic neoplasia is suspected.

11 Fine-needle aspiration of the enlarged prostate under ultrasound guidance is appropriate to try to achieve a cytological diagnosis, especially where enlargement consists mainly of solid tissue. Cytology will often provide enough evidence to differentiate between inflammation/infection, BPH, and neoplasia. There will be some overlap between these conditions cytologically and, if doubt exists, surgical biopsy should be pursued (see step 12). Aspiration should be performed cautiously and with preparation for complications where there are cystic structures or cavitations associated with the prostate. Fluid obtained should be evaluated cytologically and also should be cultured to allow differentiation between abscesses, fluid-filled cysts, and hemocysts (the last two have similar underlying pathophysiology and are usually associated with BPH). There is potential for patients with prostatic abscessation to develop local or generalized peritonitis or septicemia after aspiration. Therefore, surgical intervention and drainage should be the next option, and antibiotic therapy should be initiated once samples are obtained.

12 When the diagnosis is uncertain based on fine-needle aspiration of the prostate, or when aspiration is considered unsafe to perform, surgical exploration of the abdomen for biopsy of abnormal tissue and treatment of any cysts or abscesses is recommended.

13 In patients in which squamous metaplasia of the prostate is identified on cytology or histopathology, and in some patients with paraprostatic cysts, hyperestrogenism should be pursued. These conditions are seen most often in male dogs with functional Sertoli cell tumors (in either a normally positioned or intra-abdominal testicle) or in those given estrogen-containing drugs. Initially, estrogens will cause prostatic atrophy, but if metaplasia or cysts develop, the prostate will enlarge again and clinical signs of prostatomegaly may develop.

14 When a paraprostatic cyst is identified or when there is a very large prostatic cyst that will require surgical intervention, fine-needle aspiration is not indicated. The patient should go directly to surgery for cyst excision or marsupialization and prostatic biopsy, with or without neutering.

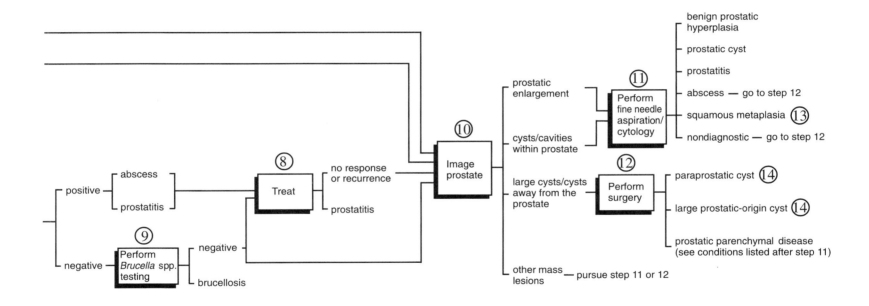

Respiratory Disorders

1 Depending on the underlying cause, nasal discharges are serous, mucoid, mucopurulent, or hemorrhagic (epistaxis). The discharge flows forward to the external nares or back to the nasopharynx and is swallowed. Patients may exhibit stertor, stridor, coughing, excessive swallowing, hemoptysis, and hematemesis (if large amounts of blood are swallowed). Young animals should be checked for congenital defects (nasopharyngeal stenosis, palatine clefts), impacted foreign material, and nasopharyngeal polyps (cats). Causes of mucopurulent and hemorrhagic nasal discharges in middle-aged or older dogs commonly include neoplasia and fungal infection. Cats also have chronic viral upper respiratory tract (URT) infections.

2 Historical questions should include the onset and duration of signs, a history of local radiation therapy, and trauma. Intranasal foreign bodies cause acute signs; patients are distressed, sneeze, and paw their faces. Fungal infections and neoplasia are more insidious, with sneezing or stertor often developing before a discharge, especially if the condition is far back in the nose. Cats with chronic URT infection may have a history of fever and oculonasal discharge as kittens and persistence or recrudescence of discharge later in life. Upper dental arcades should be evaluated for loose or painful teeth suggesting extension of a tooth root abscess into the nasal cavity. The nose and frontal sinuses should be checked for asymmetry, changes in bone density, and discomfort. The nares should be evaluated for rostral masses. The oral cavity should be checked for palate defects, enlarged tonsils, and masses. Unilateral nasal discharge suggests tooth root problems, a mass, a foreign body, or fungal rhinitis, while bilateral discharge is more frequent with upper/lower respiratory infections and allergic rhinitis, although extensive neoplasia and fungal infections may involve both sides. A wisp of cotton is held in front of either nostril to check airflow. The presence of neurological signs (depression, seizures) is important since the caudal aspect of the nasal cavity is separated from the brain only by the thin cribriform plate, which is easily disrupted by trauma, neoplasia, and infection.

3 Patients with systemic illness, coughing, weight loss, or nasal masses need thoracic radiographs for diffuse or metastatic neoplasia, pulmonary fungal infection, esoph-ageal abnormalities, or aspiration pneumonia that might cause a mucopurulent nasal discharge. Pulmonary lesions with nasal fungal infection and primary nasal neoplasia are rare.

4 Patients with a history of trauma, dental disease, facial asymmetry, and visible nasal/oral masses should have nasal/skull radiographs to check for bone destruction, dental disease, or fractures. Since radiography requires anesthesia, a minimum database of laboratory tests, FeLV/FIV tests (cats), and possibly a coagulogram should be obtained. It may be necessary to progress to tissue biopsy, rhinoscopy, dental extractions, and so on. Increased radiographic soft tissue density in the nasal cavity is either a mass or fluid. The two cannot be distinguished unless there is bone destruction (unlikely with fluid). Bony sequestrae are uncommon, developing secondary to trauma and bone devitalization.

5 Obvious nasal lesions on physical examination or radiographs require bone/soft tissue biopsy to distinguish neoplasia from infection. Nasal masses in dogs almost invariably are malignant. In young cats they may be benign inflammatory polyps. Nasal lymphoma is more common in cats than in dogs. Fungal infections can be a primary cause of nasal discharge (mainly cryptococcosis in cats and aspergillosis in dogs). Primary bacterial infection is highly unlikely. In cats with nasal masses, *Cryptococcus neoformans* titers should be evaluated, especially in the southern/southwestern United States or other endemic areas. Titers are reliable but may be negative with a localized fungal infection or in immunosuppressed patients.

6 In patients with submandibular lymphadenopathy, nodes should be aspirated or biopsied. It is unusual for nasal neoplasia to metastasize to regional nodes and for a nasal fungal infection to be diagnosed cytologically from a lymph node aspirate. Draining lymph nodes are likely to be reactive.

7 If the only abnormality is a nasal discharge, it should be characterized. Cytology and culture are rarely useful, although *C. neoformans* (cats) or canine nasal mites (*Pneumonyssoides caninum*) sometimes can be identified. Secondary bacterial infection is usually found.

8 Young cats and dogs with a mucopurulent nasal discharge, fever, an ocular discharge, or lower respiratory tract (LRT) signs probably have underlying viral disease. In cats, it is usually due to a complex of infections (herpesvirus, calicivirus, and *Chlamydia* spp.). They can have oral lesions (*Chlamydia* spp.), corneal ulcers (herpesvirus), or symmetrical distortion of the nose. FePLV infection may cause upper respiratory tract signs, although other systems are generally more severely affected. In dogs, the most common cause of nasal discharge is CDV infection. Parvovirus also may be associated with URT signs, but gastrointestinal disease is generally more significant. Infectious tracheobronchitis (kennel cough) causes coughing and, less frequently, nasal and ocular discharges.

9 Watching the patient prehend and swallow food allows assessment of these functions. Patients with swallowing abnormalities or esophageal dysfunction are predisposed to aspiration pneumonia and nasopharyngeal food impaction.

10 Epistaxis suggests neoplasia, fungal infection, severe inflammation, or rickettsial disease (because of thrombocytopenia and vasculitis). Less frequently it occurs with foreign bodies, coagulopathies (thrombocytopenia, vWF deficiency, ingestion of anticoagulants), and hypertension. These are easy to exclude from the differential list via rickettsial titers, a coagulogram, vWF measurement, and blood pressure determination. It is important to exclude coagulopathy before tissue biopsy, since this predisposes patients to epistaxis. Platelet counts less than $20–30,000/\mu l$ cause spontaneous hemorrhage, while counts of $50–80,000/\mu l$ may result in epistaxis with trauma or vasculitis (e.g., Rocky Mountain spotted fever). Rickettsial disease also causes external nasal planum lesions and other types of nasal discharge. Coagulograms are not needed in all patients with epistaxis, especially if bleeding is minor or there is evidence of an underlying nasal mass.

11 Hypertension is associated with epistaxis in humans and is a rarely documented possibility in dogs and cats.

12 Patients with serous nasal discharges should undergo an ophthalmological examination to assess for ocular inflammation and excessive tear production. Patients also should be evaluated for irritating factors in the environment that lead to rhinitis.

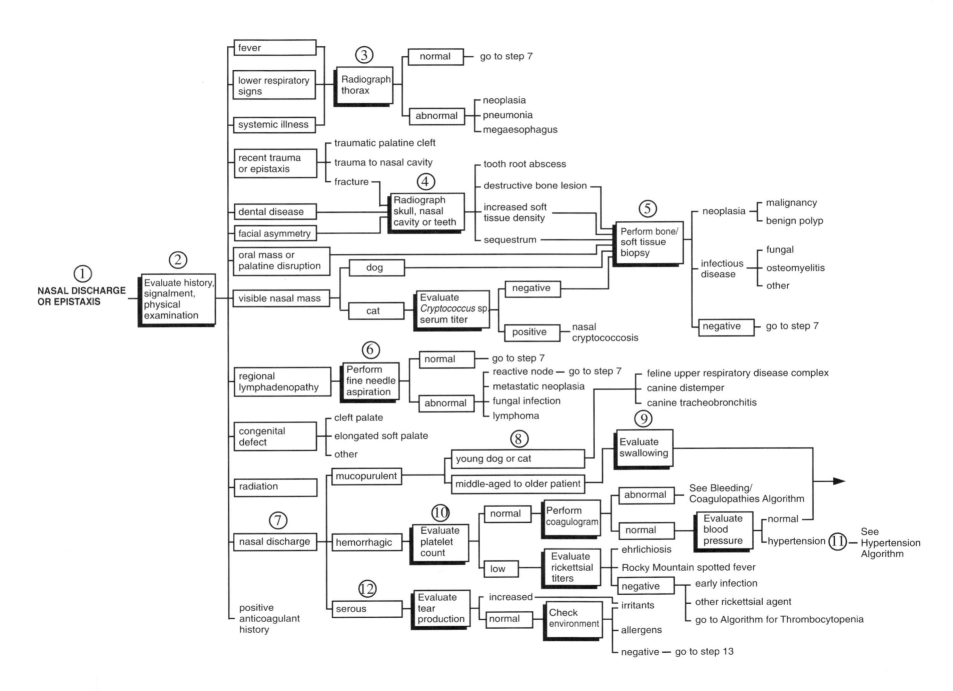

13 The next step is general anesthesia/heavy sedation to complete portions of the oropharyngeal examination that were not possible in the conscious patient. This allows identification of abnormalities previously discussed after the initial history taking and physical examination (step 2).

14 If no abnormalities are seen or if a problem needs to be investigated further, general anesthesia with tracheal intubation is required. Nasopharyngeal examination requires relatively deep anesthesia due to the sensitivity of the area and the ease with which a gag response can be stimulated. Retroflex examination of the nasopharynx can be accomplished using a bronchoscope or endoscope (depending on the size of the patient) or a spay hook and dental mirror. This allows identification of masses, structural changes, or foreign material (grass awns, other vegetation, or food in dogs and grass, bones, or sewing needles in cats). It also identifies inflammatory changes (lymphoid hyperplasia, nasal discharge). Often masses can be biopsied and polyps and foreign bodies removed by this method. Brush cytology of discharges can be performed or the caudal nasal cavities can be flushed to dislodge foreign bodies.

15 Nasopharyngeal stenosis results in partial or complete occlusion of the openings of the ventral nasal meati into the nasopharynx. It may be a congenital defect or develop as a result of trauma to the area. In cats it is most often a consequence of chronic nasal inflammation.

16 In patients with no obvious cause of a nasal discharge on retroflex rhinoscopy or those in which a cause is found but more complete evaluation is required to determine the extent of a lesion, testing should progress to nasal imaging. It is important to image the nasal cavity early on, especially before it is flushed with fluid or much bleeding occurs. This is because it is difficult to distinguish fluid and soft tissue densities radiographically and even sometimes on LT scans. Nasal and dental arcade radiographs are helpful to identify bone and soft tissue masses, fluid, destruction of fine turbinates, tooth root abscesses, frontal sinus involvement, and radiodense foreign material. They may guide the clinician to perform rhinoscopy or to explore an area surgically. CT scanning of the nose is best for identifying very focal lesions or those far back in the nasal cavity (ethmo-turbinates, sinuses, cribriform plate) that are difficult to evaluate radiographically or reach with a bronchoscope. The CT appearance of the nose may suggest whether an increased nasal/sinus density is likely to be a mass or due to a fungal infection. Fungal infections cause a lot of turbinate recession and more "open space" in the nose. A CT scan also allows diagnosis of less common conditions such as ethmoidal cysts (rare in dogs and cats) and disease involving the dental arcades. A CT scan is vital for assessment of cribriform plate damage and extension of nasal disease into the brain (or vice versa). Either a CT scan or an MRI scan is needed for radiation planning to treat nasal neoplasia.

17 Once the nasal cavity has been imaged, direct rhinoscopy may be performed in appropriately sized patients. This allows biopsy and histopathology of focal lesions and general mucosal biopsies in patients that do not have obvious focal lesions, flushing out or direct removal of foreign material, and evaluation for fungal infection (fungal granulomas/plaques) for cytology and culture. Rhinoscopy also allows identification of rare cases of canine nasal mites (*P. caninum*) and canine/feline nasal nematode infestation (*Capillaria aerophilia*). Even when a focal lesion is identified, diagnosis may prove frustrating due to the inaccessibility of some areas of the nasal cavity or because normal nasal mucosa is overlying a mass arising from bone or turbinates. If an abnormal site is identified on a CT scan or radiographs, it may also be helpful to try to aspirate the region for cytological evaluation. A needle can be directed into the lesion either through overlying bone (if damaged) or through the palate.

18 Note that benign nasal masses are extremely rare in dogs. If this is the histopathological diagnosis of a mass, further investigation and possibly surgical biopsy are indicated, as endoscopic biopsies may have obtained only reactive tissue on the edge of a malignant lesion.

19 Rostral polypoid rhinitis is a rare cause of nasal discharge in dogs (particularly young Irish wolfhounds) in association with *Rhinosporidium* spp. infection.

20 When nasal biopsies show only inflammation, with no obvious underlying cause, or are negative, it may be useful to obtain screening titers for fungal disease. How-ever, with the exception of latex cryptococcal antigen titers for cats, these titers are of questionable use. This is particularly the case for *Aspergillus* spp. titers. Patients with a confirmed nasal infection often have negative titers due to the localized nature of the infection or a poor systemic immune response.

21 Exploratory rhinotomy and sinus trephination may be considered for further diagnosis of patients with moderate to severe nasal discharge or epistaxis. The potential underlying conditions are the same as those that may be discovered by rhinoscopy (e.g., fungal infections, neoplasia). Exploratory surgery is indicated only when these conditions are not found on prior evaluation. Surgery is a relatively radical procedure associated with a significant risk of hemorrhage and turbinate damage. In cats it carries the risk of subsequent anorexia due to pain and loss of sense of smell.

22 Lymphoplasmacytic inflammatory infiltrates in the nose indicate inflammation or an allergic response. Probable underlying conditions are immune mediated, but other conditions should be stringently excluded and the environment should be evaluated for direct irritants and allergens prior to initiating immunosuppressive therapy. Antihistamines may be tried, but there is no conclusive evidence that they are useful for rhinitis in dogs and cats.

23 In cats, chronic upper respiratory disease complex and nasal turbinate damage are always underlying possibilities with chronic nasal discharge. Nasal biopsy specimens and tonsillar swabs may be obtained for virus isolation, and IFA for viral inclusions may be performed on cytology specimens.

24 When no abnormalities are found within the nasal cavity but patients have a nasal discharge, especially when it is associated with crusting or erosion of the external portions of the nose or superficial areas of the nasal septum, immune-mediated disease should be considered. Conditions affecting mucocutaneous junctions include SLE, discoid lupus erythematosus (DLE), and various members of the pemphigus complex of diseases. Further testing may include tissue biopsy and IFA, ANA titers, and evaluation for involvement of other body systems.

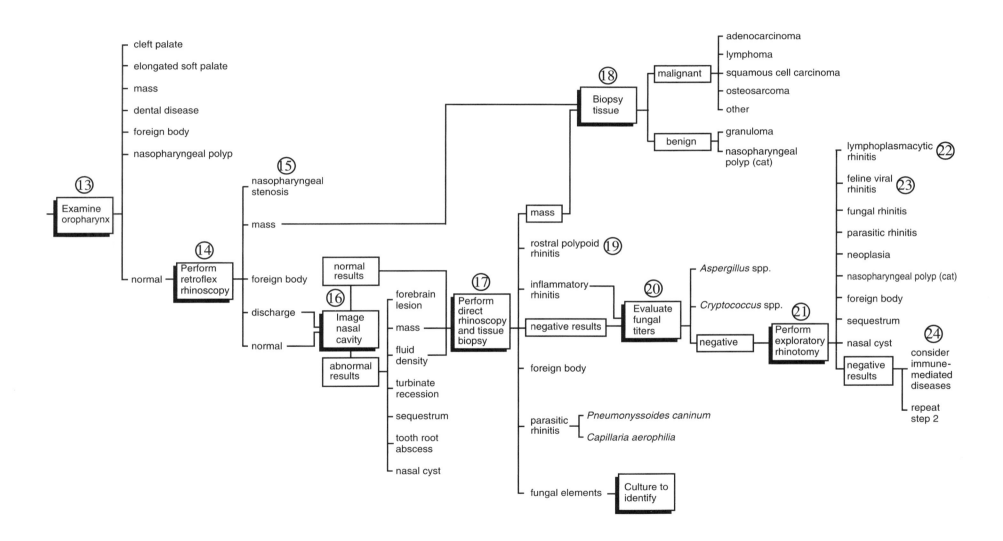

1 Stertor (snoring) and stridor (a harsh, high-pitched sound) result from turbulent airflow due to upper airway obstruction. Stertor originates in the nasal cavity/nasopharynx, while stridor develops in the oropharynx/larynx. Noise and dyspnea usually are inspiratory.

2 Young animals with stertor/stridor can have congenital defects (e.g., brachycephalic airway obstruction syndrome [BAOS], hyperplastic rhinitis in wolfhounds), infections (e.g., feline upper respiratory infection [FURI]), tonsil enlargement, or nasopharyngeal polyps (cats). Older animals can have peripheral neuropathy (idiopathic, paraneoplastic, canine hypothyroidism) or upper airway neoplasia. Historical questions include whether onset was sudden (trauma, foreign body), if problems are chronic and progressive (neoplasia, FURI), whether there has been contact with animals with similar signs, and the patient's vaccination status.

3 Physical examination determines the severity of obstruction and sometimes diagnoses the problem (BAOS, palate cleft, oronasal fistula). Bone deformity suggests aggressive processes (neoplasia, fungal infection, and sometmes chronic FURI).

4 Nasal disease causes obstruction, stertor, and sometimes discharge or epistaxis. Examination can diagnose external nares stenosis, palatine clefts, oronasal fistulae, and masses (if these are eroding into the oral cavity). Cats with acute nasal discharge and fever probably have FURI (herpesvirus I, calicivirus, *Chlamydia* spp.). In dogs it is probably infectious tracheobronchitis (*Bordetella bronchiseptica* and viral pathogens) or CDV. The latter is more serious and has a poorer prognosis.

5 Patients with oropharyngeal disease can present with both stridor and stertor. Conditions seen on examination include oropharyngeal/tonsillar masses, nasopharyngeal polyps (cats), foreign bodies, and trauma.

6 Patients with laryngeal disease and conditions affecting the cervical and intrathoracic trachea to the level of the carina present with inspiratory stridor and voice change. They can be severely compromised and cyanotic or have nonproductive, harsh coughing due to airway collapse and mucosal irritation.

7 Dog bites, vehicle trauma, and gunshots cause cervical trauma. Subcutaneous emphysema suggests extrathoracic airway damage. Radiographs should be taken for injuries interrupting the tracheal lumen and for pneumothorax, pneumomediastinum, and lung collapse.

8 Pharyngeal/retroflex nasal examination under anesthesia requires a laryngoscope, a dental mirror, and something to hold back the soft palate or an endoscope/bronchoscope. Radiographs of the caudal pharynx, larynx, and cervical regions may detect masses, some foreign bodies, emphysema (with penetrating trauma), fractures, tracheal collapse, masses, laryngeal distortion, and bone and palate abnormalities.

9 Patients with inspiratory stridor or cyanosis require light anesthesia and laryngeal examination. Premedication that might interfere with vocal cord movement should be avoided. The length of the palate and its relationship to the epiglottis should be assessed for a long soft palate. The larynx can be evaluated for masses, saccule eversion, collapse, and vocal cord paralysis. Patients with severe upper airway collapse also can have collapse of the intrathoracic trachea and mainstem bronchi.

10 If a loose/abscessed tooth or oronasal fistula is present, nasal and dental imaging (radiographs/CT scan) is helpful.

11 Congenital defects of the hard or soft palate result from failure to close during development. Acquired defects are generally in the hard palate and result from a fall. Overlong soft palates cause laryngeal obstruction.

12 Pharyngeal and nasal foreign bodies are more common in dogs than in cats and include grass blades, awns, food, sticks, toys, and fish hooks. Cats are more likely to get sharp objects (bones, needles) embedded in the pharynx.

13 Pharyngeal trauma (e.g., dog fight wounds, snake bites) leads to swelling and upper airway obstruction.

14 Upper airway inflammation can be due to FURI in cats or to kennel cough and herpesvirus in dogs. Cats can develop tonsillitis in association with FeLV/FIV. Signs include pain on swallowing, fever, hypersalivation, and anorexia.

15 Nasal/frontal sinus imaging can be via radiography, CT scans, or MRI scans. Scans show the structure of the ethmoturbinate and frontal sinuses, areas that are hard to reach endoscopically. Bone destruction is caused by tumors and fungal infection, while increased density represents tissue, blood, or mucus.

16 Vocal cord paralysis can be unilateral (due to the unusual path of the left recurrent laryngeal nerve in the neck) or bilateral. Patients present with exercise intolerance, cyanosis, and inspiratory stridor. Vocal cord paralysis can be congenital (Bouviers and Siberian huskies), result from damage to the recurrent laryngeal nerve, or result from local or generalized polyneuropathy. Polyneuropathy usually is idiopathic but can be immune-mediated, paraneoplastic, or occur with canine hypothyroidism. EMG confirms denervation/muscular problems. Other tests include an ANA titer, thyroid profiles, and evaluation for other neurological problems.

17 Laryngeal fibrosis/stenosis can develop after trauma or surgery. Disruption of laryngeal mucosa predisposes to fibrosis, scarring/webbing, and stenosis, especially in cats.

18 Laryngeal collapse is seen mainly in small-breed dogs (which are also predisposed to tracheal collapse). It is exacerbated by lower airway disease (bronchitis, asthma), which increases upper airway inspiratory pressures. It is not surgically correctable, and a permanent tracheostomy is needed to bypass the area.

19 Laryngeal hypoplasia in brachycephalic breeds occurs alone or with saccule eversion and tracheal hypoplasia.

20 Laryngitis is a nonspecific finding, mostly in dogs. Infectious tracheobronchitis causes acute laryngitis. Chronic laryngitis is seen with excessive vocalization and chronic trauma, (pulling on a leash). Inflammation causes stridor, voice change, and coughing.

21 With laryngeal trauma, radiographs identify fractures and emphysema. Hyoid bone fractures cause severe airway obstruction and dysphagia, as the larynx cannot move normally. Hyoid bone fragments can be removed surgically. Patients often recover spontaneously.

22 Laryngeal masses can be benign or malignant. They arise from muscle (leiomyoma, rhabdomyosarcoma), cartilage (chondrosarcoma), lymphoid tissue (lymphoma), or mucosa (squamous cell carcinoma).

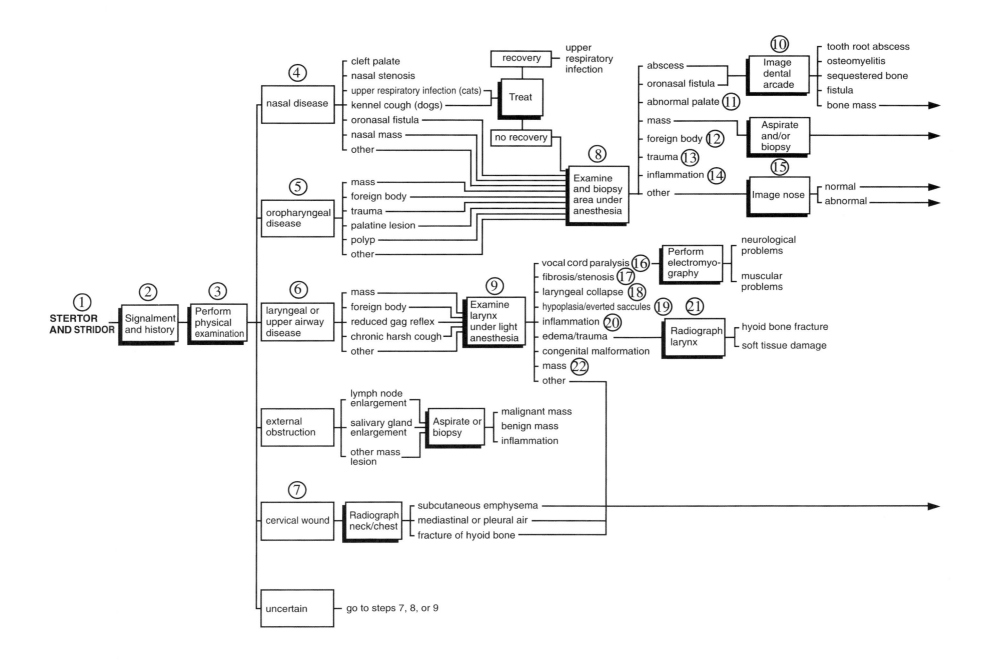

23 Tracheoscopy evaluates the larynx and the trachea to the carina. It is sensitive in assessing for tracheal collapse, masses, foreign bodies, and external airway obstruction.

24 Inflammatory polypoid lesions in cats arise from the lining of the middle ear, auditory canal, and nasopharynx. They may be very large and often result from chronic inflammation in these areas. Affected cats tend to be young, but polyps may be seen in cats of any age. Removal by gentle traction may be curative (50% of cases). If radiographs or a CT scan show middle ear involvement, traction removal is combined with ventral bulla osteotomy if appropriate.

25 Granulomas or abscesses in the oronasopharynx are generally secondary to trauma or foreign body impaction. Portions of the foreign body may still be found in the abnormal tissue. Granulomas and abscesses also develop in cats with severe pharyngitis or tonsillar inflammation secondary to FURI, FeLV, and FIV.

26 Benign tumors of the pharynx, nasopharynx, and nose are very rare in cats and dogs. Tumor types include adenoma, papilloma, fibroma, chondroma, and osteoma.

27 Malignant tumors of the pharynx, nasopharynx, and nasal cavity are much more common in dogs and cats. They include adenocarcinoma (particularly nasal), squamous cell carcinoma, lymphoma, melanoma, tonsillar carcinoma, chondrosarcoma, osteosarcoma, and fibrosarcoma (see step 31).

28 Pharyngeal mucoceles occur mainly in dogs and can cause airway obstruction. They are large, mucus-filled structures in the caudal pharynx that form from abnormalities of mucus-producing glands in these areas and not from salivary tissue. Diagnosis and therapy require surgical excision, drainage, and histopathology.

29 Unless there is an obvious destructive lesion in the bone of the nose or frontal sinuses and radiographs, representing either a tumor or osteomyelitis, the next step is direct rhinoscopy of the nasal passages to try to identify lesions in the turbinates and overlying mucosa that can be biopsied.

30 Parasitic infections of the nose, although extremely rare, have been reported in dogs and cats and can cause stertor. The most common ones are the nasal mite (*P. caninum*), which may be seen on direct examination of the nose, and the nasal nematode (*C. aerophila*), which may be found on nasal biopsy.

31 As described above, nasal masses are generally malignant in dogs and cats. They arise from the nasal planum and within the nasal cavity and paranasal sinuses. Tumor types include squamous cell carcinoma of the nasal planum, adenocarcinoma of the nasal cavity, lymphoma, fibroma, fibrosarcoma, hemangioma, hemangiosarcoma, melanoma, mast cell tumor, osteosarcoma, and chondrosarcoma.

32 Nasal mycotic infections are caused by opportunistic, saprophytic organisms. These are inhaled and become established in the noses of cats and mesocephalic and dolichocephalic dogs. Rhinoscopy generally identifies fungal plaques or granulomas within the nasal cavity and sinuses and marked turbinate recession. Biopsy and culture are required to identify the type of fungus. Surgical exploration of the sinus cavities may be needed to identify infection if it is confined to this area.

33 Rhinitis (inflammation of the nose) is caused by primary and secondary bacterial infections, viral infections, immune system overstimulation, and allergic disease. Neutrophilic infiltrates predominate with bacterial infection in dogs and with *Chlamydia psittaci* infection in cats. Secondary bacterial infections are common in patients with nasal damage/inflammation. Viral rhinitis is common in cats secondary to herpesvirus 1 and calcivirus infection, and may occur in dogs secondary to infectious tracheobronchitis and CDV infection. These conditions usually manifest with lymphoplasmacytic infiltrates. Allergic rhinitis includes lymphoplasmacytic and sometimes eosinophilic infiltrates. Lymphoplasmacytic rhinitis is a disease of unknown etiology that may be due to an abnormal immune response within the nose. Young Irish wolfhounds may develop hyperplastic rhinitis, again thought to be due to an abnormal immune response. Cats may have nasopharyngeal polyps deep in the nose instead of the nasopharynx, and in rare cases dogs may develop polypoid rhinitis secondary to infection with *Rhinosporidium seeberi*.

34 Tracheal collapse may be cervical, intrathoracic, or both. Identification of the extent of narrowing of the tracheal lumen, location of the collapsed area, and the presence or absence of mainstem bronchial collapse are important in determining how to manage the condition (surgically versus medically) and the prognosis.

35 Tracheal stenosis may be a congenital malformation (in which case it may be multifocal and segmental due to the absence or malformation of tracheal rings and stenosis at those sites) or secondary to trauma (in which case stenosis is usually found only in one location). Acquired stenosis may be the result of blunt chest trauma and tracheal stretching, penetrating wounds, and necrosis secondary to the presence of a foreign body or excessive pressure in the cuff of an endotracheal/tracheostomy tube.

36 Tracheal hypoplasia may occur alone or as part of BAOS. It is one of the conditions that are probably diagnosed more easily by radiography than assessed by tracheoscopy. Tracheal hypoplasia exists when the diameter of the trachea is less than two times the width of the third rib where the trachea crosses that rib.

37 Tracheal masses are very rare and may be benign or malignant. Squamous cell carcinoma, adenocarcinoma, and lymphoma have been reported, as have chondromas and granulomas secondary to parasitic infestation (with *Oslerus osleri*). Parasitic infestation of the trachea is most commonly seen in kenneled dogs, particularly greyhounds, and young animals.

38 Tracheitis (inflammation of the trachea) may be noninfectious (due to environmental irritants, chronic coughing, allergic airway inflammation) or infectious (tracheobronchitis in dogs, FURI). It generally manifests with mucosal swelling (edema and irritation, sometimes with a mucoid or mucopurulent discharge).

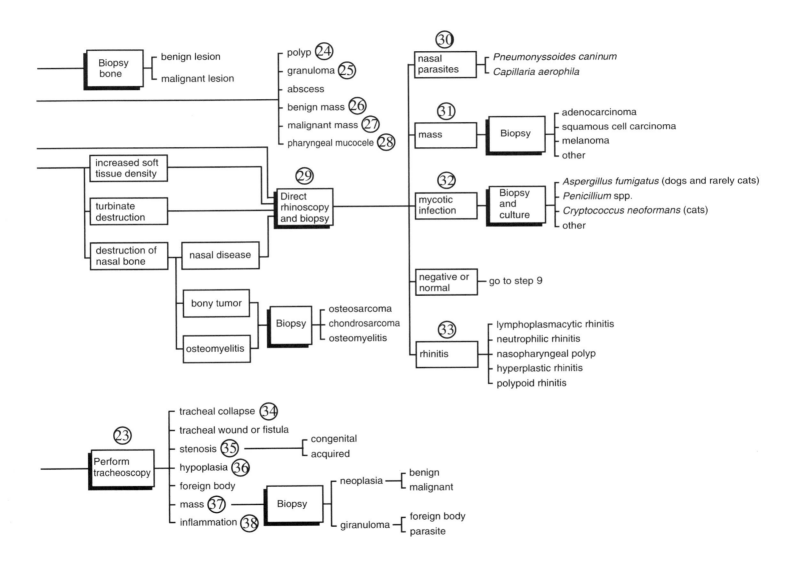

1 Dyspnea is labored breathing. It is assessed by the respiratory rate, rhythm, and character. It can result from systemic, respiratory, or cardiovascular disease. It usually occurs secondary to disorders that interfere with pulmonary gas exchange (decreased RBC number/hemoglobin-carrying capacity, airway obstruction, infiltrative lung disease, cardiac dysfunction causing pulmonary edema or inadequate pulmonary blood flow). Occasionally, dyspnea is caused by weakness/paralysis of respiratory muscles or occurs as a compensatory response to hyperthermia or severe metabolic acidosis.

2 Some specific causes of dyspnea, common in certain breeds, are related to the patient's age or other disease processes (e.g., BAOS in brachycephalic dogs and short-faced cats, collapsing trachea and mitral insufficiency with subsequent heart failure and pulmonary edema in older small-breed dogs). Knowing the vaccination, travel, and environmental history is helpful in increasing the index of suspicion for infectious diseases (fungal pneumonia, CDV pneumonia, toxoplasmosis), trauma, or toxin exposure (pulmonary hemorrhage from warfarin exposure). Obese pets can be dyspneic due to excessive intrathoracic fat or displacement of the diaphragm by excessive intra-abdominal fat (pickwickian syndrome). Try to ascertain whether dyspnea is associated with inspiration, expiration, or both. Dyspneic patients with inspiratory stridor or stertorous respiration usually have upper airway obstruction (stenotic nares, laryngeal paralysis, collapsing trachea, tracheal obstruction). Increased expiratory effort is associated with lower airway obstruction (bronchitis, pulmonary edema, neoplastic masses, or pneumonia). If the depth of breathing is decreased (rapid, shallow breathing), lung expansion probably is restricted. Restrictive breathing patterns are associated with pneumothorax, pleural effusion, diaphragmatic hernia, fractured ribs, and alveolar or pulmonary interstitial infiltrates. Decreased breath sounds often are associated with pneumothorax and pleural fluid. If both breath and heart sounds are decreased ventrally but breath sounds are heard dorsally, consider pleural effusion.

3 In endemic areas, *Dirofilaria immitis* infection should be excluded early on in dyspneic dogs and cats.

4 Cervical spinal cord and peripheral neuromuscular diseases cause weakness/paralysis of respiratory muscles. Quadriparesis and quadriplegia usually are presenting signs.

5 Dyspnea, hyperpnea, or tachypnea can be a response to hyperthermia. Other intrathoracic causes of dyspnea that produce fever (e.g., pneumonia) should be excluded via thoracic radiographs.

6 Patients with anemia severe enough to cause dyspnea have pale mucous membranes.

7 Most patients with dyspnea due to cardiac disease have physical examination abnormalities, including arrhythmias, tachycardia, pulse deficits, cardiac gallop rhythms/murmurs, jugular pulses/distended jugular veins, weak peripheral pulses, slow capillary refill times, crackles, or muffled heart sounds. If no signs of cardiac disease are found, suspect respiratory disease as the cause of dyspnea.

8 Crackles are snapping sounds of short duration caused by fluid accumulation or by popping open of airways plugged with mucus. Crackles associated with heart failure usually are heard dorsally and caudally. With severe heart failure, crackles are more generalized. Crackles also occur with chronic obstructive pulmonary disease and neurogenic pulmonary edema.

9 Flail chest occurs in trauma patients when several ribs on both sides of the point of impact are fractured and intervening rib segments lose continuity with the remainder of the thorax. The fractured segment moves inward during inspiration and outward during expiration, compromising respiration.

10 Some patients require emergency treatment before further testing is performed. If the respiratory pattern and thoracic auscultation suggest pleural effusion or pneumothorax, thoracocentesis should be considered when there is no strong evidence of coagulopathy. Needle thoracocentesis is best performed with a small-gauge butterfly catheter attached to a three-way stopcock and syringe at the sixth to eighth intercostal spaces just below the level of the costochondral junction. Aspiration of either side usually drains the contralateral hemithorax adequately because the mediastinum in dogs and cats usually is fenestrated.

11 If the possibility of inspiratory stridor has been eliminated and the patient is stable, thoracic radiographs are the most useful diagnostic test for evaluation of dyspneic patients.

12 A variety of lungworms cause dyspnea/coughing, both as a result of the parasites themselves and due to the inflammatory reaction they induce. A fecal examination for parasite ova should be performed.

13 If pulmonary infiltrates, hilar lymphadenopathy, or masses are found on thoracic radiographs, fine-needle aspiration can be attempted for cytological evaluation. Aspiration is most easily performed with fluoroscopic or ultrasound guidance. If diffuse pulmonary disease is found, either bronchoscopy or "blind"-needle aspiration of the lung with a small-gauge needle can be performed. Pneumothorax is a potential complication of lung aspiration.

14 If thoracic radiographs are unrewarding or inconclusive, check the hemogram and serum chemistry profile. With bacterial bronchopneumonia there may be leukocytosis with a left shift and degenerate neutrophils. Eosinophilia suggests pulmonary parasites, *D. immitis* infection, or allergic bronchitis. Hypokalemia can cause impaired ventilation and dyspnea.

15 If a cause of dyspnea has not been found, abnormal arterial partial pressures of oxygen and carbon dioxide increase the suspicion of pulmonary thromboembolic disease, a condition that rarely causes radiographic changes.

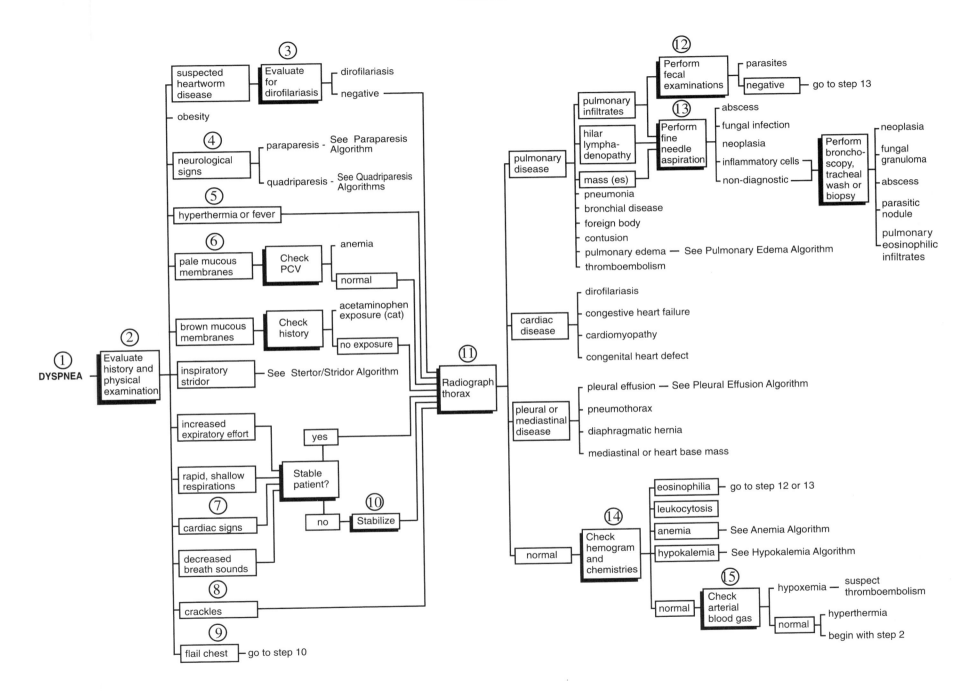

1 Coughing is a reflex defense mechanism that removes foreign material and exudate from the respiratory tract. Almost any disorder of the upper or lower respiratory system can cause coughing by stimulating cough receptors. Heart disease also triggers coughing by causing pulmonary edema or left mainstem bronchial/tracheal compression. Cats cough less than dogs, except with parasitic or allergic airway disease.

2 Coughing after eating/drinking suggests laryngeal dysfunction. Nocturnal coughs occur with cardiac insufficiency, pulmonary edema, or psychogenic conditions. If the cough is dry, hacking, or goose honk–like, consider tracheitis, tracheal collapse, and compression of mainstem bronchi by left atrial enlargement or masses. Infectious tracheobronchitis or chronic bronchitis in dogs causes a productive cough and gagging. Cats with bronchial disease have episodic coughing, expiratory wheezes, and dyspnea. Hemoptysis (coughing blood) occurs with pulmonary disease (e.g., neoplasia, pulmonary thromboembolism, *D. immitis* infection, foreign body, fungal pneumonia, or coagulopathy). A soft, moist cough suggests pneumonia, parasitic or allergic disease, pulmonary thromboembolism, or edema.

3 Since coughing occurs with both respiratory and cardiac disease, a thorough physical examination is needed to allow the two to be distinguished.

4 Stertorous respiration, inspiratory dyspnea, or coughing after eating suggests upper airway disease (mass, infectious tracheobronchitis, foreign body, laryngeal dysfunction, or collapsing trachea). The last is seen mainly in middle-aged and older small/toy-breed dogs presenting with a goose honk cough. If infectious tracheobronchitis is suspected (step 6), treat the condition before pursuing further testing.

5 Lateral and ventrodorsal thoracic and lateral cervical radiographs taken on expiration and inspiration can sometimes show collapse of different portions of the trachea and mainstem bronchi along with some tracheal foreign bodies and masses and cardiac enlargement.

6 Infectious tracheobronchitis in dogs is caused by *B. bronchiseptica* and several viruses. The condition occurs at any age and in any breed, especially those exposed to affected dogs in boarding kennels, shows, and veterinary clinics. A dry or occasionally productive cough can be elicited on tracheal palpation or with exercise/excitement.

7 If the cough is associated with inspiratory stridor or voice change, examine the vocal folds under light anesthesia for laryngeal paralysis.

8 When coughing does not resolve and is localized to the upper airways, fluoroscopy or tracheoscopy is the next step. The former does not require anesthesia.

9 Tracheoscopy requires injectable anesthesia and a bronchoscope. It is sensitive for identifying tracheal/mainstem bronchial collapse. If a mass is found, biopsy can be attempted. If not, go to step 12 or 18.

10 Coughing associated with expiratory dyspnea, hemoptysis, crackles, or wheezes suggests lower airway disease (pneumonia, pulmonary edema, bronchial disease, asthma, or pleural effusion).

11 If examination detects a heart murmur, arrhythmia, pulse deficits, or jugular pulses, suspect cardiac disease and evaluate thoracic radiographs, an echocardiogram, and an ECG.

12 Evaluate dogs from endemic areas for *D.immitis* infection via a Knott's test or an antigen test. Antibody detection is sensitive for exposure in cats. A cough is relatively common with *D.immitis* infestation in both species and is due to thromboembolic disease, right heart failure, or allergic pulmonary infiltrates.

13 Thoracic radiographs are valuable for evaluating lower airway coughs. If neoplasia is suspected, left and right lateral and ventrodorsal radiographs should be taken to assess for discrete masses and lymphadenopathy.

14 Transthoracic needle aspiration/biopsy of focal masses and lymph nodes can be done from plain radiographs or with ultrasonographic/fluoroscopic guidance. Complications include pneumothorax, hemothorax, or abscess rupture and pyothorax.

15 Thoracotomy is an invasive technique, but it obtains large tissue samples and allows excisional biopsy and examination of other lung lobes/lymph nodes.

16 Lungworms cause coughing, wheezing, and respiratory distress due to the parasites themselves and the inflammatory reaction induced. Most are diagnosed by identifying eggs and larvae in feces or tracheal wash fluid. Circulating eosinophilia and eosinophilic bronchitis are present. Other parasites also can affect lung tissue (e.g., *Toxocara* spp. larvae)

17 Tracheal lavage fluid can be obtained for cytological analysis and culture. The patient is sedated, the area over the midcervical trachea is shaved and aseptically prepared, and a large-gauge catheter is introduced between the tracheal rings and positioned at the level of the carina. Five to 20 ml warm saline is instilled then reaspirated.

18 If a diagnosis is not achieved with the tests previously described, then proceed to fine-needle aspiration of the lung (for primary parenchymal disease) (step 14) or anesthesia for bronchoscopy and bronchoalveolar lavage (for primary airway disease).

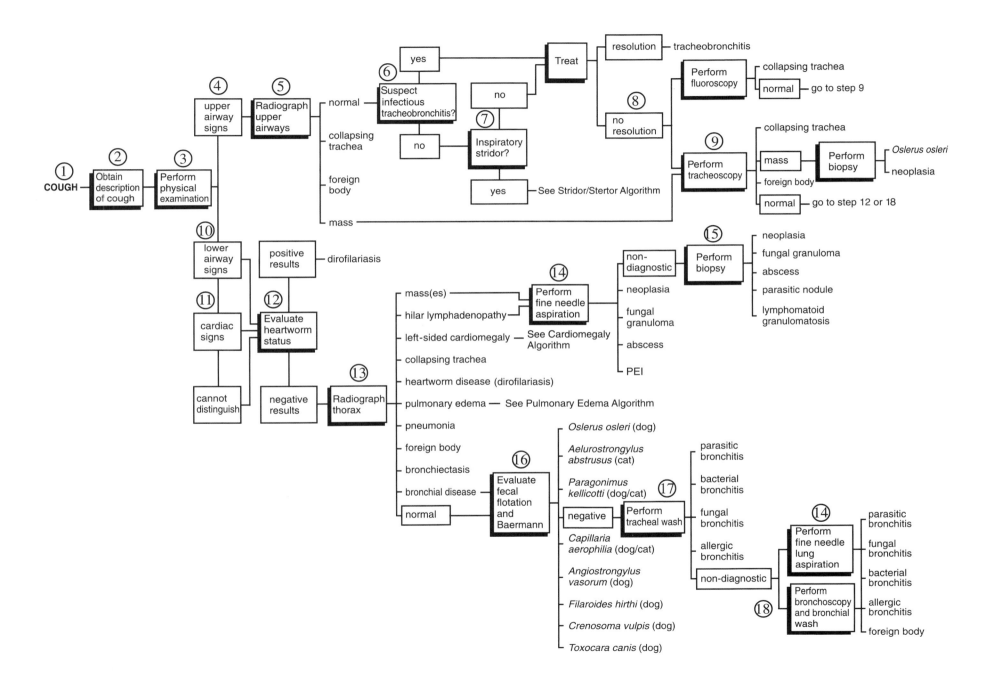

1 Cyanosis is a blue tint to skin/mucous membranes caused by excessive desaturated Hb in capillary blood.

2 Cyanosis can be central or peripheral. Central cyanosis (CC) occurs with desaturation of systemic arterial Hb and affects mucous membranes and skin. Administration of oxygen alleviates CC caused by cardiac or respiratory disease. Peripheral cyanosis (PC) is due to local desaturation of Hb, often caused by peripheral circulatory problems (vasoconstriction, arterial/venous obstruction).

3 Methemoglobin (Mb) is a normal product of Hb oxidation and usually is present at low concentrations. Methemoglobinemia results from exposure to oxidant chemicals that increase the rate of heme iron oxidation. It also can be congenital due to an enzyme deficiency that reduces the rate of Mb reduction. Acetaminophen is a common oxidant causing excessive Mb production, especially in cats. Blood becomes brown colored, and mucous membranes are "muddy" and cyanotic. Other oxidants that increase Mb in blood, especially in cats when metheme reduction is slow, include nitrates, nitrites, topical benzocaine, and methylene blue.

4 Young patients presenting with CC often have a congenital heart defect, causing right-to-left shunting of blood past the lungs, or congenital methemoglobinemia. Congenital heart defects usually have associated murmurs. If arterial hypoxemia is present, there is cyanosis of all mucous membranes except when cyanosis is due to a right-to-left shunting patent ductus arteriosus (PDA). In such cases, there is cyanosis of caudal mucous membranes/nail beds only. Because the defect occurs after the arterial branches from the aorta to the cranial portions of the body, oral mucous membranes remain pink. In adult/older patients with CC, chronic pulmonary disease, heart failure, or pulmonary neoplasia is likely.

5 Weak excursions of the thoracic wall can indicate muscle weakness, peripheral neuromuscular disease, or CNS disease affecting the cervical spinal cord/brainstem. Other neurological signs should also be seen.

6 Pulmonary crackles and wheezes indicate pulmonary edema, pneumonia, asthma, or chronic bronchitis.

7 Muffled heart and lung sounds suggest disease of the pleural space (pleural effusion or pneumothorax).

8 Subcutaneous emphysema is accumulation of air under the skin. Disruption of upper airways (from the nose to the intrathoracic trachea) is likely.

9 If methemoglobinemia is suspected to be the cause of hypoxemia, evaluate the color of a venous blood sample for a brown tinge. Also evaluate the PCV since polycythemia (PCV > 60%) is a result (but not a cause) of severe, chronic hypoxemia and congenital heart disease resulting in anatomic shunts. Mucous membranes will be dark red with polycythemia.

10 Since most cases of CC and some cases of PC involve cardiopulmonary disease, thoracic radiographs are important. Pulmonary disease causing CC usually is associated with obvious parenchymal changes.

11 Thromboembolic disease often affects pulmonary vessels (PTE). Patients are acutely dyspneic. Thoracic radiographs usually are normal but occasionally show mild pleural fluid lines or hyperlucent zones due to loss of blood flow. Arterial blood gas analysis or scintigraphy (ventilation-perfusion scans) confirms the diagnosis of PTE.

12 Cardiac causes of CC or PC can be associated with changes in heart size/shape. Enlargement of the right ventricle or the main, lobar, or peripheral pulmonary arteries suggests *D. immitis* infection.

13 Arterial blood gas analysis distinguishes CC (decreased partial pressure of carbon dioxide [$PaCO_2$] due to hyperventilation) from PC (normal $PaCO_2$)

14 Alveolar hypoventilation leads to hypercapnea and respiratory acidosis. Patients with CC have decreased plasma pH, slight bicarbonate elevation, and reduced partial pressures of oxygen (PaO_2). Causes include pleural effusion, airway obstruction, severe pneumonia, pneumothorax, and PTE.

15 Ventilation-perfusion mismatch (VPM) implies adequate pulmonary ventilation and inadequate perfusion or vice versa. The end result is hypoxemia. Ventilation usually is sufficient to remove CO_2. Any interstitial or alveolar disease can cause VPM (pulmonary edema, neoplasia), as can PTE.

16 Cold exposure causes vasoconstriction and a blue tint to the extremities. In shock compensatory mechanisms redistribute blood flow to vital organs, leading to peripheral blanching and mild cyanosis.

17 Absent/weak femoral pulses occur with thrombosis, particularly in cats with cardiomyopathy (*saddle thrombus*). Other causes include septic emboli and hypercoagulability. Rear limb tissue is cold and cyanotic.

18 Nephrotic syndrome results in loss of ATIII via the kidneys and a hypercoagulable state. Affected animals develop thromboemboli, particularly in pulmonary and femoral arteries.

19 In cold hemagglutinin disease, patients have high titers of an immunoglobulin that binds RBCs at temperatures below 98.6°F. Agglutination reduces the blood supply to colder portions of the body (the extremities) and causes gangrenous necrosis (e.g., of the ear and tail tips) in cold weather.

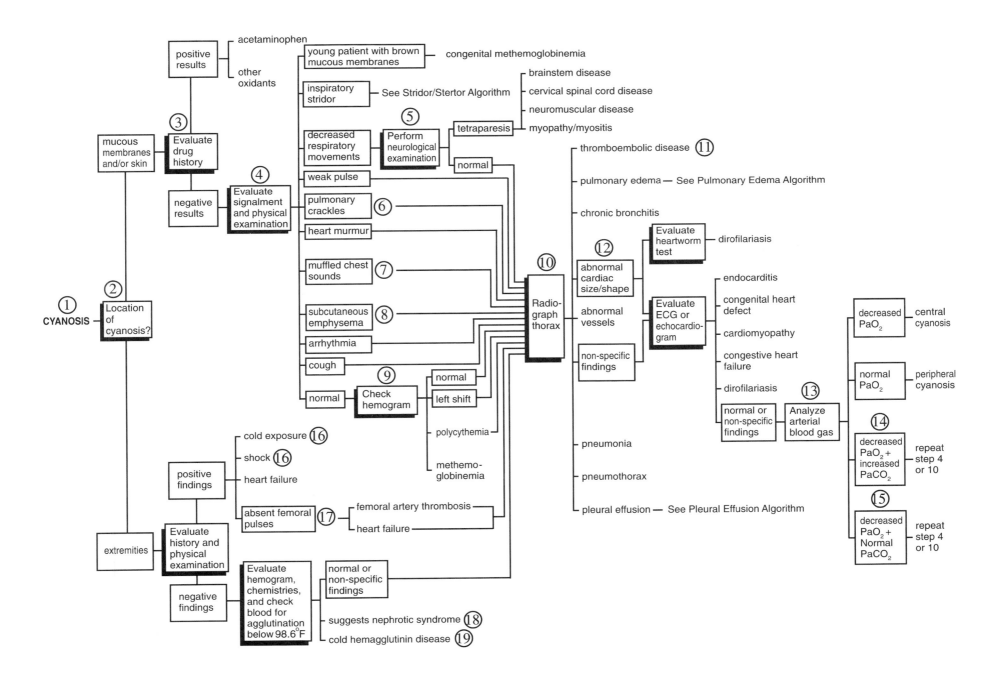

1 Pleural effusion is accumulation of fluid within the pleural space. This is the usually microscopic space between the visceral pleura (the membrane overlying the lungs) and the parietal pleura (the membrane lining the thoracic cavity). Alterations in conditions within the thoracic cavity change fluid dynamics across the pleural space. Under normal circumstances, fluid passes from the parietal surface of the pleura to the visceral surface. Hydrostatic and oncotic pressures in the systemic circulation favor pleural fluid formation at the parietal surface. Hydrostatic and oncotic pressures in the pulmonary circulation favor pleural fluid absorption at the visceral surface. Conditions that alter this delicate balance lead to pleural fluid accumulation. Patients with pleural effusion usually present with varying degrees of dyspnea and tachypnea. They may or may not be cyanotic, depending on the degree of compromise. Sometimes a fluid line can be auscultated in standing patients. Radiographs of the thorax are likely to be the most useful diagnostic step to prove that pleural effusion exists. However, it should be noted that many patients are so severely compromised by the condition that initially only lateral views should be taken, and patients that struggle should be allowed to rest for as long as is necessary between views. Ventrodorsal thoracic radiographs compromise already poor lung function and are unnecessary to document large amounts of fluid. The lateral view allows the clinician to determine the extent and location of the fluid and the best site for thoracocentesis. All other radiographs can be taken after thoracocentesis, when the patient is more stable and when films can be of more use in determining the underlying cause of fluid accumulation.

2 Since the single most useful early diagnostic test in patients with pleural effusion is likely to be thoracocentesis, it is important to exclude underlying coagulopathy as a cause of pleural fluid accumulation. Coagulopathy is probably the only direct contraindication to thoracocentesis. Exclusion initially is via evaluation of the patient's history (drug administration, known or potential exposure to anticoagulants, likely environment for anticoagulant rodenticides, possibility of malicious poisoning, a poorly supervised patient, a history of liver disease, or neoplasia). If necessary, coagulation times should be evaluated (marked prolongation of the PT and PTT is suspicious for anticoagulant exposure). The other condition that needs to be excluded is DIC, in which

228

there also will be low platelet counts and increased fibrin degradation products (FDPs).

3 Thoracocentesis is a useful diagnostic and therapeutic step in a patient with documented or suspected pleural effusion. Use of a relatively small-gauge needle or butterfly catheter, three-way stopcock, and extension set allows removal of most fluids for analysis and relief of dyspnea. In extremely dyspneic patients, care should be taken not to lacerate visceral pleura, lung tissue, or intercostal vasculature (running at the back of every rib) during the procedure. If thoracocentesis is negative, the suspected pleural effusion may be an artifact secondary to fat accumulation within the thorax, a mass lesion, or a skin fold seen on radiographs, and other causes of dyspnea or tachypnea should be sought. However, failure to retrieve fluid also may be due to the presence of a very thick exudate. Fluid associated with pyothorax can require a very large-gauge needle or thoracostomy tube for drainage. It also is possible that fluid is compartmentalized (loculated). This often happens with chronic effusions, especially when there is irritation of pleural surfaces (e.g., pyothorax, chylothorax). If this is suspected, ultrasound guidance may be used to locate pockets of fluid. Analysis of the fluid obtained allows categorization of the type of pleural effusion formed. Note that there can be overlap between the cellularity and protein contents in these categories (e.g., modified transudates and exudates). Also, the same underlying condition can cause different types of effusion (e.g., neoplasia can result in the formation of either an exudate or a modified transudate). In addition, different conditions can cause the formation of the same type of fluid (e.g., chylous effusions form due to right-sided heart failure, trauma, and intrathoracic neoplasia).

4 Exudates are relatively high in protein (total protein > 3.5 g/dl) and have high concentrations of WBCs (often > 5000/mm^3). When the exudate is serosanguinous or sanguinous, the PCV should be assessed. If the PCV approaches that of peripheral blood (>20%), trauma, coagulopathy, or a bleeding intrathoracic mass should be suspected.

5 A coagulogram, including platelets and FDPs, assesses the coagulation status (see step 2). If it is abnormal, the signalment (young animal, breed known to have

coagulopathies) and history (previous bleeding episodes, documented factor deficiency) may be used to determine whether it is likely to be a congenital coagulation disorder. Usually patients bleed due to factor VIII, factor IX, or severe vWF deficiency. If platelets are low and FDPs are present, DIC is likely and an underlying cause (e.g., neoplasia, sepsis, splenic torsion) should be sought. If there is a history of exposure to anticoagulant rodenticides or if this is a possibility, a PIVKA (products of vitamin K antagonism) test can be considered for confirmation.

6 If the coagulogram is normal in a patient with hemothorax and there is no history of trauma or if there is evidence of DIC, neoplasia should be suspected. Further imaging of the thorax for mass lesions is required, and a number of techniques may be employed. Thoracic radiographs require drainage of pleural fluid and lung reexpansion to be useful (further thoracocentesis is not recommended in patients suspected to have DIC). Thoracic ultrasound prior to fluid drainage can image masses, but care must be taken not to mistake collapsed lung tissue for a mass. Thoracic CT or MRI scans can be performed whether or not fluid has been removed.

7 Patients with a large number of lymphocytes on cytology or milky-appearing fluid should be evaluated for chylous effusion. Note that chylous effusions can be modified transudates as well as exudates and that if the patient has not eaten recently, fluid may not be grossly milky in appearance. Fluid should be evaluated cytologically for chylomicrons, and fluid triglyceride and cholesterol concentrations should be compared with those of peripheral blood (fluid triglycerides should be higher than in peripheral blood, and cholesterol should be lower). Alternatively, feed a high-fat meal, such as cream, if the patient will eat it, and see whether the fluid turns milky. Chylous effusions are associated with trauma, intrathoracic neoplasia, right-sided heart failure, thrombosis or tearing of the thoracic duct secondary to jugular catheter placement, or they may be idiopathic. The last is most common.

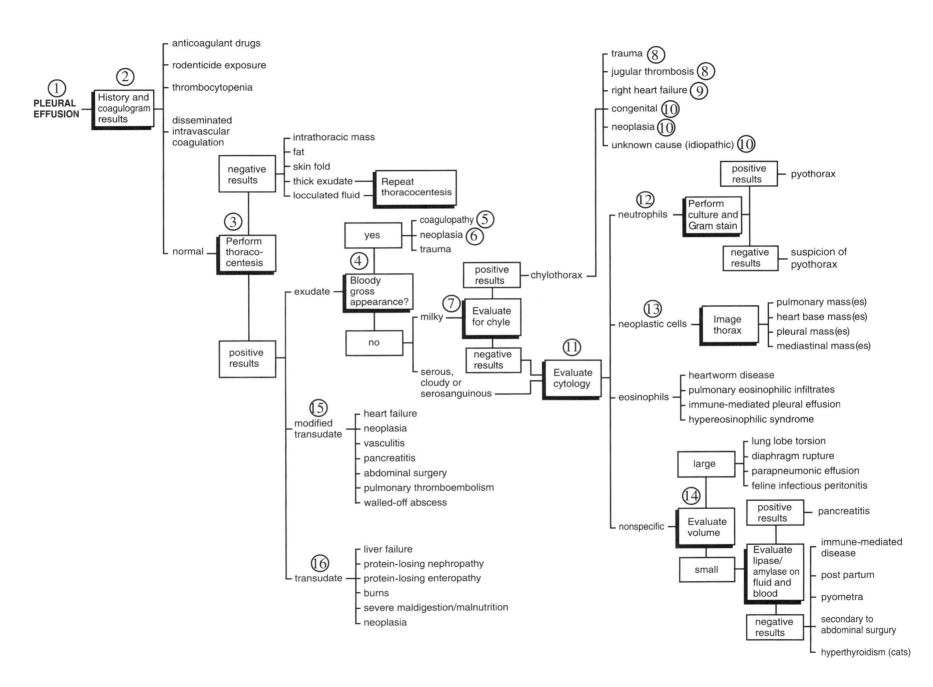

8 The history should be evaluated for trauma (especially to the chest) or for jugular catheter placement (usually within the last 10–14 days). Thoracic duct lacerations can resolve over time, provided that the pleural fluid is kept drained. Jugular vein thrombosis and concurrent thoracic duct occlusion also can resolve with time, especially if heparin is given to prevent clot extension. Thrombolytic agents (streptokinase or urokinase topically on the clot or systemic tissue plasminogen activator) also can be administered. Prior to the use of such agents, venous angiography (via a jugular catheter placed in the left jugular vein well above the site of the suspected laceration or thrombus) should be performed. Lymphangiography also can document thoracic duct rupture or occlusion (see below).

9 If cardiac disease (right-sided or biventricular heart failure) is suspected based on the history and physical examination, an echocardiogram should be obtained. Physical examination findings that suggest right-sided heart failure include evidence of severe primary pulmonary disease, tricuspid or pulmonic heart murmurs, increased jugular pulses, and hepatojugular reflux. Pleural effusion secondary to right-sided heart failure is most commonly seen in cats. Dogs tend to develop abdominal effusions.

10 In a patient with a negative history of trauma or cardiac problems, suspect underlying disease, particularly intrathoracic neoplasia or abnormalities of the thoracic duct (either congenital or acquired) as the cause of chylothorax. Check the signalment (congenital defects manifest in young animals, while older ones tend to develop neoplasia, although lymphoma can be seen in young animals). The history should be evaluated for previously identified underlying diseases. Consider imaging techniques for the thorax, including radiography following thoracocentesis, ultrasound with fluid still present, or CT/MRI scanning. Alternatively, a contrast study (lymphangiography) can be performed. This requires a surgical approach to the abdomen and cannulation of a lymphatic vessel, usually within the mesentery. This is not a particularly easy technique to perform, but lymphatic visualization can be improved by feeding a high-fat diet prior to surgery.

11 If the PCV of the fluid does not approach that of peripheral blood and the fluid is not chylous, cytology is the next step in determining the underlying cause of a thoracic exudate. All cytology findings should be interpreted in light of the peripheral WBC count since this can influence fluid cellularity to some extent (e.g., an eosinophilic pleural effusion may be less important in a patient with marked peripheral eosinophilia).

12 When large numbers of neutrophils are present in an exudate, the cells should be evaluated for bacterial or fungal inclusions and for whether cells are degenerate or nondegenerate. Degenerate neutrophils are more likely to be associated with septic effusions (i.e., pyothorax), and this finding should be followed by a Gram stain and culture to look for bacteria and fungal elements. Depending on the underlying infection, specialized culture techniques may be needed (e.g., for *Actinomyces* spp. and *Nocardia* spp.). Septic effusions may be the result of penetrating chest wounds (usually bites in cats), foreign bodies (usually inhaled), esophageal rupture, parapneumonic effusions, or ruptured pulmonary abscesses.

13 Occasionally, pleural effusions contain neoplastic cells. However, it is very important to try to differentiate clusters of neoplastic cells from activated mesothelial cells. The latter will shed into any pleural effusion and can have a highly atypical appearance. Finding lymphoblasts or acinar arrangements of carcinoma cells is relatively definitive for neoplasia, and only the location of the mass lesion then needs to be discovered. This usually involves thoracic ultrasound or thoracic radiography following drainage of the effusion.

14 Sometimes the cellularity of the exudate is relatively nonspecific (i.e., nonchylous, nonsanguinous, nonseptic, nonneoplastic). At this stage, it is important to look at the fluid volume. With large effusions, look for mechanical reasons for fluid formation. These include lung lobe torsion in large-breed dogs (look at the position of the bronchi on radiographs), diaphragmatic rupture (especially with liver entrapment), parapneumonic effusion, and FIP in cats. Smaller effusions may be associated with pancreatitis, pyometra, abdominal surgery, hyperthyroidism (without congestive heart failure) in cats, and immune-mediated problems (polyarthritis, SLE, and pulmonary granulomatosis).

15 Modified transudates occupy a gray area between exudates and transudates in terms of their composition (protein and cellularity). There also is a great deal of overlap between underlying conditions that cause modified transudates and exudates, especially the less specific types of exudate (i.e., those other than blood, pus, or chyle). Many conditions that lead to serous or serosanguinous exudates also cause modified transudates (e.g., heart failure, neoplasia, and abscesses), and much of the same diagnostic algorithm should be followed. Note that pulmonary thromboembolic disease occasionally causes small amounts of pleural effusion, usually a modified transudate, and should be considered in patients with severe dyspnea but only mild pleural effusion. Vasculitis (which has a large number of underlying causes) is a relatively common cause of modified transudate formation in the pleural space.

16 Transudates are effusions with low protein content (<2 to 2.5 g/dl) and cellularity. They form because there is insufficient plasma oncotic pressure to hold fluid in the vasculature or to allow fluid reabsorption by blood vessels or lymphatics. The most common causes of transudate formation in the pleural space include failure of albumin production (in liver failure), protein loss from the body (protein-losing nephropathy, protein-losing gastroenteropathy, frank hemorrhage, or severe burns leading to cutaneous protein loss). It may also be seen with severe maldigestion or malnutrition, some types of neoplasia, and any condition that causes lymphatic obstruction.

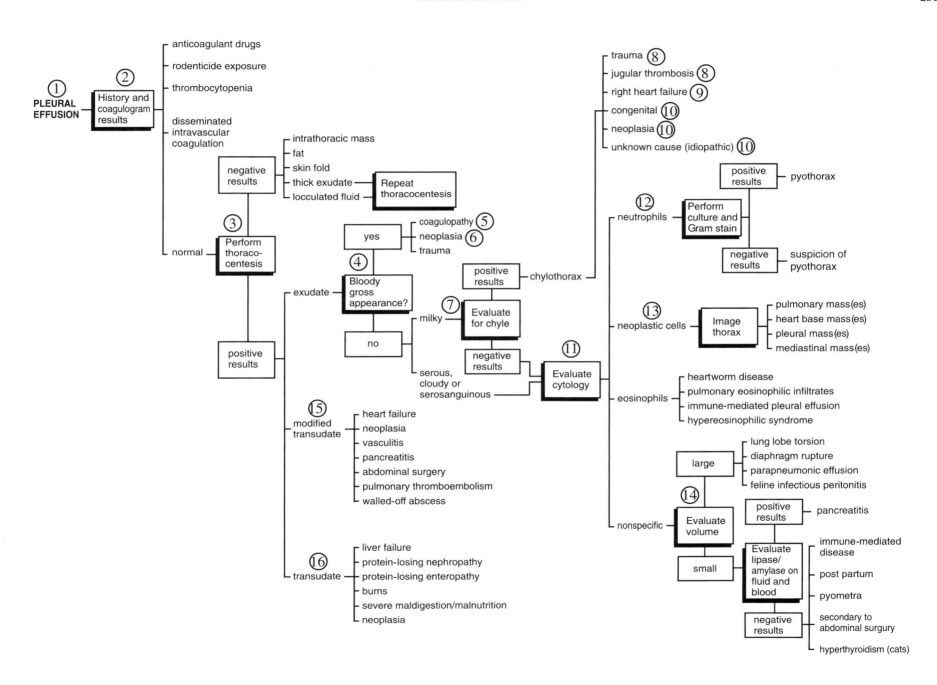

1 Pulmonary edema is accumulation of fluid within interstitial and alveolar lung spaces. It is not a primary condition but rather a manifestation of another disease process such as heart failure. There are two recognized forms of pulmonary edema: cardiogenic and noncardiogenic. Cardiogenic edema is more common. Pathophysiological mechanisms for pulmonary edema include increased hydrostatic pressure, decreased plasma oncotic pressure, increased capillary membrane permeability, lymphatic dysfunction, and increased negative intrapleural pressure. Dogs and cats frequently develop pulmonary edema as a result of increased hydrostatic pressure from left-sided heart failure.

2 Common clinical signs of pulmonary edema include coughing, cyanosis, exercise intolerance, and dyspnea. Patients should be evaluated for signs of cardiac disease such as tachycardia, pulse deficits, heart murmurs, arrhythmias, and distended jugular veins (the last seen more often with right-sided heart failure). Note that cats can have significant heart disease without having murmurs or arrhythmias. On thoracic auscultation, pulmonary edema may sound like crackles or pops, but breath sounds also can be normal. Crackles in a dorsal or caudal location are most often associated with heart failure.

3 The diagnosis of pulmonary edema is confirmed via thoracic radiography. Cardiogenic edema is associated with initial development of an interstitial pattern in the perihilar area that progresses to an alveolar pattern. Noncardiogenic pulmonary edema has more of an alveolar pattern from the start, especially in the dorsocaudal lung fields. In cats, pulmonary edema can be asymmetrical and multifocal in distribution, making it difficult to distinguish the two types of edema radiographically. Edema sometimes can be confused with pneumonia. The latter usually has a more anterior and cranioventral distribution and is usually more severe in one lung than the other. If focal or generalized cardiomegaly is seen, then cardiogenic pulmonary edema should be suspected. However, right-sided cardiac enlargement can develop secondary to pulmonary hypertension in noncardiogenic pulmonary edema.

4 Since cardiogenic pulmonary edema is common, finding an enlarged heart on radiographs or signs of cardiac disease on physical examination should lead the clinician to evaluate the heart via echocardiography.

5 If the heart appears normal on thoracic radiographs or if its size cannot be determined, cats should undergo echocardiography anyway. Cats often do not have signs of cardiac disease radiographically because of the high incidence of hypertrophic/restrictive cardiomyopathy (HCM/RCM). With HCM, cardiac muscle enlargement occurs inward, reducing ventricular volume and cardiac output. In RCM, changes in the cardiac muscle/endocardium reduce diastolic filling of the heart. Backward failure and pulmonary edema can occur with both conditions. Enlargement of the cardiac silhouette is a very late development.

6 In dogs and cats without echocardiographic changes, review the history and physical examination to exclude causes of noncardiogenic pulmonary edema. These include upper airway obstruction, laryngeal paralysis, electrical cord bites, neurological disease, and trauma. Upper airway obstruction need only be transient to cause noncardiogenic pulmonary edema. Noncardiogenic pulmonary edema is rare in cats.

7 Upper airway obstruction manifests as stertorous or stridorous respiration, inspiratory dyspnea, cyanosis, coughing, gagging, or collapse.

8 BAOS is found in all brachycephalic dog breeds, but especially the English bulldog. Persian and Himalayan cats also can be affected. Stenotic nares, elongated soft palate, everted laryngeal saccules, and hypoplastic trachea all can be present and cause upper airway obstruction and secondary laryngeal collapse. High environmental temperatures and excessive panting exacerbate the condition.

9 Dogs with congenital laryngeal paralysis usually are less than 1 year of age. Commonly affected breeds are the Bouvier des Flandres, Siberian husky, Irish setter, Dalmatian, and bull terrier. Acquired laryngeal paralysis occurs most often in large-breed dogs, especially older males. The condition generally is due to a peripheral neuropathy, although occasionally cervical trauma is the cause. Often underlying causes of peripheral neuropathy cannot be determined. The diagnosis is made by direct examination of the larynx without sedation. During inspiration, one or both arytenoid cartilages and vocal folds do not abduct. Cats rarely are affected.

10 If there are no signs of upper airway obstruction, evaluate the oral cavity for signs of a burn wound caused by biting a live electrical cord. Inquisitive puppies and kittens are affected most often.

11 Once upper airway obstruction and electrical cord bites have been discounted, review the history for any possibility of head trauma or seizures within the past few days. These could cause neurogenic (noncardiogenic) pulmonary edema. Perform a neurological examination for changes in behavior, mentation, proprioception, or cranial nerve deficits that suggest a CNS disorder.

12 If neurological signs are absent, evaluate the serum albumin concentration. Hypoalbuminemia causes decreased plasma oncotic pressures. However, it is unlikely that hypoalbuminemia alone could cause pulmonary edema, although it can be a contributing factor in conjunction with other predisposing problems. Excessive fluid administration resulting in vascular overload in a patient with hypoalbuminemia can cause pulmonary edema. The serum albumin concentration is usually less than 1.8 g/dl in these cases, and subcutaneous edema often develops prior to pulmonary edema.

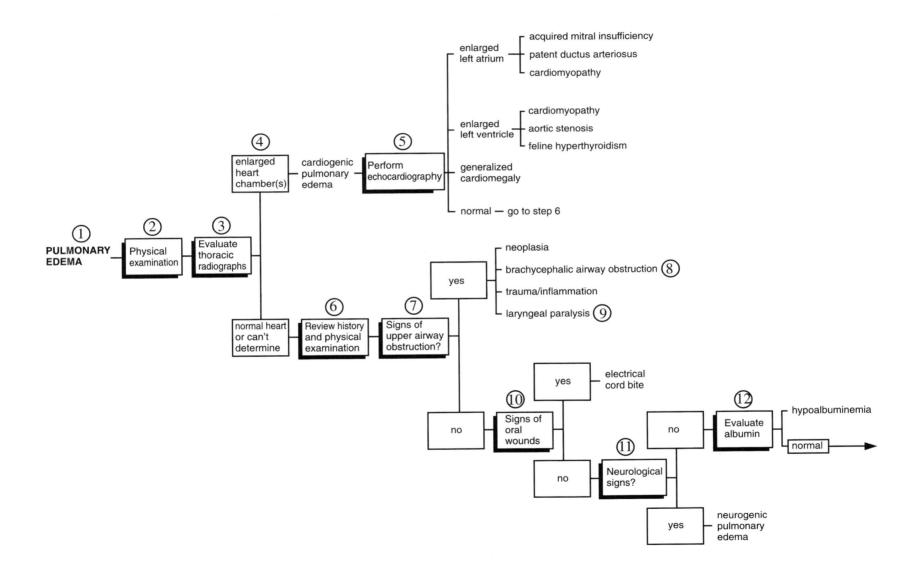

13 Several systemic diseases may be associated with noncardiogenic pulmonary edema and respiratory signs and have been collectively described as acute respiratory distress syndrome (ARDS). The syndrome may be acute (sudden onset of clinical signs) or chronic (development of signs over several days). The most common causes of ARDS reported in dogs and cats are pancreatitis, sepsis, endotoxemia, and aspiration pneumonia, as well as parvovirus infection (specifically in dogs).

14 If not done previously, echocardiography may be indicated in patients with negative findings to exclude subtle cardiac disease that may not be apparent on thoracic radiographs.

15 If the heart is normal on echocardiography, evaluate for liver disease via the history and physical examination and by measuring liver enzymes on a serum chemistry screen. Other liver function tests may become necessary. Exactly how liver disease causes pulmonary edema in the absence of hypoalbuminemia is unknown.

16 While an arterial blood gas evaluation is useful for identifying the extent of pulmonary dysfunction and assessing the response to therapy, it does not allow specific diagnosis of the underlying cause of pulmonary edema.

17 If all tests are normal to this point, then edema is presumed to be of neurogenic origin. If the neurological examination is normal to this point, the abnormality is located either in the peripheral nerves to the thorax or within an area of the brain that does not result in obvious mentation changes, cranial nerve abnormalities, or gait deficits. To pursue the problem further, a CT or MRI brain scan and spinal fluid analysis are required.

18 Pulmonary thromboembolic disease (PTE) very, very rarely causes pulmonary edema. If it is present, edema/alveolar densities usually are very mild, especially when compared to the severity of clinical signs and hypoxemia on blood gas analysis. PTE is due to obstruction of pulmonary arteries and arterioles by blood clots, emboli of bacteria, foreign material, air, fat, or parasites. Hyperlucent zones (due to loss of the regional blood supply) and mild alveolar pulmonary infiltrates (edema or hemorrhage) are seen rarely on thoracic radiographs. The diagnosis can be difficult to make without using ventilation and perfusion scanning with radioisotopes.

19 Inhalation of hot smoke damages the mucous membranes of the upper respiratory tract and leads to laryngeal edema. Inhalation of incomplete products of combustion into the bronchi/bronchioles allows them to combine with mucous to produce acids and alkali. These damage the airways. Noxious fumes can damage the lungs when plastics, rubber, or other synthetic products burn. In smoke inhalation, severe pulmonary changes usually do not develop until 16–24 hours after the event. Thoracic radiographs show edema, atelectasis, pleural effusion, or early pneumonia.

20 When sepsis is identified, there often is no known underlying cause. Where a cause is identified, the patient may have preexisting infection, have undergone surgery, have an indwelling thoracostomy or gastrostomy tube or central venous catheter, or have suffered a penetrating injury into a body cavity. Patients also may have an underlying disease that causes immunosuppression and predisposes them to systemic infection (diabetes mellitus, hyperadrenocorticism, systemic viral infection). Certain therapies also predispose patients to systemic infection (chemotherapeutic drug administration, glucocorticoids, and intravenous nutrition). Common clinical findings in septic patients include tachypnea, fever, tachycardia, hyperemic mucous membranes, and melena and bloody diarrhea. Laboratory abnormalities include respiratory alkalosis, leukocytosis, neutrophilia with a degenerative left shift or neutropenia, elevated liver enzymes, and hypoalbuminemia.

21 Acute severe pancreatitis causes severe vomiting, abdominal pain, marked depression, hypotension, and shock-like symptoms. Cellular membrane destruction causes release of proenzymes and activated trypsin, which leads to release of bradykinin and other substances that cause hypotension. Other biochemical reagents and toxic substances are activated or released, including myocardial depressant factors and intestinal toxins. Electrolyte imbalances also can contribute to abnormal pulmonary function.

22 Respiratory complications of acute uremia include pulmonary edema, pneumonia, uremic pneumonitis, pleural effusion, and PTE. Pulmonary edema can result from excessive fluid administration and volume overload in patients with ARF. Once administered, an excessive fluid load can be difficult or impossible to correct in an oliguric patient.

23 DIC is a complex syndrome caused by systemic coagulation and fibrinolysis. The hemorrhagic phase of acute DIC causes signs of petechiation, ecchymotic hemorrhages, and bleeding from multiple sites. Bleeding often is less obvious or absent in thrombotic or chronic compensated DIC. The condition has been associated with ARDS, resulting in noncardiogenic pulmonary edema.

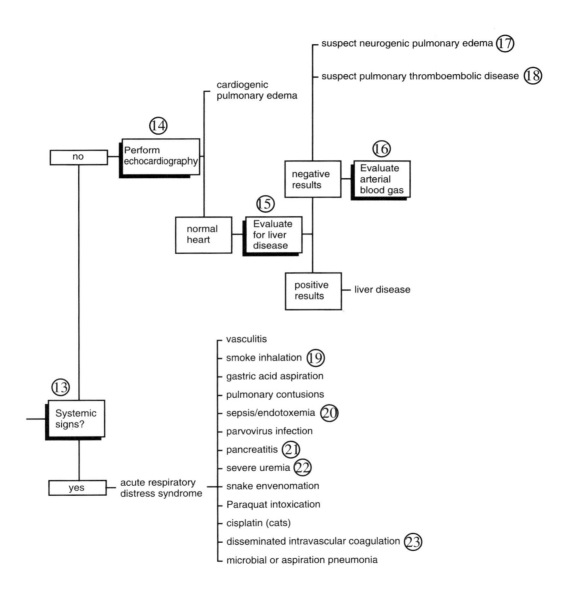

Cardiovascular Disorders

1 Tachycardia is a rapid heart rate, usually greater than 160 beats per minute (BPM) in both cats and dogs. Heart rates greater than 180 BPM may be physiological in small dogs and puppies. Rates greater than 210 BPM may be physiological in cats. Causes of tachycardia include primary cardiac disease, hypoxia, sepsis, drugs, toxins, metabolic abnormalities, and autonomic nervous system imbalances.

2 Clinical signs may or may not be present with tachycardia. If the arrhythmia is very rapid, the animal may collapse as a result of decreased ventricular filling in diastole and forward pump failure (low output failure). Other signs of heart failure (coughing, dyspnea, exercise intolerance) also can be found with tachycardia. Tachycardia can result in pulmonary edema if the arrhythmia is fast enough. This is due to inadequate length of diastole, reducing ventricular filling and causing backward failure.

3 Drugs that might cause or contribute to a rapid heart rate include digitalis, atropine, glycopyrrolate, thyroxine, and catecholamines. While digitalis is sometimes used to break atrial tachycardia or slow ventricular response rates in atrial fibrillation, it can cause a variety of tachyarrhythmias, especially if toxic serum concentrations are reached. The most common arrhythmias due to digitalis are atrioventricular (AV) nodal blockade (see the algorithm for bradycardia) and extrasystoles from delayed afterdepolarizations. Since gastrointestinal disturbance usually precedes arrhythmias, digoxin should be discontinued or the dose reduced when gastrointestinal signs occur. Doxorubicin can produce cardiotoxicity, dilated cardiomyopathy, and tachyarrhythmias.

4 An ECG should be evaluated to determine the type of tachycardia present.

5 Ventricular tachycardias are common. They originate below the AV node, in the bundle of His, the distal Purkinje fibers, or the ventricular muscle itself.

6 Ventricular premature complexes (VPCs) are early ventricular beats that occur before the next projected normal heartbeat. They are characterized by wide, bizarre QRS complexes without an associated P wave. They can occur in pairs, in runs (three or more in a row), or as a bigeminy (VPCs alternate with normal sinus beats). A positive QRS deflection indicates a right ventricular focus, whereas a negative QRS deflection indicates a left ventricular focus. Pulse deficits may be detected in association with VPCs. Underlying causes are numerous and include primary cardiac disease, splenic conditions, endotoxemia, and drugs.

7 Ventricular flutter is an extremely fast, bizarre, and unstable arrhythmia that is only one step above ventricular fibrillation. Causes include severe conditions such as myocardial trauma, anoxia, hypotension and shock, and electrolyte imbalances. Intravenous lidocaine or procainamide should be used immediately to treat the arrhythmia.

8 Ventricular fibrillation is an uncoordinated, chaotic rhythm synonymous with cardiac arrest. It can be preceded by ventricular extrasystoles with the R on T phenomenon, sustained ventricular tachycardia, and then ventricular flutter. Treatment with direct-current countershock may reverse it.

9 Four or more VPCs in a row define ventricular tachycardia. Uniformly shaped (monomorphic) complexes are more benign than multiformly shaped (polymorphic) ones and do not need to be treated unless there is hemodynamic compromise (poor peripheral perfusion, pulse deficits), especially if the underlying cause is known and is being treated. Polymorphic complexes denote an unstable rhythm that needs to be treated with parenteral drugs.

10 If the tachycardia is severe enough to cause collapse, pulmonary edema, or cardiogenic shock (pallor, slow refill time, hypothermia, weakness), the arrhythmia should be treated before pursuing other diagnostic testing.

11 Supraventricular tachycardias originate above the AV node and include those arising from the sinus node, atrial muscle, or AV junctional tissue.

12 Atrial flutter is characterized by a rapid, sustained, and regular series of atrial depolarizations without a rest phase between P waves. It is an uncommon tachycardia resulting in atrial rates that frequently are faster than 300 BPM. If vagal stimulation (see step 14) fails to convert the arrhythmia, intravenous digitalis, beta-blockers, or calcium channel blockers can be tried. The underlying causes of atrial flutter are similar to those of atrial fibrillation.

13 Atrial fibrillation is characterized by a rapid, irregularly irregular rhythm, absence of P waves on the ECG, and fibrillation waves in the baseline. Most cases are associated with left ventricular dysfunction due to stretching of the left atrial muscle, leading to electrical abnormalities and formation of a new pacemaker focus. It is appropriate to use digoxin first to slow the heart rate by blocking the AV node. Common causes of atrial fibrillation include chronic mitral regurgitation, dilated and restrictive cardiomyopathy, and congenital heart defects. An idiopathic form occurs in large-breed dogs with a normal left ventricle.

14 Atrial and junctional tachycardias are difficult to differentiate, and if an exact location cannot be determined, the problem is called a *supraventricular tachycardia*. The ECG findings include a heart rate so rapid that P waves are difficult to see. Vagal maneuvers (carotid sinus or ocular compression) can stop these arrhythmias. Causes usually are related to a structural cardiac lesion causing atrial distention (hemangiosarcoma, myocarditis, endocarditis, cardiomyopathy), hypoxia, or digitalis toxicity. Such tachycardias should be treated if sustained, if there is a history of collapse or weakness, or if there is structural heart disease that would be compromised by tachycardia.

15 Sinus tachycardia is characterized by a rapid heart rate with discernible P waves of normal size and shape, followed by normal QRS complexes. It is caused by sympathetic stimulation of the sinoatrial (SA) node and is a normal physiological response to fever, pain, excitement, or other causes of adrenergic release. It also is seen with drugs that block the parasympathetic nervous system, hyperthyroidism, and pain. It requires no treatment unless it is extremely rapid or sustained. Addressing the underlying cause of the sympathetic stimulation is usually sufficient. Vagal maneuvers only temporarily slow the heart rate rather than abolishing the arrhythmia.

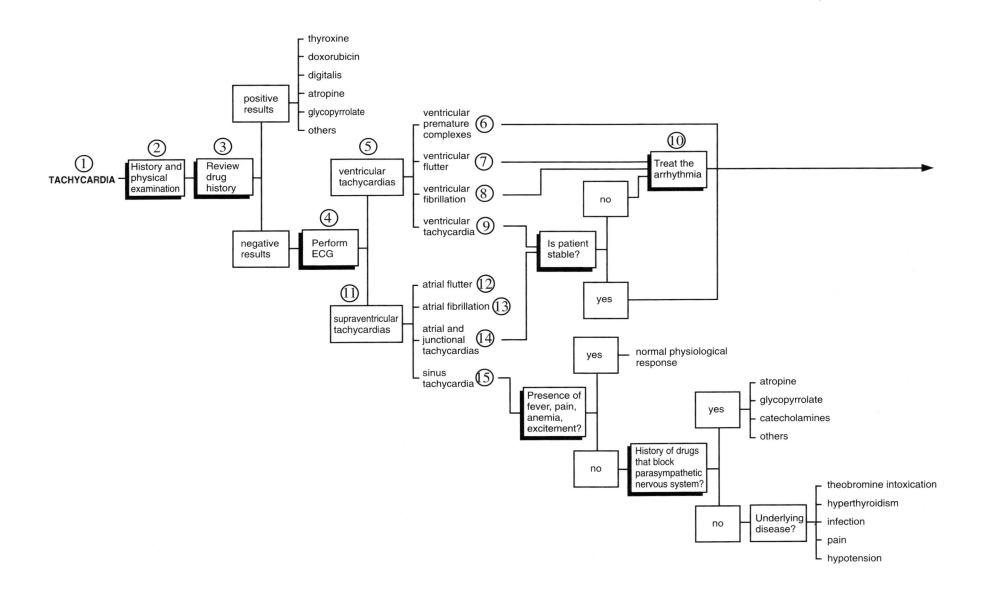

16 Once the patient has been stabilized, thoracic radiographs should be evaluated for primary pulmonary problems and changes in the cardiac silhouette that suggest underlying cardiac disease or causes of hypoxia.

17 Radiographic signs of *D. immitis* infestation include enlargement of the right ventricle and main pulmonary arteries and a dilated, tortuous, or blunted appearance of the caudal lobar arteries. The severity of changes seen on radiography is related to the adult worm burden, the duration of infection, and a variety of host-parasite interactions. In general, arrhythmias are uncommon in dogs with *D. immitis* infestation.

18 If thoracic radiographs show pulmonary disease and no evidence of cardiac enlargement, a blood gas analysis may be valuable to determine if the arrhythmia is related to hypoxia.

19 If the PaO_2 is normal in the face of tachycardia, a normal heart size, and normal thoracic radiographs, evaluate a minimum database, looking for signs of hypokalemia, hypomagnesemia, sepsis, endotoxemia, renal failure, hypocalcemia, or hypercalcemia.

20 If the results are normal, consider Lyme myocarditis or thyrotoxicosis.

21 If thoracic radiographs show a normally sized or enlarged heart, an echocardiography is recommended to evaluate cardiac function and either primary myocardial changes or those that may have developed secondary to the tachycardia (e.g., ventricular dilation as a result of incipient failure). An echocardiogram also can provide more information about the severity of cardiac dysfunction associated with cardiomegaly and *D. immitis* infestation.

22 Dilated cardiomyopathy (DCM) is associated with ventricular dilation, poor cardiac contractility, and congestive heart failure. Atrial fibrillation has been reported in as many as 75–80% of DCM cases. Other common rhythm abnormalities include ventricular tachycardia and VPCs. Large and giant breeds of dogs are predisposed to DCM (German shepherds, Great Danes, Doberman pinschers, Saint Bernards, and Irish wolfhounds). Most are males and young to middle-aged. Boxers and English and American cocker spaniels can also have DCM. Dilated cardiomyopathy in cats is usually but not always associated with taurine deficiency and is now very rare since feline dietary requirements for taurine have become known.

23 Hypertrophic cardiomyopathy (HCM) is a rare disease in dogs but is found commonly in cats, mostly in middle-aged males. It is characterized by left ventricular inward hypertrophy. Biatrial enlargement and mild to moderate right ventricular hypertrophy may also be found. The ECG changes vary, but ventricular and supraventricular arrhythmias have been noted. Two common conditions that cause left ventricular hypertrophy are hyperthyroidism and systemic hypertension. These must be excluded before idiopathic HCM is diagnosed. Serum thyroid concentrations should be evaluated in cats over about 7 years of age.

24 Restrictive cardiomyopathy (REM) in cats is due to myocardial or endomyocardial fibrosis that restricts ventricular filling in diastole. The endomyocardial form has been associated with endomyocarditis, potentially related to viral infection. The causes of the myocardial form are not known. The most characteristic echocardiographic finding is a very dilated left atrium.

25 Mitral valve disease, the most common heart disease in dogs, is characterized by a thickened, distorted mitral valve resulting from endocardiosis. The valve fails to close in systole, causing regurgitation of blood into the left atrium. It affects mostly old small-breed dogs and, rarely, cats. Acquired tricuspid, aortic, and pulmonary valvular diseases are less common. Arrhythmias associated with valvular disease include sinus tachycardia, atrial or VPCs, and atrial fibrillation.

26 Most congenital cardiac defects are detected during routine vaccination visits. A heart murmur is the most common abnormality. Most cases are asymptomatic when first examined, and patients do not develop clinical signs until heart failure or arrhythmias occur. Atrial fibrillation and other tachycardias have been noted with patent ductus arteriosus and pulmonic stenosis. German shepherds have idiopathic ventricular arrhythmia which may cause sudden death.

27 Pericardial diseases include constrictive pericarditis, pericardial effusion, intrapericardial masses or cysts, and congenital pericardial defects. Arrhythmias associated with pericardial disease vary from sinus tachycardia to supraventricular and ventricular arrhythmias. Common ECG findings include elevation of the ST segment and reduced QRS voltages. Electrical alternans (beat-to-beat changes in the QRS voltage or ST segment) can be seen with pericardial effusion. Echocardiography is the most sensitive and specific noninvasive method for detecting pericardial effusion.

28 Common cardiac neoplasms include hemangiosarcoma of the right atrium (common in German shepherds and golden retrievers) and aortic body tumors (chemodectoma, nonchromaffin paraganglioma). Aortic body tumors occur most commonly in aged, brachycephalic dog breeds. Most cardiac neoplasms result in pericardial effusion.

29 Pheochromocytomas are often functional endocrine tumors that arise from the adrenal medulla. Clinical signs result from excessive production of catecholamines and local tissue invasion of the tumor. Clinical signs are variable but include panting, dyspnea, weakness, exercise intolerance, irritability, cyanosis, cutaneous flushing, collapse, and abdominal distention. Cardiac abnormalities are seen in a significant number of canine patients with pheochromocytomas. These include cardiac murmurs, tachycardia, ventricular fibrillation, and other arrhythmias. Catecholamines can directly cause myocarditis or conduction abnormalities, probably as a result of catecholamine-induced vasoconstriction and secondary myocardial ischemia.

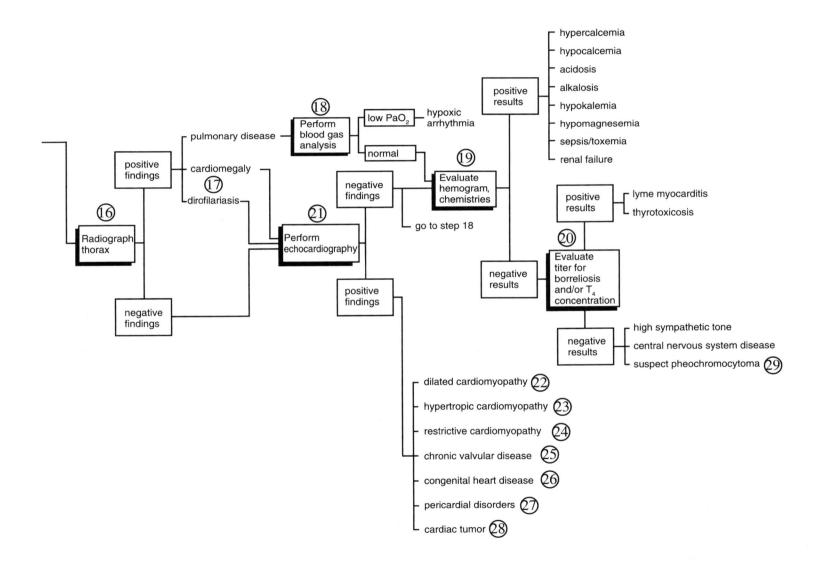

1 Bradycardia means a slow heart rate, usually below 60 BPM for dogs and below 120 BPM for cats. Bradycardia occurs either because the SA node in the heart does not fire when it should or because impulse conduction is blocked at the AV node. Bradycardia also may be due to idiopathic ventricular rhythms (slower than normal sinus rates).

2 Animals with bradycardia may not be symptomatic. Symptomatic animals may be lethargic or show intermittent weakness, collapse, or syncope, especially during exercise or stress. They often are not capable of increasing cardiac output by increasing the heart rate. Since some drugs slow the heart rate (cardiac glycosides, calcium channel blockers, beta blockers, quinidine, procainamide, narcotics, xylazine, and other anesthetics), a drug history is imperative. Some metabolic disturbances such as hypocalcemia, hyperkalemia, hypothermia, and hypothyroidism also can slow the heart rate. In an athletic, highly conditioned dog, a slow heart rate can be within normal limits.

3 If bradycardia is detected, an ECG should be done to identify the type of bradyarrhythmia. Some bradyarrhythmias are normal or not significant enough to require further diagnostic testing. Some are transient or related to other disease states. Others require more thorough evaluation.

4 Ventricular asystole usually occurs either just before cardiopulmonary arrest or after repeated attempts at resuscitation. It is an end-stage event.

5 AV nodal blockade is the result of problems with conduction of impulses through the AV node from the atria to the ventricles. The causes of AV nodal blockade are diverse and vary to some extent with the degree of blockade. There are three degrees of AV nodal blockade. First-degree blockade is the mildest, with an extended P-R interval (greater than 140 msec in dogs and 80 msec in cats). The heart rate is not usually affected significantly. First-degree blockade is usually due to excess vagal tone and is readily abolished by exercise or anticholinergic drugs. Second- and third-degree AV blockade can cause bradycardia. Second-degree blockade may be physiological (again due to excessive vagal tone) or pathological (due to damage to or fibrosis of the AV nodal tissue). The former type is readily abolished by atropine or exercise and does not cause clinical signs. Third-degree AV blockade is always due to damage to the AV node and total abolition of impulse conduction through that node. Causes include endocarditis, Lyme myocarditis, traumatic myocarditis, cardiomyopathy, endocardiosis, and fibrosis.

6 There are two types of second-degree heart blockade: Mobitz type I and Mobitz type II. In Mobitz type I, the P-R interval lengthens progressively until a P wave occurs with no subsequent QRS complex. It is considered a normal finding and often is related to excessive vagal tone or the negative chronotrophic effects of digitalis, antiarrhythmic drugs, or α_2-stimulating anesthetics. In Mobitz type II blockade, the P-R intervals are longer than normal and do not extend, but periodically the QRS complex disappears. There is often a pattern to the blockade such as three P waves for every two QRS complexes. Second-degree blockade does not require treatment unless the animal is symptomatic, but Mobitz type II can progress to third-degree AV nodal blockade with worsening of the underlying disease process.

7 In third-degree AV blockade, no conduction occurs between the atria and ventricles. As a result, there is no association between P waves and QRS complexes. The QRS complexes appear at regular intervals at a rate determined by the escape pacemaker, a ventricular escape rhythm of about 40 BPM. Most patients are symptomatic and require artificial pacemaker implantation. The causes of third-degree AV blockade include aortic stenosis, ventricular septal defect, cardiomyopathy, myocardial fibrosis, bacterial endocarditis, digitalis intoxication, hyperkalemia, and Lyme disease (borreliosis).

8 Sick sinus syndrome also has been called *bradycardia-tachycardia syndrome* because paroxysmal tachycardia may alternate with bradycardia. In this condition, the diseased tissue is in the sinus node of the heart (fibrosis with vascular disturbances such as microcoronary arteritis), affecting the normal cardiac pacemaker rate and rhythm. Although it has been associated particularly with minia-ture schnauzers (especially females), other breeds can be affected. Onset usually occurs in middle or old age, and there is an association with chronic mitral valve disease. Patients usually are symptomatic and the condition often does not respond well to medical therapy, requiring artificial pacemaker implantation.

9 Persistent atrial standstill is a rare condition. It can be the result of fibrosis of the atrial muscle secondary to chronic mitral regurgitation or muscular dystrophy in springer spaniels. Other possible causes include hypothermia, digitalis intoxication, and hyperkalemia.

10 Sinus arrest, or SA nodal blockade, is characterized by a long pause after a PQRS complex. The pause is greater than twice the distance between two normal PQRS complexes. A junctional or ventricular escape beat usually follows the pause and prevents asystole. High sympathetic (i.e., vagal) tone, caused by respiratory, neurological, or gastrointestinal disease, is a common cause. Other differentials include being a brachycephalic breed of dog, drug toxicity, cardiomyopathy, electrolyte imbalance, atrial disease, vagal nerve injury, and neoplasia.

11 Primary ventricular rhythms generally are slower than sinus or junctional rhythms. Accelerated idioventricular rhythms are a subset of ventricular tachycardia, with a rate between 70 and 160 BPM, positioning it between an idioventricular rhythm (<70 BPM) and ventricular tachycardia. Slower accelerated idioventricular rhythms occur in response to bradycardia and are a type of ventricular escape beat that is faster than the usual 20–70 BPM. The arrhythmia is uncommon but may be seen in shock, gastric dilation and volvulus, digitalis intoxication, with general anesthesia, and with cardiomyopathy.

12 Hyperkalemia and hypocalcemia have been associated with either sinus bradycardia or problems with AV nodal conduction. Hypothyroidism (in dogs) has been associated with sinus bradycardia and a reduction in the amplitude of P and R waves. Such changes are reversible with appropriate hormone replacement therapy.

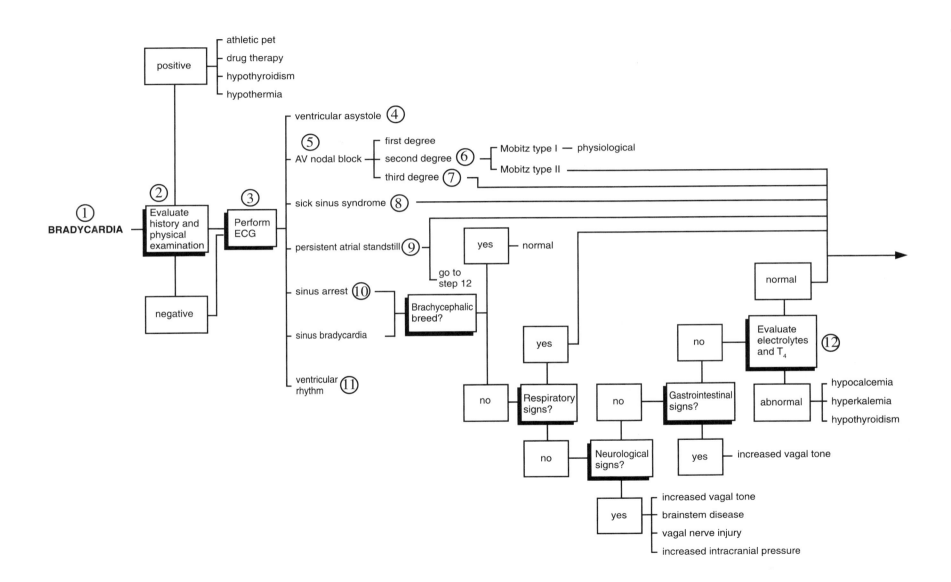

13 Thoracic radiographs help to evaluate the size and shape of the heart, the state of the pulmonary vasculature and pulmonary tissue, and the presence of intrathoracic masses.

14 Generalized cardiomegaly or isolated chamber enlargement in a dog or cat with a bradyarrhythmia should be followed by echocardiography to further characterize the state of the heart muscle.

15 Leukocytosis with a left shift in the presence of bradycardia may be caused by bacterial endocarditis. Echocardiography is one of the most specific tests for endocarditis, but lesions must be at least 2 mm thick to be seen.

16 Lyme disease is caused by the spirochete *Borrelia burgdorferi*. Two ticks (*Ixodes dammini, I. pacificus*) are vectors for the organism. A positive titer for the disease can represent clinical disease, past exposure, or relatively recent vaccination against the disease. In rare cases, Lyme myocarditis causes a variety of arrhythmias (ventricular extrasystoles, second- and third-degree AV blockade) and signs of congestive heart failure (pulmonary edema, ascites, pleural effusion).

17 An echocardiogram may reveal an intracardiac reason for the bradyarrhythmia (e.g., cardiac mass lesions, ventricular septal defects, cardiomyopathy). It also may indicate severe underlying cardiac disease such as a mass or myocardial failure, where pacemaker implantation is not warranted because the underlying condition is severe, progressive, and irreversible.

18 Aortic stenosis is associated with a crescendo-decrescendo murmur auscultated near the left third to fourth intercostal space and radiating to the carotid arteries. Breeds predisposed to this congenital defect include Newfoundlands (known to be an inherited defect), golden retrievers, German shepherds, rottweilers, and boxers. Most frequently the condition is subaortic stenosis, characterized by an obstructive, fibromuscular band below the aortic valve in the left ventricular outflow tract. Sometimes the condition involves failure of the aortic valve leaflets to separate properly during development (true aortic stenosis). If left ventricular pressure becomes high enough as a result of this obstruction of the outflow tract, left ventricular baroreceptors are stimulated to cause reflex vasodilation, bradycardia, and syncope. Radiographic changes associated with aortic or subaortic stenosis include left ventricular enlargement and poststenotic aortic dilation. Echocardiography can determine the degree of left ventricular hypertrophy.

19 Most ventricular septal defects (VSDs) are located in the septum between the ventricles, but some may involve the AV valves and atrial septum. They usually cause volume overload to the left side of the heart as a result of shunting of blood to the right side of the heart and overcirculation of blood back to the left side of the heart. Clinical signs of left heart failure include cough, exercise intolerance, and lethargy. Development of these signs depends on the size of the defect. Many dogs and cats are asymptomatic for VSD. Although thoracic radiographs may show left ventricular and atrial enlargement, echocardiography offers the most definitive means of diagnosis.

20 Bacterial endocarditis causes destruction and proliferation of the endocardium (the valves or the endocardial wall). The condition results from microorganisms colonizing the endocardium, commonly affecting the valves. Ventricular premature beats and tachyarrhythmias are more commonly encountered than bradyarrhythmias. Commonly isolated organisms include beta-hemolytic *Streptococcus, Staphylococcus intermedius, Escherichia coli, Corynebacterium* spp., and *Pseudomonas* spp. A heart murmur, fluctuant fevers, hyperglobulinemia, and glomerulonephritis are frequent clinical signs. Murmurs are heard especially in patients in which an infective lesion renders a valve incompetent. Mitral and aortic valves are most commonly affected. Positive blood cultures are good supportive evidence of bacterial endocarditis but often need to be taken during a "fever spike." Urine cultures also can be useful. Echocardiography is one of the most specific tests for identifying endocarditis "plaques," but lesions must be at least 2 mm thick to be seen.

21 Atrial masses include hemangiosarcoma of the right atrium and aortic body tumors. Both can result in pericardial effusion and bradyarrhythmias. Hemangiosarcoma is common in German shepherds and golden retrievers. Aortic body tumors include chemodectoma and nonchromaffin paraganglioma and occur most commonly in aged, brachycephalic breeds of dog.

22 Cardiomyopathies most frequently cause tachyarrhythmias due to heart failure and sympathetic autonomic nervous system overstimulation. However, occasionally they can cause SA arrest and third-degree heart blockade.

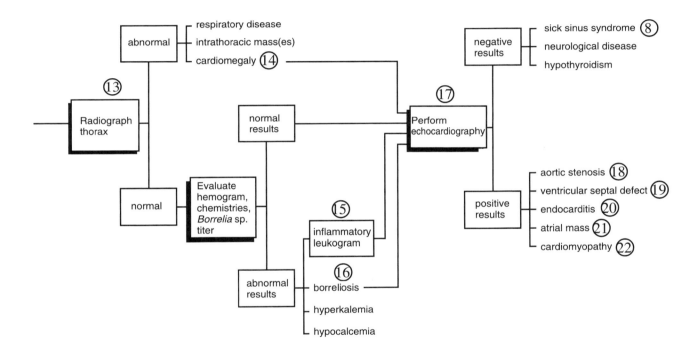

1 Systemic hypertension is elevation of systolic and diastolic blood pressures (greater than 180 and 100 mm Hg, respectively). Hypertension can be primary (idiopathic) or secondary to conditions such as renal or cardiac disease, glucocorticoid excess, diabetes mellitus, toxemia of pregnancy, and thyrotoxicosis. Common causes of hypertension are hyperadrenocorticism in dogs and chronic renal failure and hyperthyroidism in cats. Many dogs and cats show no clinical signs until acute blindness develops as a result of retinal edema, hemorrhage, and detachment. Other clinical signs include left ventricular hypertrophy, renal failure, seizures, cerebrovascular accidents (strokes), and dementia.

2 Indirect blood pressure is measured with a blood pressure cuff of suitable width (40% of the circumference of the limb) and a transducer (usually an ultrasonic Doppler flow detector) on the artery distal to the cuff. The cuff is inflated to occlude arterial flow and then released gradually until a pulse is detected in the artery (systolic blood pressure). When the flow of blood stops being pulsatile and becomes continuous, that is the diastolic blood pressure. Assessment of diastolic pressure is subject to a great deal of operator variation. Direct blood pressure is measured with an arterial cannula connected to a pressure transducer. This method is more accurate but is stressful for conscious patients, resulting in more false-positive results. Patients with borderline systolic pressures (up to 200 mm Hg) should be tested with the owner present, over a more prolonged period, and in a quiet, dark room or at home.

3 Once hypertension has been documented, a minimum database of laboratory tests helps to determine the underlying causes. The hemogram will show polycythemia (leading to hyperviscosity and hypertension). A serum chemistry profile indicates elevated ALP (suggesting steroid induction of the isoenzyme in hyperadrenocorticism), renal failure, or hyperglobulinemia (which also causes hyperviscosity and secondary hypertension). A baseline serum thyroid (T_4) concentration is appropriate for cats to diagnose hyperthyroidism and for dogs on thyroid supplementation. Canine hypothyroidism also may be considered (it is a rare cause of arteriosclerosis and hypertension).

4 Patients with low serum K^+ and increased Na^+, with no evidence of renal dysfunction, may have inappropriate aldosterone secretion by the adrenal medulla (hyperaldosteronism), which is confirmed via serum aldosterone assay. It has not been documented in veterinary patients.

5 Elevated ALP in dogs (rarely in cats) with any of the following—a "pot-bellied" appearance, thin skin, visible cutaneous vessels, hepatomegaly, PD, PU, polyphagia, and increased blood vessel fragility—suggests hyperadrenocorticism and warrants ACTH stimulation or low-dose dexamethasone suppression testing. Prior to testing, the history should be evaluated for exogenous glucocorticoid administration. An ACTH stimulation test is the preferred test due to its specificity. If it is positive, consider further testing to differentiate various forms of hyperadrenocorticism. If it is negative in patients with suspicious clinical signs, consider more sensitive, less specific tests (low-dose dexamethasone suppression test, urine cortisol/creatinine ratio determination).

6 Azotemia in conjunction with low urine specific gravity indicates renal failure. If this is present, consider abdominal ultrasound for pyelonephritis, polycystic renal disease (cats), renal dysplasia, and other structural changes. Renal artery blood flow can be evaluated via color flow Doppler; however, this technique may not be sensitive enough to detect rare cases of renal artery stenosis. If appropriate, look for underlying causes of renal disease (urine culture, ANA titer, *Leptospira* spp., and rickettsial titers, screening for FIP). Consider renal biopsy to conclusively determine the underlying conditions (glomerulonephritis, amyloidosis, chronic inflammation), as this may influence the therapy and prognosis. However, many veterinary patients have severe renal disease by the time hypertension is detected, limiting therapeutic options to blood pressure control.

7 Hypoalbuminemia and proteinuria in a patient with hypertension but without overt renal disease should raise the suspicion of glomerular problems (glomerulonephritis, amyloidosis). The urine protein/creatinine ratio should be measured. An elevated cholesterol concentration (nephrotic syndrome) may suggest amyloidosis or other forms of renal disease.

8 Hypertensive patients with hypercalcemia may have hyperparathyroidism or renal failure (see the algorithm for hypercalcemia)

9 If resting T_4 concentrations are high-normal or midrange, and clinical signs of other illness exist, consider T_3 suppression testing or measurement of free T_4 by equilibrium dialysis (*not* an analogue assay) to determine if serum T_4 concentrations are artifactually suppressed and the patient is actually suffering from hyperthyroidism.

10 In patients whose laboratory tests are inconclusive, echocardiography evaluates for underlying heart conditions that cause hypertension (e.g., HCM in cats, chronic mitral regurgitation and cardiac overload in dogs). Some patients with essentially normal hearts will have secondary changes (e.g., mitral regurgitation and left atrial enlargement, left ventricular hypertrophy) resulting from excessive systemic blood pressure.

11 Common (and some rare) causes of hypertension in dogs and cats have been excluded at this point. Further testing is needed to differentiate primary hypertension from a number of very uncommon disorders. The history should be evaluated for estrogen administration, pregnancy toxemia, and licorice ingestion/toxicity. Renal angiography and measurement of the plasma renin concentration are required to diagnose renal artery stenosis. A CT or MRI scan diagnoses intracranial masses. Pheochromocytoma is a rare catecholamine-secreting tumor of the renal medulla. Clinical signs are related to catecholamine release (peripheral vasoconstriction, sinus/ventricular tachycardia, rear limb weakness, collapse, shock, sudden death). About 50% of cases are not suspected antemortem. In a patient with appropriate clinical signs, consider an ECG for cardiac arrhythmias (caused by the excitatory effects of catecholamines) and abdominal ultrasound for adrenal masses (medullary tumors deep within the gland may be invisible). Other tests include the phentolamine blocking test (temporarily antagonizes catecholamine release, reducing blood pressure), the clonidine response test (will not suppress catecholamine production by pheochromocytomas), or measurement of the 24-hour plasma/urinary catecholamine ratio. Circulating plasma catecholamine concentrations are not useful, especially since tumors are intermittent secretors.

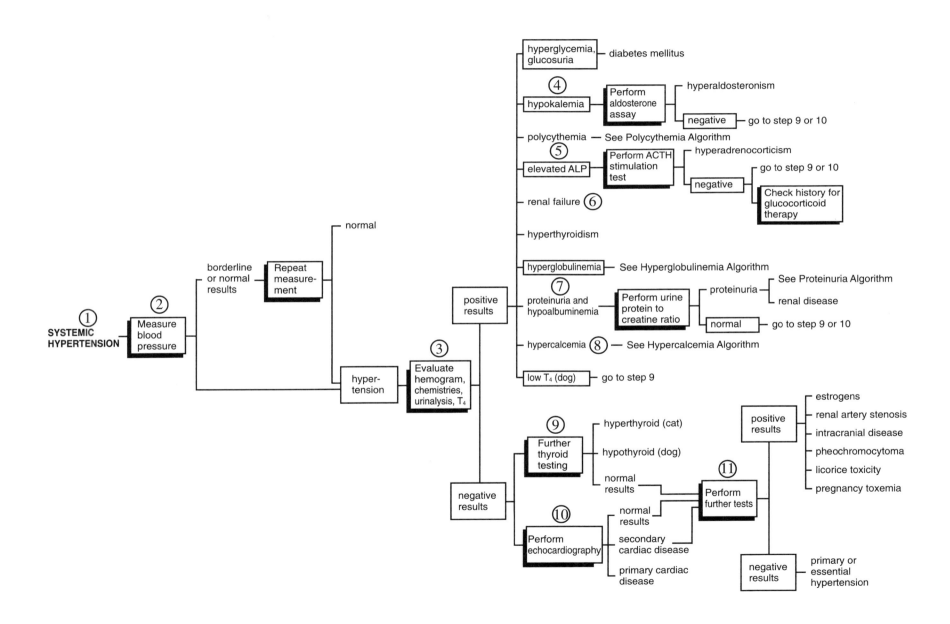

1 Cardiomegaly is enlargement of the cardiac silhouette. Enlargement may be due to overload of individual chambers (left atrium in chronic mitral insufficiency [MI]), heart muscle disease (e.g., DCM), pericardial effusion, or masses. Cardiomegaly is rare in cats because of a low incidence of acquired valvular disease and because HCM is the most common myocardial problem in this species. Cardiac muscle hypertrophy occurs inward, and changes in heart size develop only very late in the condition.

2 Doberman pinschers, cocker spaniels, and boxers are predisposed to DCM. Small-breed dogs are likely to have left atrial enlargement secondary to MI. German shepherds and golden retrievers are predisposed to pericardial bleeding from heart-base hemangiosarcoma. Certain congenital cardiac defects are seen in specific breeds and may result in cardiomegaly secondary to volume overload (e.g., subaortic stenosis, patent ductus arteriosus). Cats and Chinese shar-peis are predisposed to congenital pericardioperitoneal diaphragmatic hernia. The dietary history may be important (step 19). A history of drug therapy should be obtained for agents that affect the myocardium (step 21). Radiation therapy also may damage the heart muscle. Preexisting conditions that may result in enlargement of the cardiac silhouette include hemangiosarcoma (which may arise from or metastasize to the heart base) and FIP virus infection (which may cause pericardial effusion). Patients with cardiomegaly may be asymptomatic or have a history of exercise intolerance, weakness, collapse, cough, pallor, or dyspnea. On physical examination there may be tachycardia, poor or variable pulse quality, heart murmurs, jugular pulses (with right heart failure), or muffling of heart sounds. The last may suggest pericardial or pleural effusion. Localization of murmurs suggests an underlying cause of cardiomegaly (e.g., pulmonic or subaortic stenosis, MI, etc.).

3 Thoracic radiographs should be evaluated to determine overall heart size, focal chamber enlargement, and vascular and pulmonary patterns. In dogs, cardiomegaly is present when the heart covers more than three and a half rib spaces on a lateral radiograph or occupies more than two-thirds of the thoracic cavity on the ventrodorsal view (in both dogs and cats). In cats, cardiomegaly is present when the width of the heart covers more than three rib spaces on the lateral radiograph. Other radiographic findings that suggest cardiomegaly include elevation of the carina, displacement of the intrathoracic trachea to run parallel with the vertebral column (note that this may be normal in breeds such as bulldogs), splitting of mainstem bronchi by left atrial enlargement, or increased sternal contact of the heart due to right atrial enlargement. In dogs, there is considerable breed-related variation in the radiographic appearance of the heart. Although the test of choice for patients with cardiomegaly is echocardiography, this test is not always immediately available to the clinician. Nor is it necessary for all patients. For example, isolated left atrial enlargement associated with a left-sided systolic regurgitant heart murmur in an older canine patient does not necessarily require an echocardiogram to identify MI. A globoid appearance of the cardiac silhouette is suggestive of pericardial effusion. However, this cannot always be distinguished from generalized cardiomegaly in patients with DCM. Occasionally, a heart-base mass is seen radiographically.

4 An ECG may provide information about the causes of cardiomegaly seen on radiographs. Decreased complex size may suggest pericardial effusion in patients with a globoid cardiac silhouette, especially if accompanied by electrical alternans (variable complex size). Small complexes also are seen in obese and hypothyroid patients and those with pleural effusion. Increases in complex height or width, arrhythmias, or shifts in the mean electrical axis may suggest specific chamber enlargement or underlying myocardial disease. The ECG is unlikely to provide definitive results, and while positive findings are helpful, negative ones do not preclude underlying disease.

5 Disruption of the diaphragm line and abnormal gas shadows around the heart suggest traumatic diaphragmatic hernia or pericardioperitoneal diaphragmatic hernia (usually congenital). Pericardioperitoneal diaphragmatic hernia is a relatively common congenital defect in dogs and cats. It may be detected in young animals but also may be found in mature/aged patients without signs of clinical problems. Clinical signs accompanying either form of diaphragmatic disruption may include gastrointestinal problems due to bowel entrapment in the hernia, coughing, dyspnea, and pleural effusion. Cats appear less likely to be symptomatic or have entrapped organs in the hernia sac. Ultrasound of the chest/abdomen may help to confirm herniation.

6 Thoracic radiographs may show pulmonary patterns suggestive of metastatic neoplasia (e.g., from heart-base tumors), chronic small airway disease which may cause pulmonary hypertension and right-sided cardiomegaly (cor pulmonale), or pulmonary edema (suggesting left-sided heart failure). They also may show caudal vena cava dilation or pleural effusion that may be the result of right-sided heart failure.

7 Cranial mediastinal masses may obscure the cranial border of the heart and suggest cardiomegaly. Thoracic ultrasound can differentiate these two problems.

8 Pulmonary arterial dilation, tortuosity, and "pruning" in the periphery are common with *D. immitis* infestation, particularly in dogs. This condition also may lead to right-sided cardiac enlargement and, on occasion, pleural effusion. An occult heartworm test (for *D. immitis* somatic antigens) for dogs on preventive medication or examination of a peripheral blood smear for microfilaria in those not on preventive medication allows diagnosis of *D. immitis* infestation as a cause of right-sided cardiomegaly.

9 Feline patients may require an antibody test to determine exposure to heartworms since they are not a primary host for *D. immitis* and may not have sufficient female heartworms (three or more) to be positive on the antigen test. Testing for microfilaremia is unlikely to be positive in feline patients even if they are not on heartworm preventive medication, as many infections are sterile.

10 Canine patients with clinical and radiographic signs of heartworm disease that do not test positive for *Dirofilaria* spp. rarely may have a similar infestation with *Angiostrongylus vasorum*, a parasite of the pulmonary artery and right ventricle in dogs. The larvae may be found in feces using the Baermann technique or on bronchoalveolar lavage.

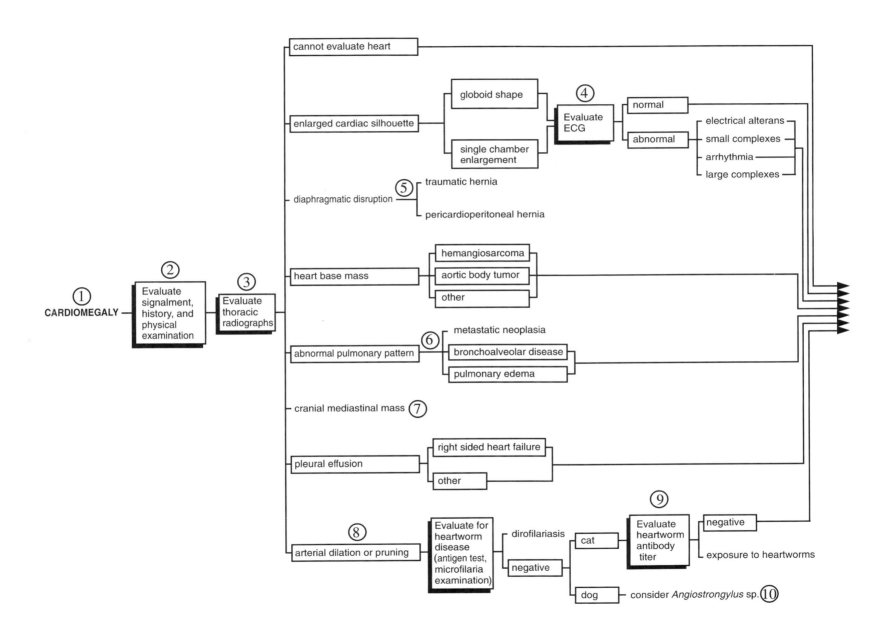

11 Although all tests previously described are helpful in diagnosing the underlying causes of cardiomegaly, echocardiography is the single most useful diagnostic test. In most instances, it will provide answers about the pericardium, presence of mass lesions, cardiac contractility, chamber dimensions, and valvular integrity. In the hands of a skilled operator, it also allows diagnosis of congenital defects, restrictive cardiomyopathy, and *D. immitis* infestation. In some instances it must be combined with bubble studies, selective arteriography, or, rarely, myocardial biopsy to confirm the diagnosis.

12 Pericardial thickening may be focal or diffuse. If focal, it may be neoplastic or due to benign cystic structures (pericardial/epicardial cysts). Generalized thickening may represent diffuse neoplasia (lymphoma, mesothelioma) or inflammation (infectious or immune-mediated pericarditis).

13 Pericardial effusion characteristically produces a very globoid appearance to the heart radiographically that is difficult to distinguish from cardiomegaly except by echocardiography. Pericardiocentesis is needed to assess the fluid formed and potentially to diagnose the underlying cause. Pericardial effusions may be sanguinous (e.g., with a bleeding hemangiosarcoma or left atrial rupture), suppurative, suggest FIP, contain neoplastic cells (e.g., lymphoma or mesothelioma), or may be transudates/modified transudates (e.g., in patients with congestive heart failure or hypoalbuminemia). Prior to pericardiocentesis, the coagulation status may need to be checked, although pericardiocentesis may need to be performed as an emergency procedure. It is important to look for left atrial/pericardial masses before fluid drainage, as fluid may outline the mass.

14 Congenital valvular abnormalities range from poorly formed or distorted valve leaflets and failure of separation of leaflets (valvular stenosis) to abnormalities of vessel walls associated with the valves (subaortic stenosis).

15 Endocardiosis is a change in heart valves with aging (particularly AV valves) resulting from chronic structural (myxomatous) degeneration and fibrous nodule formation. The underlying causes are not known, but heredi-

tary factors appear to contribute. It is relatively common in dogs, especially in small breeds.

16 Infective endocarditis results from colonization of heart valves by bacteria, destroying the valves. Bacteremia is the most common underlying cause and arises from a variety of sources (wounds, cutaneous infections, abscesses, pyelonephritis, etc.). Mitral and aortic valves are the most common sites for endocarditis.

17 Tricuspid insufficiency (TI) may be a primary valvular problem (acquired or congenital) or may result from pulmonary hypertension and right-sided cardiac overload.

18 Primary DCM is a relatively common heritable condition in dogs. Underlying subcellular problems are suspected. It is unusual in cats (DCM used to be common in association with taurine-deficient diets in cats). DCM is a relatively common acquired disease in dogs, affecting 0.65% of purebred dogs, 5.8% of Doberman pinschers, and 6% of Scottish deerhounds.

19 Cats on unusual/home-cooked diets that are deficient in taurine (either due to the ingredients or to processing) or those on urinary acidifiers causing potassium depletion (which may reduce taurine stores) are predisposed to develop DCM. Dogs and cats on vitamin E- and selenium-deficient diets also may develop cardiac muscle problems.

20 Inflammatory myocarditis is more likely to cause cardiac arrhythmias than chamber dilation. However, arrhythmias may lead to myocardial failure (due to forward pumping problems and volume overload). Some forms of myocarditis cause primary cardiac muscle problems (e.g., parvovirus infection in puppies between 3 and 10 weeks of age, *Trypanosoma cruzi* infection in young dogs in the southern United States, *Neospora* spp. in dogs and *Toxoplasma* spp. in cats).

21 The drug history is important in the initial evaluation of patients with cardiac problems/enlargement of the cardiac silhouette. Doxorubicin, a chemotherapeutic agent, has specific toxicity to heart muscle that may result in DCM, especially in dogs. Although toxicity generally

manifests at higher (cumulative) doses, it may develop idiosyncratically at lower doses and may be immediate or delayed many months post-therapy. Furazolide and ionophore toxicoses also cause myocardial damage. Drugs such as cocaine, amphetamines, digoxin, and catecholamines cause arrhythmias and severe tachycardia, failure of cardiac filling, secondary cardiac overload, chamber dilation, and cardiomegaly. Avocado ingestion has been reported to cause cardiac muscle problems in dogs.

22 Cardiac muscle hypertrophy may result in enlargement of the cardiac silhouette. This is not always the case, especially in cats with HCM when hypertrophy occurs inward and is rarely detectable on thoracic radiographs. Cardiac muscle hypertrophy in the absence of systemic hypertension can be the result of an increase in cardiac workload (e.g., left-to-right shunts causing cardiac overcirculation, heart valve abnormalities leading to blood flow in the wrong direction, and secondary to pulmonary hypertension). Initially, muscular hypertrophy and increased fractional shortening develop because of circulatory overload. Only later do chamber dilation and reduction in fractional shortening occur. This condition eventually results in congestive heart failure. There is a great deal of overlap between the acquired and congenital valvular conditions that cause cardiac enlargement due to chamber hypertrophy and dilation. Cardiac muscle hypertrophy also may occur without increased cardiac workload. It may result from acromegaly, a condition in which excessive amounts of circulating growth hormone cause general hypertrophy of soft tissues, including heart muscle. On occasion, it may result in congestive heart failure. In dogs, the condition is seen most commonly in females as a result of excessive serum progestogen concentrations. These may develop because of prolonged metestrus or administration of progestogens for estrus prevention. Progestogens increase mammary growth hormone production, resulting in clinical signs of acromegaly. In cats, acromegaly is generally caused by a pituitary tumor. Cardiac muscle hypertrophy also may be seen as an idiopathic and probably heritable condition in dogs (with diminution of the left ventricular chamber due to inward hypertrophy and moderate radiographic signs of enlargement of the left ventricle and atrium). Rarely, cardiac muscle infiltration (e.g., by a diffuse tumor) results in enlargement of the heart.

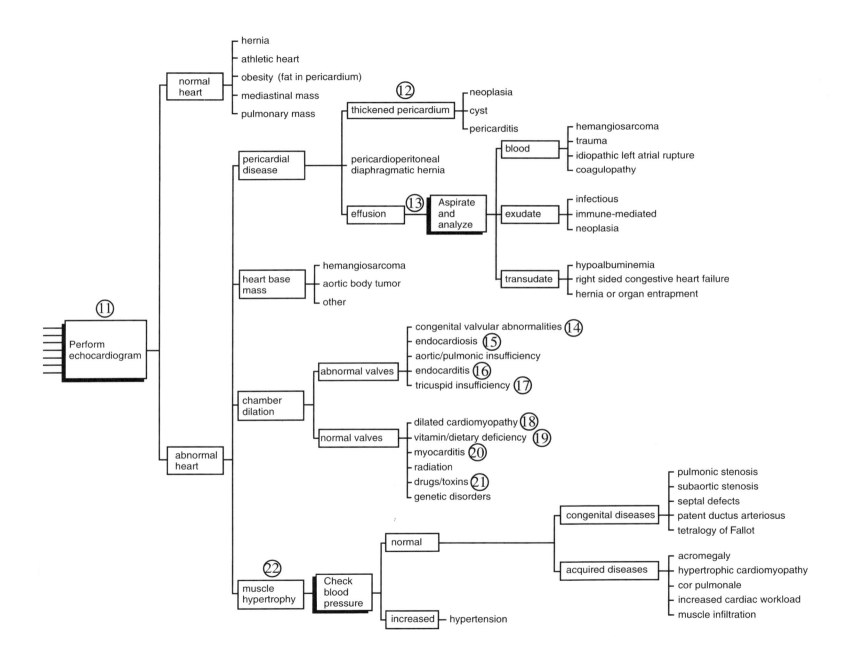

Index

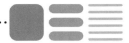

Note: Page numbers followed by f refer to figures.